15.29

Classic Texts in Health Care

D0294398

Classic Texts in Health Care

Edited by

Lesley Mackay BSc PhD

*Lecturer, School of Healthcare Studies, University of Leeds, UK; Honorary
Senior Research Fellow, Department of Applied Social Science, Lancaster
University, UK*

Keith Soothill BA PhD

Professor, Department of Applied Social Science, Lancaster University, UK

Kath Melia BNurs (Manc) PhD

Professor, Department of Nursing Studies, University of Edinburgh, UK

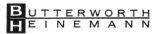

OXFORD BOSTON JOHANNESBURG MELBOURNE NEW DELHI SINGAPORE

Butterworth-Heinemann
225 Wildwood Avenue, Woburn, MA 01801-2041
Linacre House, Jordan Hill, Oxford OX2 8DP
A division of Reed Educational and Professional Publishing Ltd

℞ A member of the Reed Elsevier plc group

First published 1998

British Library Cataloguing in Publication Data
A catalogue record for this book is available from the British Library

Library of Congress Cataloguing in Publication Data
A catalogue record for this book is available from the Library of Congress

ISBN 0 7506 2738 7

UCSM

613.7042 UEA

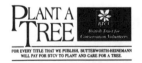

PLANT A TREE

BTCV
British Trust for
Conservation Volunteers

FOR EVERY TITLE THAT WE PUBLISH, BUTTERWORTH-HEINEMANN
WILL PAY FOR BTCV TO PLANT AND CARE FOR A TREE.

Typeset by David Gregson Associates, Beccles, Suffolk
Printed and bound in Great Britain by Biddles Ltd, Guildford and King's Lynn

Contents

Part II   Professions   129

Part III   How Far Have We Come? Or Fifty Years of the National Health Service   275

viii   Contents

Preface

We have found that developing a set of readings is rather like a 'mystery train journey'. One starts off by having some hazy idea of the likely destination but, as the journey progresses, one begins to think that perhaps one may arrive somewhere else. If the destination of the mystery train journey is indeed somewhere different, then the question soon arises as to whether the surprise is a pleasurable one. Ultimately, of course, our readers will make the decision about this book and we shall then be able to assess whether our work has been worth while and we have indeed reached the right destination.

Compiling this collection of Classic Texts has been both interesting and rewarding. Interesting in that we have discovered that remembered texts are not always saying what we thought they were, some having been simplified in our memories, others embellished. And the task has been rewarding, reminding us of the enduring quality of much of the work which has been undertaken in the study of health and health professionals. Inevitably, we have not found room for all of our favourite texts and decisions have had to be taken to include and exclude which have not been easy.

We hope this collection will be a window into the world of health research: to medical sociology, to the sociology of health and illness, to the experiences of patients and the lay perspective as well as to research into professions and to the environment in which they work. But we should like to emphasize that these texts are excerpts, 'tasters' if you like, from which we would hope the interested reader will be motivated to turn to the original texts. Our aim has been to raise issues, some of which are being neglected today, to re-emphasize the importance of previous work and to help the reader make connections between the present and the past. The authors of these texts make reference to a wide range of sources and issues. These are well worth pursuing. What is surprising is how many of issues facing those who work in and use health services have been encountered before. There is no need to reinvent the wheel – look and see what has been done before, how the issues have been perceived and approached.

As editors we have been keen, almost with missionary zeal (!), to proclaim classic work from an essentially sociological tradition which is well-written. While what constitutes 'well-written' must be, to some extent, subjective, the work that we have chosen often tackles complex issues and ideas but does not unnecessarily complicate. We present extracts which go beyond 'the flavour of the month'. However, we are aware that new agendas on health are appearing ever more rapidly, so we have peered into the crystal ball and chosen some relatively recent work which we feel are classics in the making.

The titles of the three parts of this book go beyond being a convenient way to divide up the book. We believe that the cornerstones when considering health care in Britain are to think about the patient, the health professionals and what we have accomplished over the last half century in health care. It cannot be denied that the early hopes of the National Health Service have not always been realized. However, an understanding of the issues and the dynamics of health care provided by these Classic Texts shed some light on the impossibility of meeting some of those post-war aspirations. The message for the future might be: we neglect at our peril the work of the past.

L.M., K.S. and K.M.

Editors' note

While every effort has been made to trace the copyright holders of any material included in this work which is not the work of the authors, this has not always been possible. The publishers would like to hear from anyone who has information which may lead to the identification of the copyright holder/s for any material for which we were unable to obtain permission for use and will endeavour to make the appropriate amendments at our earliest opportunity.

Introduction

Keith Soothill, Lesley Mackay and Kath Melia

The remarkable rise of interest in health and illness among social scientists has been a phenomenon of the second half of the twentieth century. This book is in part a celebration of the half century since the Second World War when the importance of studying social science in order to understand many of the issues of health and illness has been more fully recognized. Celebration is itself important, for it enables persons who were not party to the events to begin to understand the past and to begin to grasp the reasons for present preoccupations which have some earlier origins.

The past provides the building blocks of the future. In moving forward, there is a need either to reject some strait-jackets of the past which has trammelled development or to learn what has been achieved to avoid, in a familiar phrase, 'reinventing the wheel.' These possibilities are not mutually exclusive and, in studying health and illness, one wants to point out to a future generation some traps which have been identified in the past and to remind of some points of liberation.

Prior to the Second World War, there had certainly been interest in the social determinants of mortality, but this was an interest pursued with much more vigour and rigour by statisticians and social reformers than by professional social scientists. Indeed, prior to the 1930s, only the work of sociologist, Emile Durkheim stood out as offering a distinct theoretical contribution when he looked at the causes of the differences among social groups regarding deaths of a very particular kind – namely suicide (Durkheim, 1952). Of course, the implicit influences of cause and effect were described in the work of Marx and Engels of the health of working men, women and children, but prior to the Second World War there were really no sustained sociological analyses of medicine, of its institutions and its activities. The burgeoning of interest came after the war and even then, in Britain at least, the major developments came later.

In the early 1980s Jefferys asked why was there such a late development in Britain of an interest in the sociology of medicine.[1] One of the crucial points is to understand the tremendous complacency and euphoric assumptions made in the immediate post-war years. The launching of the

National Health Service was, of course, one of the genuine accomplishments of the immediate post-war Labour governments (1945–51). It raised all sorts of hopes that the benefits of health, at least, would be available to all.

In a parallel area, the sociology of education, the work of Halsey and colleagues (1957) on social mobility and education had a profound impact. Perhaps this was partly in recognition of the fact that the upper middle classes in Britain had quite evidently opted out to the public school system. On the other hand, the development of the sociology of health or medicine was more hesitant in the first decades after the war. The basic questions being raised about education were not being raised about health. There was not the feeling that the health care system was a major determinant of social stratification. In other words, the questions were not being asked about the relationship between health and social class.

The sociology of medicine later widened into and overlapped with other areas: the sociology of health and illness, the sociology of the professions, and issues of social policy. While there may be some dispute about some of the detail, there is quite substantial agreement of the phases of development. However, we attempt in the next section a bold framework to try to encompass the whole period.

Fifty years of research into health and illness (1945–95)

It is a daunting task to summarize 50 years of research in a few paragraphs but for the study of health and illness it is remarkably simple, dividing quite comfortably into two quarter centuries. From the end of the Second World War to the early 1970s (1945–70), the medical doctor was placed at the centre of the illness nexus. This was the outcome of the remarkable influence of the theorizing of the American sociologist, Talcott Parsons (1951, 1975) who dominated social scientific thinking in the two decades after the war. His structural-functional approach gradually became recognized as being 'medico-centric'. By the end of the 1960s the influence of Parsons was waning.

From the early 1970s the shift over the past 25 years has been in two major directions. First, there began an increasing stress on the importance of thinking about 'health' rather than just 'illness'. Secondly, there has been an increasing focus on the importance of the lay person's view. These two pathways converge but they are analytically distinct and so can be considered separately. While many would embrace the charge that developments in the past quarter of a century have been towards becoming 'lay-centric', we briefly mention the dangers. We tentatively suggest that a more robust framework is needed for the twenty-first century.

Although no longer fashionable, the contribution of Talcott Parsons was seminal. He is now most remembered for his theoretical analysis of the sick role and of the role of the physician as an agent of social control. This is part of a development of considering health and illness within a deviance framework. Essentially Parsons argued that there are four features of the sick role. Briefly, illness is first viewed as involuntary – hence the occupant of the sick role cannot be held responsible for his condition; secondly, the occupant of the sick role is exempted from his usual work, family, civic and other obligations – the extent of his exemptions depends upon the nature of his illness condition; thirdly, the sick role is conditionally legitimate – in other words, he is expected to do what he can to restore his health; fourthly, he is expected to seek competent help in his efforts to restore his health. Most descriptions of Parsons are phrased in the masculine mode and his lack of interest in gender is just one flaw. In this traditional conceptualization of the relationship between physician and patient, a fundamental flaw identified in the 1970s was the assumption that the interests of physician and patient are harmonious. Gerson (1976), for example, argued that in most contemporary medical settings the relationship between physician and patient may be fraught with inherent contradictions. Gerson argues that this inherent conflict is generated by the fact that illness is simultaneously the physician's work and a disabling of the patient's self. Thus, practising medicine is the work of the physician, and he must necessarily be as much concerned with the conditions of his work as with the particular medical condition of particular patients. However, from the perspective of the patient, illness is not work in the sense of 'making a living', it is grossly uncomfortable, often painful, often embarrassing, even a terrorizing experience involving the fundamental character of the self.

Parsons' approach adopted the perspective of the physician. Gerson argues that a major task of medical sociology is to analyse the inherent contradictions of the physician–patient relationship and to investigate how these are managed by everyone concerned. These include not only patient and physician, but the enormous complex of commitments and obligations to colleagues, relatives and friends which both have in their surrounding social arrangements. In fact, we argue that this task or agenda of how these varieties of relationships are managed has been somewhat neglected in the past two decades and should become more explicitly the main focus of research in the next quarter of a century. There are two important factors which tended to mask the inherent conflict of interest between physician and patient according to Gerson.

The first was the fact that medical care was increasingly being provided in very large complex settings. Sometimes the patient was simply overlooked and nobody really noticed. So, for example, with the enthusiasm surrounding the complex technology of heart transplant operations, there were press conferences in which the surgeons came close to saying: 'It was a very successful operation, but the patient died.'

The second feature was that many illnesses are short term and relatively inconsequential in their 'social side-effects' to the patients, and traditional medical sociology had tended to focus, rather arbitrarily, on these relatively short-term acute conditions. In fact, such conditions are highly routinized in medical practice and understood by the general public. In broad terms, there is a relatively smooth and efficient processing of conditions which fit rather neatly into the framework of the traditional sick role paradigm. However, when one moves on to the catastrophic, long-term and chronic illnesses, different issues come into play. Such illnesses may severely affect or curtail (or even eliminate) the normal activities of patients and they often require complex and continuing management quite different from the acute conditions.

It is, in fact, from sociological studies of such diseases – catastrophic, long-term and chronic illnesses (e.g. Davis, 1963; Glaser and Strauss, 1966, 1968) – that the notion of illness as politics rather than deviance clearly emerges. The argument is that the process of managing such illnesses requires a different order of skills and procedures on the part of both patient and staff.

Not only must such patients become medically quite sophisticated to learn how to live with their illness or disability, but they must also learn how to deal with a whole set of different and complex bureaucracies which are notably idiosyncratic in their procedures. Similarly, physicians in such circumstances must reconcile themselves to 'managing' rather than 'curing' the illness. There is a loss of autonomy for the physician to a whole set of other specialists and disciplines. The doctor has to learn how to manage quite extensive and intimate relationships with patients and their relatives on a continuing basis. Furthermore, it is increasingly clear that there are a whole set of ethical dilemmas which are challenging for the physician – what is the precise definition of death, when should scarce resources be used or withheld, and so on.

The major difficulty with Talcott Parsons' framework is that it is 'medico-centric'. It places the figure of the doctor at the centre of health care processes. The approach overestimates the therapeutic impact of the physician and medical institutions (Gallagher, 1976). Correspondingly, it underestimates the potential therapeutic impact of the family and other lay supportive systems in the community. In fact, what the Parsons' formulation overlooked was the impact of the patient's social relationships and the patient's customary physical environment upon his disease and his treatment. Traditionally, physicians had been deficient in recognizing and coping with this.

The towering figure replacing Parsons in the early 1970s as the pivot of medical sociology was Eliot Freidson. Some of Freidson's notable achievements in the early 1960s have been summarized by McKinlay (1977): providing the first useful overview of the state of knowledge in the sub-field (Freidson, 1961–62), the first to challenge the then prevailing Parsonian formulation of the sick role (Freidson, 1961), introducing the concept of a 'lay referral system' (Freidson, 1960), highlighting elements of conflict in the physician-patient relationship (Freidson, 1962), describing how patients relate to medical organizations (Freidson, 1963a) and speculating on the changing role of hospitals in modern society (Freidson, 1963b). Freidson's main canon of work is contained in a trilogy which appeared in the 1970s – *Profession of Medicine* (1970a), *Professional*

Dominance (1970b), and *Doctoring Together* (1975) – in which, as McKinlay points out, Freidson draws together his various contributions and elaborates a substantial argument concerning the dominant position of physicians within the institution of medicine in particular and, more generally, their unique position within the broader society.

Medical training is lengthy and during this period medical students are 'socialized' to become physicians. This area had been usefully probed in some earlier work brought together by Robert Merton and his co-editors in *The Student Physician* (1957). Merton sought to demonstrate that during training students develop conceptions of themselves as doctors, absorbing enough knowledge and gaining in confidence so that they can deal with patients without too much anxiety. Howard Becker and his colleagues (1961) stressed that the students' perspective on their educational experience differs from that of their medical teachers.

During medical training students do, of course, gain command over specialized knowledge and skill. While all physicians share roughly the same basic technical education, they do not practise in the same way (Freidson). In the few systematic studies of medical practice that have been made, the association between medical education and subsequent performance is at best weak.

While undoubtedly important and insightful in a whole variety of ways, Freidson can still be regarded in some ways as a transition figure. He provided crucial insights to challenge the Parsonian approach and also gave some substantial hints of what was to come. Nevertheless, his work had an intrinsically medical focus, with his attempts to clarify the sociological characteristics of the medical profession. However, the agenda was changing.

In a review published in 1978, Stacey widened the agenda for the field of medical sociology (see Chapter 7). She noted how the origins of medical sociology rested in the rather practical concerns of medical practitioners and health administrators. Stacey proposed a sociology of health and illness rather than of medicine as a way of breaking free of medical dominance in the research enterprise. More specifically, Stacey wanted to see a sociology surrounding the problems of health, illness and of suffering. Hence, she was beginning to articulate the task of medical sociology to be patient-oriented rather than doctor-oriented.

The reorientation of medical sociology was taking place during an era which was also crucial for nursing. Nursing in the course of its self-conscious efforts to create a body of knowledge for the discipline took a greater interest in social scientific findings, particularly relating to the social context of illness. In fact, the psychosocial dimension of the patient had become increasingly important since the 1950s and 1960s (see Armstrong, Chapter 37). A series of nursing reports called for the move of nursing into higher education and latterly there were moves to develop nursing as a research-based profession (Lancet, 1932; Athlone, 1938; RCN, 1964; DHSS, 1972; UKCC, 1986). Certainly nursing began to be on the move in ways which would eventually challenge the hospital as the main focus of nursing activity. The shift complemented the wider moves towards a more patient-oriented perspective.

One effect was to introduce the importance of prevention. Also, the process of becoming ill before crossing the threshold of the doctor's surgery came under scrutiny. This related directly to Freidson's notion of a 'lay referral system'. With the focus increasing on the patient, there was a corresponding move from interest in the hospital to the community and the way in which patients were selected for hospital attention (see Stimson and Webb, Chapter 11).

As issues of health promotion and health education came to have an increasing influence, the direct importance of medicine was implicitly challenged. In fact, important challenges came from within the house of medicine itself. In the mid-1970s, Thomas McKeown, Professor of Social Medicine at Birmingham University, made a major impact (see Chapter 3) by proposing – with a considerable weight of evidence – that the total contribution of medical and surgical interventions to reductions of mortality has been small compared with the impact of environmental 'public health', political, economic and social measures. In fact, what becomes clear from McKeown's work is that in the past the impact of medicine has been more on disability than on death. So, while not minimizing the value of clinical medicine, especially in reducing the consequences of those diseases which cannot be prevented, McKeown's work was an important reminder that medical care is but one factor in determining the health of a population.

McKeown's work was part of a general shift in recognizing the importance of social causes of illness, but around the same time there was renewed interest in what was meant by 'health'. In 1975 Kelman (see Chapter 1) pointed out that 'perhaps the most perplexing and ambiguous issue in the study of health since its inception centuries or millennia ago, is its definition'. In fact, as Kelman stresses, the first scientific approach to health originated with the development of the machine model of the human body. With this conception, 'health' came to be regarded as the perfect working order of the human organism. Kelman argues that the methodologies that developed from this view consider illness to be both natural (biological) and occurring on an individual basis. It then follows that treatment is pursued essentially on an individual basis using surgical or chemical means of treatment. This approach relegates the recognition and implications of social causes of illness to secondary importance.

While an appreciation of the social basis of many diseases and ill-health has a long history, the great thrust in the recognition of the social basis of many diseases and ill-health came with the publication of the Chadwick Report in the mid-nineteenth century (Chadwick, 1843). The report showed that the gross inadequacy of water supplies, drainage and facilities for the disposal of refuse in big towns were the biggest sources of disease. The study of epidemics – or epidemiology – had begun in earnest. However, the environmentalist approach to health is clearly in conflict with the biological and individual orientation of the classical school which still underpins much of modern medicine.

The second major shift over the past 25 years has been an increasing focus on the importance of the lay person's view. This has developed from various directions. So, for example, important contributions by feminists from the 1970s onwards have emphasized the importance of women controlling their own bodies and the dangers of 'medicalizing' some everyday activities in people's lives. In brief, 'medicalization' involves the notion that health professionals, usually doctors, tend to offer biomedical or technical solutions to what are inherently 'normal' aspects of everyday life. As Nettleton (1995) stresses, it is in relation to childbirth that the concept of medicalization has been most fully developed. Certainly the control of pregnancy and childbirth has been taken over by a predominantly male medical profession and 'because childbirth is defined as a "medical problem" it becomes conceptualized in terms of clinical safety, and women are encouraged to have their babies in hospital' (p. 28).

The women's movement has made health a central plank of their platform in identifying causes of women's subordination. The focus on the control of female sexuality which has variously existed in both religious and secular Western patriarchal societies (Turner, 1987) also relates to an increasing interest in the sociology of the body over the past decade or so (see, for example, Lawler, 1991). Curiously, until comparatively recently the body has been of little interest to social scientists although, of course, issues relating to health, medicine and illness may closely involve considerations of the body. As Nettleton stresses, 'feminist sociologists were the first to recognise and make explicit the significance of the body for social theory. Feminist analyses of women's bodies have revealed the extent to which medical and scientific descriptions of the biological basis of bodies are socially constructed, and may be used for ideological purposes such as maintaining gender inequalities' (Nettleton, 1995, p. 101). In fact, the argument is that this regulation and control of women's bodies have been particularly evident in recent developments in the field of the new reproductive technologies (NRTs).

However, the problems confronting women in relation to health care are just part of a wider debate about health inequalities which highlight that various social groups seem to be getting a bad deal. In the 1970s work began to identify the problems of women, while work developing from the mid-1980s began to identify some of the problems of ethnic minorities in relation to the provision of health care. However, the main debate which proved to be something of a watershed in the early 1980s related directly to the question as to why the health status of the working class continued to be lower than that of the rest of the population (see Chapter 51).

Soon after the arrival of the Thatcher government in 1979 there were reports coming in which were set off by the previous Labour administration. Of course, one mechanism of a government to deal with a potentially thorny issue is to set up a committee of enquiry or a Royal Commission which will report when everyone has forgotten about the contentious issue. In 1977 the then Labour government set up a Working Party, chaired by Sir Douglas Black, Chief Scientist at the DHSS and president of the Royal College of Physicians.

The Black Report was published in 1980 and regarded as so alarming that the government certainly tried to bury it by publishing only a few copies and releasing it just before a national holiday. However, despite the attempts to submerge it, the Report was soon described by the *British Medical Journal* and many others as 'the most important medical report since the War', although its principal recommendations have never been implemented.

In essence, the Black Report showed considerable class differentials in health. It showed, for example, that 'men and women in occupational class V [that is, the unskilled] had two and a half times greater chance of dying before reaching retirement age than their professional counterparts in occupational class I' (Townsend and Davidson, 1982, p. 51). Moreover, 'class differences in mortality are a constant feature of the entire human life-span' (p. 51), being most marked in infants and children. In infants, for example, 'the most marked class gradients are for deaths from accidents and respiratory diseases' (p. 52). Among adults, 'the rates of death from accidents and infectious diseases show steep class gradients, but equally an extraordinary variety of non-infectious diseases like cancer, heart and respiratory diseases also show marked class differences' (p. 56).

The government strongly rejected the report. The main bone of contention was about the explanations for the differences and what to do about trying to narrow the gaps rather than any major challenge to the 'facts'. In essence, the epidemiological debate since the early 1980s has been between those who emphasize the importance of the lifestyle or behaviour of individuals, and those who stress the importance of the socioeconomic environment. Despite some considerable political battles between the medical profession and the government in relation to the implementation of some of the major health reforms, almost unnoticed has been an alliance forged between the government and the medical profession in trying to tackle health problems.

The crucial point to recognize is that the ideology of medicine individualizes problems rather than laying bare the social causes of ill-health. The individualization of illness has been one of the crucial ingredients of the health policies of the 1980s and early 1990s. In many ways the individualization of illness is pernicious, for it shifts interest away from the complexities of the causation of illness and disease. Crawford (1977 – see Chapter 13), in a powerful article, was one of the first to recognize the dangers of blaming the victim.

The individualists form an essentially conservative group, as they see the problem of health differences being solved within the existing class structure – for example, by members of the working class changing their lifestyle so that it more closely matches that of the healthier social classes. In contrast, the environmentalists generally form a more radical group in terms of positing solutions to health differences, seeing the need for a change in the way that society is structured. Each group emphasizes different aspects of the economic system.[2] The conservative group stresses the process of consumption: for example, social differences in smoking, diet and exercise. The radical group is more likely to stress the process of production: for example, social differences in exposure to dangerous work systems and industrial chemicals. In essence, the battle is about the importance of cultural versus structural factors in the explanation of health inequalities. Considering cultural factors favours the reflection on the ways that people behave, while a focus on structural factors favours greater emphasis on where people are placed within the social system. The two approaches with their main focus of concern and their main solution to contemporary health problems is shown in Table 1. Increasingly the focus moved from sociology to health policy.

While Table 1 provides a summary of the main difference between the approaches at the beginning of the 1980s, the emphasis on the production process by some radical critics was somewhat undermined by the sudden increase in unemployment in the early 1980s which shifted the focus away from the production process to the question of how unemployment may affect health.

One year after the Black Report, a report by Fagin (Fagin and Little, 1984) was produced – again only a few copies were published in the first instance. Fagin's report catalogued the consequences of long-term unemployment and produced reminders of research from earlier times of high unemployment in the 1930s: depression, headaches, asthmatic attacks, loss of appetite, family tensions, financial worries. Significantly, the report focused on the family; in fact, husband, wives and children all displayed signs of distress as a result of the breadwinner's unemployment. The government blandly asserted that there was little to worry about in relation to the health of the unemployed. Nevertheless, studies using the annual General Household Survey (GHS) have consistently shown that unemployed men and women are more likely to report health problems than those who are employed. The explanations for these differences are various. Some assert the physiological impact of the stress of being unemployed, others highlight that unemployment may lead to a loss of material resources, while the possibility exists that a process of health selection may be taking place in

Table 1   Contrast between two different types of health model

	Main focus of concern	Main solution to health problems
'Radical' health model	On production process	Changing socioeconomic environment
'Conservative' health model (also known as the 'lifestyle model')	On consumption process	Changing behaviour

so far as those who are already unhealthy are the very ones who are more likely to lose their jobs.

Some commentators have stressed that there are interesting parallels between the controversy over the impact of unemployment on health and the developing concern over the links between smoking and cancer. The early research which first brought out these links generated much academic debate on methodology and validity. Slowly then, and for some people, fatally slowly, the links became more widely accepted as the pile of research evidence grew. Those who resisted the evidence in the smoking and cancer controversy were, of course, big business, while with unemployment and the claims of structural factors influencing ill-health it has been the government who have resisted some of the growing and compelling evidence of links. For reasons which have already been mentioned, the government have pursued a health programme which largely focuses on cultural factors affecting health and an appeal to behavioural change as the main solution. Although perhaps linked rather insidiously to 'the ideology of victim-blaming', the government have over the past decade or so placed much greater emphasis on the importance of the patient, the consumer, the client, the customer – in short, the lay person.

Certainly it is a noble aspiration to place the lay person more appropriately centre stage. It is a battle which has neither been easy nor completed. One needs to recognize that there are various aspects to the battle. Historically, lay persons, whether as patients or as informal carers, have often had a bad deal from health professionals. Put simply, many of their concerns have not been taken seriously. But, to be fair, there have been moves forward. Perhaps a decade ago patients may have been given the same time at an outpatients' clinic as a dozen others and expected to wait around the whole day until called. Nowadays there is a greater recognition that patients do have other lives to lead and appointment times are generally taken more seriously by participants. However, these are just minor improvements to service delivery. There is still some way to go. Nettleton (1995) stresses why the study of lay health beliefs is of value to health care practice:

- An understanding of lay conceptualizations may provide insights into matters which may be dangerously 'written off' as 'incorrect' knowledge by professionals. Such discrepancies may lead to misunderstandings.
- An understanding of people's ideas about health maintenance and disease prevention is crucial to the effectiveness of health education and health promotion programmes. Lay health beliefs may act as powerful mediators.
- The study of health beliefs may contribute to our knowledge of informal health care. In fact, most health care work is carried out by lay people either in the form of self-care or caring for relatives and health workers.

Indeed, perhaps the most important insight is provided by Stacey (1988) – see Chapter 7 – that we are all health workers. While such a cry is heart-stirring stuff, one needs to begin to operationalize such compelling thoughts. In other words, how do we put such thoughts into practice?

Moving towards the twenty-first century

So, to summarize the 50 years since the Second World War, it is clear that doctors and medicine dominated the theorizing of the first 25 years, with accompanying accusations of health care being 'medico-centric', while there emerged over the next 25 years a shift to make the lay person the centre of attention. The latter task has not been completed, and there is still much to do before the patient, the consumer, the client (or whatever is the current label for the lay person) is the centre of professional activity, but we need to ask what does being 'lay-centric' mean? What are the goals and what are the dangers?

Certainly there are some fundamental questions which need addressed. In a market economy the customer may always be right, but is this necessarily the case in health care? Should the lay person be at the centre of the stage, beyond representing the simple, symbolic, but often unrecognized, truth that the interests of the lay person should be paramount? However, we still need to confront the issue of how are the interests of the lay person best served (Figure 1).

In the current year, starting the third quarter since the Second World War and coming to the fiftieth year anniversary of the founding of the National Health Service, we are arguing that there needs to be a new conceptualization of working relationships. Indeed, we argue that there are risks with an over-emphasis on lay conceptions and further suggest that such an over-emphasis may lead to charges of being 'lay-centric' in ways which

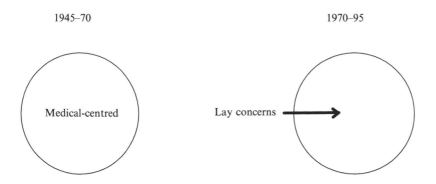

1945–70   1970–95

Medical-centred   Lay concerns

Figure 1   From 'medico-centric' to 'lay-centric'

distort. In other words, while tempting, it may be unwise to regard the voice of the user as sovereign. We maintain that while lay health beliefs and expressions of need are undoubtedly important, it may be inappropriate for lay persons to hold the centre of the stage quite so totally, just as many would hold that it may be unwise for students to decide how to run a university.

In reality we maintain that there needs to be an honest recognition that health professionals and others working in areas of health and illness with lay persons must work together. In brief, while Parsons too readily assumed a consensus of values and more recent theorists (see Freidson, Chapter 44) have stressed the potential conflict in, say, lay-professional interactions, the source and nature of conflict needs to be examined in a more constructive manner. So we are arguing that at the centre – which draws all groups together – must be the appropriate delivery of services and a focus on 'good practice', rather than the priorities of any particular group.

In looking forward towards the twenty-first century this Introduction provides a framework which captures some crucial issues of the moment while indicating how one can use the past to understand some of the pieces of the current jigsaw puzzle which needs to be put together. Hence, some themes will be identified which are taken up in various parts of the book. In each part we present some extracts from both some Classic Texts and perhaps some which are less well-known but which have, we believe, been influential. First, however, we need to clarify why we have decided to present the extracts in their original rather than just telling readers about them, as usually happens in a normal text.

We believe the original words are important. So, for example, it is unwise to try to understand the development of the theatre without reading some of the powerful words of Shakespeare to begin to appreciate his lasting impact on theatre. While it is impossible to gauge fully his impact on the original audiences in the Globe, the words still live on the contemporary stage. However, an even more crucial point in failing to read the original and simply relying on other people telling you about Shakespeare is that interpretations of Shakespeare may serve the ends of the interpreter and not the vision of the original. A fascinating reminder from the area of nursing that the words and work of distinguished people tend to be interpreted by the prism of a particular age is included in Chapter 35, which considers how the vision of Florence Nightingale is variously interpreted and exploited to serve the particular preoccupations of a particular time period. Hence, there may be a failure to capture the important breakthrough which Nightingale made at the time.

Another problem is that stories get distorted in the telling. The famous party game of Chinese whispers where a spoken message becomes distorted as it is passed from person to person around a circle also happens, albeit in perhaps less dramatic form, in academic circles as well. Famous names of the past are called upon to justify a contemporary stance or attitude. Margaret Thatcher's persistent claim of carrying the mantle of Winston

Churchill told us much more about Margaret Thatcher than what Churchill really stood for. Our task has been to identify some crucial themes, some important authors, and to reveal what really was said. As de Tocqueville (1856) has suggested, 'history is a gallery of pictures in which there are few originals and many copies'. This book is an opportunity to sample some originals in writings about health care in the past 50 years.

Notes

1. The paper, Doctors' orders: the past, present and future of medical sociology', presented by Margot Jefferys at the British Sociological Association conference at Lancaster University in 1980, has been influential as a major source for some of the ideas presented here. Her insights provide a useful framework for the earlier period under discussion.
2. This distinction was highlighted in some unpublished work of Neil Burdess in the early 1980s.

References

Armstrong, D. (1982) The fabrication of nurse–patient relationships. *Social Science and Medicine*, **17**(8), 457–460

Becker, H., Geer, B., Hughes, E. C. and Strauss, A. L. (1961) *Boys in White: Student Culture in Medical School*, University of Chicago Press, Chicago

Chadwick, E. (1843) *Report on the Sanitary Conditions of the Labouring Population of Great Britain*, HMSO, London.

Davis, F. (1963) *Passage Through Crisis: Polio Victims and their Families*, Merrill, Indianapolis, IN

Department of Health and Social Security (1972) *Report of the Committee on Nursing*, Cmnd 5115 (The Briggs Committee), HMSO, London.

De Toqueville (1856) *L'Ancien regime* (cited in *The Oxford Dictionary of Quotations*, 4th edn), Oxford University Press, Oxford, 1992)

Durkheim, E. (1952) *Suicide: A Study in Sociology*, Routledge and Kegan Paul, London (originally published as *Le Suicide*, 1897)

Fagin, L. and Little M. (1984) *The Forsaken Families: The Effects of Unemployment on Family Life*, Penguin, Harmondsworth (the original report was published as Fagin, L. (1981) *Unemployment and Health in Families: Case Studies Based on Family Interviews: A Pilot Study*, DHSS, London

Freidson, E. (1960) Client control and medical practice. *American Journal of Sociology*, **65**, 374–382.

Freidson, E. (1961) *Patients' Views of Medical Practice*. Russell Sage Foundation, New York

Freidson, E. (1961–62) The sociology of medicine; a trend report and bibliography. *Current Sociology*, **10–11**(3), 123–192

Freidson, E. (1962) Dilemmas in the doctor–patient relationship. In *Human Behavior and Social Processes* (A. Rose, ed.), Routledge and Kegan Paul, London

Freidson, E. (1963a) Medical care and the public: case study of a medical group, *Annals of the American Academy of Political Social Science*, **346**, 57–66

Freidson, E. (1963b) *The Hospital in Modern Society*, Free Press, New York

Freidson, E. (1970a) *Profession of Medicine*, Dodd Mead, New York

Freidson, E. (1970b) *Professional Dominance*, Atherton Press, New York
Freidson, E. (1975) *Doctoring Together*, Elsevier, New York
Gallagher, E.B. (1976) Lines of reconstruction and extension in the Parsonian sociology of illness. *Social Science and Medicine*, 10, 217–218
Gerson, E. M. (1976) The social character of illness: deviance or politics? *Social Science and Medicine*, 10, 219–224
Glaser, B. G. and Strauss, A. L. (1966) *Awareness of Dying*, Aldine, Chicago
Glaser, B. G. and Strauss, A. L. (1968) *Time for Dying*, Aldine, Chicago
Halsey, A. H., Martin, F. M. and Floud, J. E. (1957) *Social Class and Educational Opportunity*, Heinemann, London
Lancet (1932) *The Final Report of the Lancet Commission on Nursing*, HMSO, London
Lawler, J. (1991) *Behind the Screens: Nursing, Somology and the Problem of the Body*, Churchill Livingstone, Edinburgh
McKinlay, J. B. (1977) The business of good doctoring or doctoring as good business: reflections on Freidson's view of the medical game *International Journal of Health Services*, 7(3), 459–483
Merton, R., Reader, G. and Kendall, P. (eds) (1957) *The Student Physician: Introductory Studies in the Sociology of Medical Education*, Harvard University Press, Cambridge, Mass.
Ministry of Health and Board of Education (1938) *Interdepartmental Committee on Nursing* (Chair: The Earl of Athlone), HMSO, London
Nettleton, S. (1995) *The Sociology of Health and Illness*, Polity Press, Cambridge
Parsons, T. (1951) *The Social System*, Free Press, Glencoe, Ill
Parsons, T. (1975) The sick role and the role of the physician reconsidered. *Health and Society* (The Millbank Memorial Fund Quarterly), Summer, 257–273
Stacey, M. (with Homans, H.) (1978) The sociology of health and illness: its present state, future prospects and potential for health research. *Sociology*, 12(2), 281–307
Townsend, P. and Davidson, N. (1982) *Inequalities in Health*, Penguin, Harmondsworth
Turner, B. (1987) *Medical Power and Social Knowledge*, Sage, London
United Kingdom Central Council (1986) *Project 2000: A New Preparation for Practice*, UKCC, London

Part I Health – Some Fundamental Issues

The topic of health has always been an emotive and political one, and questions of health are now perhaps more firmly back on the political agenda than ever before. It is, of course, tempting to be seduced into thinking that the major contemporary issues are necessarily the most important ones. Indeed, politicians are adept in developing a debate on terms that they wish to embrace rather than confronting more fundamental issues which may need to be addressed. This first part aims to focus on some of these fundamental issues in studying health.

One soon recognizes that little is new. As **Kelman** points out, 'perhaps the most perplexing and ambiguous issue in the study of health since its inception centuries or millennia ago, is its definition'. J. P. Donleavy in *The Ginger Man* (1955) finds health easy to define: 'When you don't have any money, the problem is food. When you have money, it's sex. When you have both, it's health.' In reality, it is less easy than that and simply assuming that 'health' is the absence of illness simply dodges the issue. In fact, Kelman argues that the definitional problem is crucial to the determination of healthcare policy. He suggests that health is primarily socially, rather than strictly biologically, determined. Hence, this means that we cannot view 'health' as independent of the form of society in which it is studied. This insight lays the foundation of a materialist or radical epidemiology, which has gained support among some sociologists (e.g. Stark, 1997). They argue that since the advent of capitalist industrialization, the primary determinants of death and illness in the West have shifted gradually from infectious and communicable disease – spread by unhealthy conditions such as malnutrition, overcrowding or inadequate sanitation – to a rather different set of problems, such as cancer, heart disease, hypertension, stroke, mental illness and drug addiction.

Doyal places issues of health within a wider context and considers the relationship between the biological and the social, between health, illness and society. She focuses on some of the possible effects of capitalist development and reminds us that ill-health cannot be attributed simply to capitalism in any crude sense. However, an important point emphasized is that, under capitalism, health tends to be defined in an individualistic way. Doyal goes on to explain how the functional and individualistic definition of health forms the background against which medicine itself is defined as essentially curative.

Certainly, since the late eighteenth century medicine has had an increasingly central role in dealing with sickness. **McKeown** made an early plea for the reappraisal of the role of doctors, stressing that doctors have always tended to overestimate the effectiveness of their intervention and to underestimate the risks. Perhaps the most recent challenge to the effectiveness of the house of medicine has been the arrival of AIDS. **Strong**, writing in the context of the recognition of AIDS as a problem, focuses on how a major outbreak of novel, fatal epidemic disease can quickly be followed by plagues of fear, panic, suspicion and stigma. The parallels in the reaction to AIDS to the reaction to the Black Death in the Middle Ages are striking. Strong argues that what he terms as epidemic psychology is indeed a permanent part of the human condition. Influenced by the French intellectual, Michel Foucault, whose politically as well as philosophically motivated examinations of obscure historical materials were aimed at diagnosing the present, **Armstrong** probes what he terms as the rise of 'surveillance medicine'. He notes how the medical focus began to leave the exclusive domain of the hospital and to penetrate into the wider population. An increasing emphasis on comprehensive health care links closely with the development of medical surveillance.

After defining and understanding, measuring health is equally controversial. **Bowling** usefully identifies some of the problems in trying to measure health outcomes, or consequences, of care. She indicates that most existing indicators reflect a 'disease' model. However, she notes that a person can feel ill without medical science being able to detect disease. Certainly an area which is increasingly being recognized as crucial is the lay perspective and Bowling stresses the importance of taking account of an individual's self-assessment. Doctors alone cannot measure patients' quality of life.

Stacey provides an early and important challenge to the recent tendency to speak of patients as health service consumers. Whether called 'customers', 'clients', 'consumers' or the more traditional term of 'patients', what do people think of medical care? **Calnan** identifies three interrelated elements that shape the way lay people evaluate medical care.

Why people decide to seek professional medical help in the first place is a crucial issue. **Robinson** provides a vivid account of how the social context is important in deciding whether or not it is appropriate to visit the doctor. People of different occupations, class or family status have differential expectations about what signs or symptoms it is appropriate to ignore, live with, treat or consult about. **Gerson** challenges the traditional assumption that the interests of physician and patient are indeed harmonious. He suggests that this only happens in a limited set of circumstances and often the relationship of physician and patient is much more fraught. **Stimson** and

Webb look at the process of consultation with the general practitioner and write about the contact between patient and doctor from the point of view of the patient. **Doyal** and **Elston** usefully remind us of the importance of women as consumers and producers of health care. In other words, women constitute the majority of NHS patients and make up the majority of health workers.

There is much greater emphasis nowadays on persons taking responsibility for their own health. **Crawford** talks powerfully of the ideology and politics of victim blaming. The argument that if we adopt lifestyles which avoid unhealthy behaviour we can prevent most diseases is certainly easier for some rather than others. **Blaxter's** work has provided the evidence that healthy lifestyles have the most effect when the social environment is good; rather less, if it is already unhealthy. In a ringing phrase, 'unhealthy behaviour does not reinforce disadvantage to the same extent as healthy behaviour increases advantage'. In other words, if you are living in a seriously disadvantaged situation, that is going to have the most effect on your health – or ill-health. The extract here stresses how the effects of, say, class or income or area of residence on health is much more complex than is usually recognized. **Fagin** and **Little** focus on the effects of unemployment on family life and probe the causal link between unemployment and health. Again, while the evidence suggests that there is an association between health and unemployment, the link is far from straightforward.

While we have stressed the apparent permanence of so many of the problems and that the house of medicine has perhaps not done so well as is so readily claimed, it is also important to emphasize the possibilities and realities of change. **Field** focuses on the shift over the past two or three decades in the attitudes of health care professionals towards the care of dying people. This has been welcomed, but he also reminds that 'an endemic feature of hospital care is the neglect of the patient as a person'. **Goffman's** classic work provides a framework by which we can understand that hospitals share significant similarities with other establishments for which Goffman provides the generic term 'total institution'. He shows what we are up against when we engage with total institutions. So, for example, he demonstrates how total institutions are incompatible with some other crucial elements of society, such as the family.

While Goffman focuses on the staff–inmate split in a variety of contexts, **Jeffery** concentrates more specifically on the ways that staff evaluate patients. At bottom, it seems, patients tend to split between good or interesting, and bad or rubbish. **May** and **Kelly** also discuss the range of patient typifications employed by health care personnel. However, they go further and suggest, from their own work looking at psychiatric nursing, that it is from their dealings with patients, in part at least, that a sense of professional identity emerges. **Stannard**, focusing on the increasingly important topic of how to deal with 'old folks', identifies the social conditions for patient abuse in a nursing home and provides a persuasive

account of how supervisory and professional staff may, perhaps unknow-
ingly, collude in the continuance of abuse.

The section ends where we all must end – that is, with death. **Sudnow**
maintains that the likelihood of 'dying' and even of being pronounced 'dead'
can be said to be partially a function of one's place in the social structure. He
further suggests that if you anticipate having a critical heart attack, it may be
wise to keep yourself well-dressed and your breath clean!

Reference

Stark, E. (1977) The epidemic as social event. *International Journal of Health
    Services*, 7(4), 681–705

Chapter 1

The social nature of the definition problem in health

Sander Kelman

Perhaps the most perplexing and ambiguous issue in the study of health since its inception centuries or millennia ago, is its definition. Currently, most curricula in the study of public health devote a certain, nominal, amount of time to the issue, reviewing definitions offered by earlier writers, but the conclusion is always that the definitions have virtually no operational or empirical significance, and, more importantly, that the definition question is not problematic to the empirical analysis of epidemiology, health care institutions, and health care policy. In general the issue is obviated by assuming, either implicitly or explicitly, that 'health' is the absence of illness.

[Here] it is argued that through adoption of the appropriate theoretical approach and the derivation of suitable analytical categories, the definition problem can be seen as operational, nontrivial, and highly problematic to the determination of health care policy. More concretely, the article attempts to isolate the social basis of the definition of health.

Thomas Kuhn (1962) in his now-celebrated book. *The Structure of Scientific Revolutions*, argues that the principal characteristic of any field of scientific inquiry during any particular epoch in its development is the fundamental *paradigm* (postulate) that organizes the practice of 'normal science' during that epoch. Hence, astronomy, some 500 years ago, passed from the paradigm of geocentrism to that of heliocentrism and beyond.

The first apparent scientific paradigm for health originated with the development of the machine model of the human body (since the mind or soul was relegated to a separate compartment). With this conception, 'health' came to be seen as the perfect working order of the human organism, likening the human organism to an automaton (a self-propelling machine) (Rossdale, 1965). Moreover, the methodologies of pathology and diagnostics that developed from this view (and continue to dominate in the practice of medicine, today) consider illness to be both natural (biological) and occurring on an individual basis. Treatment, therefore, is pursued on an individual bio-chemo-surgical basis, relegating the recognition and implications of social causes of illness to secondary importance, though even this secondary recognition must be viewed as 'ad hoc modification' (Kuhn, 1962, p. 78) in the face of the next paradigm to be discussed.

Although the recognition of the social basis of many diseases and ill health goes far back in medical history, the greatest boost probably came with the publication of the Chadwick Report in England and the Shattuck Report in the United States in the mid-19th century. Since that time there has been a great deal of writing on social epidemiology and the environmentalist approach to health, and this represents the second major paradigm in the discussion of health, for it is clearly in conflict with the biological and individual orientation of the classical school, still very much the predominant methodology. Yet the purpose of this paper is to show that even if their differences could be resolved, the substance of 'health' is still not defined.

Whereas the advances of the social epidemiology school over the science of its predecessor lie in the area of etiology, it still suffers from the implicit assumption that 'health' itself is biologically, not socially, determined, that the substantive meaning of 'health' is not a variant.

[While t]he etiology of heart disease and stroke is recognized, even in the leading medical journals, to be bound up in the social organization and dynamics in which its victims live (Eyer, 1975), yet this view does not receive coherent formulation and application to cure. Despite the available evidence, the bio-individual school formulates the causes as genetic, while the social epidemiological school extends the assignments of etiology only a few steps further to diet, smoking, obesity, or 'life style', that is to things that mediate the ultimate social causes. Both schools agree on treatment as well: administration of screening, chemotherapy, and heart operations to mitigate the effects of hypertension, the proximate cause.

Similarly, cancers are today recognized to result, in 60–90 per cent of the cases, from artificially created, environmental carcinogens (Bernstein, 1975), yet the prescribed treatment is ex post radiation, chemotherapy, and surgical removal rather than environmental prevention. Although, 'normal' mental illness (depression, chronic anxiety, etc.) is similarly recognized to result from adverse social organization (Fromm, 1955), again, the prescribed treatment is some combination of drugs, psychotherapy, transcendental meditation, and other forms of instrumental, victim-blaming 'cures'.

Such scientific emphasis on attempted cure, rather than prevention, might be scientifically justifiable in terms of the limited state of our understanding of the etiology of these diseases *were there also a major and visible discussion and research effort directed toward the social reorganization necessary to prevent these leading causes of illness and death.* In its absence, however, the inevitable conclusion must be that there are at least two fundamental and conflicting notions or dimensions of 'health': *experimental* and *functional.* The former may be defined as freedom from illness, the capacity for human development and self-discovery, and the transcendence of alienating social circumstances. Given the above treatment modes, it falls in the face of the latter: the 'state of optimum *capacity* of an individual for the effective performance of the roles and tasks for which he has been socialized' (Parsons, 1972, p. 117). The two are quite different concretely, in terms of the respective 'health' policies that they imply,

Moreover, they are substantially in conflict given that health policies established upon the experimental definition of 'health' would suggest the elimination of those social conditions that give rise to illness, whereas policies established upon the functional definition may merely suggest either the intervention between the social stressors and their associated pathogenesis (as through drugs) or the ex post treatment of those illnesses (as through surgery).

To return to the point of departure, it will be argued that a new paradigm in the science of health must be adopted: one that recognized that health behavior, in any society, is socially determined even to the extent that 'health' itself is primarily socially, rather than strictly biologically, determined; it is largely a socially determined category predicated upon the particular characteristics and dynamics of the society under investigation.

The materialist approach to the study of health

The development of this third paradigm (that 'health' itself is socially defined) can begin with the axiom that human beings are the basis of both the forces of production (physical ingredients of production, such as labor, resources, and equipment) and the relations of production (division of labor, legal, property, and social institutions and practices) in any society, and that therefore 'appropriate human organismic condition' (i.e. 'health') can only be understood in the concrete context of the particular mode of organization of production and the dialectical relationship between the productive forces and relations (Baran and Hobsbawm, 1972).

In Western culture the first, and still most prominent, paradigm is that of the machine model of the body and the germ theory of disease. Because of its inability to incorporate emotional and psychosomatic processes, and the social, rather than individual, causes of illness into its paradigm, it yields logically to the social epidemiology paradigm. Both, however, are limited in their capacity to generate a notion of organismic integrity, i.e. 'health', since both view 'health' as independent of the form of society in which it is studied. Given contemporary practices concerning stress, cancer, and other environmentally induced illnesses, 'health' is something other than the lack of organismic breakdown, the definition implied by both of these paradigms. Instead, a functional dimension must be recognized as part and parcel of a definition of health which purports to describe accurately health behavior in contemporary capitalist society.

[An] appropriate definition of health must recognize the inherent contradictions, in such a society, between functional and experiential health, on the one hand, and within the social determination of experiential health itself, on the other.

References

Baran, P. and Hobsbawm, E. (1972) The method of historical materialism. In *The Capitalist System* (R. Edwards, M. Reich and T. Weisskopf, eds), pp. 53–56. Prentice-Hall, Englewood Cliffs, N.J.

Bernstein, P. J. (1975) Carcinogens. *Boston Sunday Globe*, p. A-4. January 19

Eyer, J. (1975) Hypertension as a disease of modern society. *International Journal of Health Services*, 5(4), 539–558

Fromm, E. (1955) *The Sane Society*. Fawcett, Greenwich, Conn.

Kuhn, T. (1962) *The Structure of Scientific Revolutions*, University of Chicago Press, Chicago

Parsons, T. (1972) In *Patients, Physicians, and Illness* (E. Gartly Jaco, ed.), Ed. 2, pp. 107–127. Free Press, New York

Rossdale, M. (1965) Health in a sick society. *New Left Review*, no. 34, 82–90

Reprinted by permission of the Baywood Publishing Co., Inc., New York. Sander Kelman (1975) The social nature of the definition problem in health. *International Journal of Health Services*, 5(4), 625–642. © 1976, Baywood Publishing Co.

Chapter 2

Health, illness and capitalism
Lesley Doyal (with Imogen Pennell)

The first question we need to consider is the relationship between the biological and the social, between health, illness and society. Most discussions
of medical care have, until recently, taken ill health for granted, and have
rarely questioned its social or economic origins. While people are now
coming increasingly to accept that social and economic factors do have
some importance in causing ill health, they argue that this has nothing to
do with capitalism. Rather, it is assumed that it is industrialization itself
which tends to destroy health, and hence that there is nothing much we can
do about it. Thus, poor health for some is seen as a necessary consequence
of economic growth, which is itself assumed to be a desirable goal for
everyone. It is certainly possible to argue (probably correctly) that the advantages to be gained from industrial production must always involve, to a
greater or lesser extent, the destruction of human and physical resources.
Yet the nature and extent of that destruction will reflect the priorities of the
society in which the production takes place. Thus if ... it is ultimately profit,
rather than a concern to improve overall living standards, which is the most
important determinant of economic and social decision-making in capitalist
society, this will be reflected in various ways in patterns of health and illness.

While the development of capitalism may have facilitated an improvement
in the general health of the population (as measured, for example, in life-
expectancy rates), the health needs of the mass of the population continue to
come into frequent conflict with the requirements of continued capital
accumulation. This produces contradictions which are ultimately reflected in
historical changes in patterns of morbidity and mortality. In contrast, while
we cannot specify in advance a utopian blueprint for a socialist health
policy, we can assume that under socialism profit would no longer be the
criterion for making decisions about production or consumption. Very
different goods could then be manufactured, possibly using alternative
technologies, with labour organized in less damaging ways, and income
more equally distributed. While it would be absurd to suggest that all
disease would be abolished under socialism, we can assume that a real
concern for the health of the population would be reflected in planning and

decision-making. Thus, through analysing the social production of health and illness in capitalist countries we can learn more about the nature of capitalism itself, as well as becoming aware of what needs to be avoided in future if a 'healthier' society is to be created.

Of course, not all aspects of capitalist development have been equally harmful – a fact which is often forgotten. Indeed, the development of the forces of production made possible by industrial capitalism has formed the basis for a tremendous improvement in average life expectancy for people in the developed world. After the initial period of industrialization, the level of subsistence rose dramatically, with better food, clothing and housing for the working class, as well as a gradual decline in the length of the working day. All these developments have been important in improving general standards of health – although class differences still remain. However ... that same process of the development of the forces of production had at least two other dimensions to it. First, it was ultimately dependent on a particular mode of economic and social exploitation of the underdeveloped world, which was damaging to the health of third world populations. Secondly, while it removed certain threats to health in the developed world, the development of industrial capitalism itself created *new* health problems, many of which are only now becoming apparent. Thus the relationship between capitalist development and health has been a contradictory one. ...

It is a commonplace of left wing rhetoric that 'capitalism causes disease', but a generalized statement of this kind, uniformly applied to all ill health in all places and at all times, has very little theoretical or political content. We are not helped in our attempt to understand the varieties and circumstances of ill health under capitalism by being told that all people in capitalist societies are 'sick'.

_____

... [I]t is obviously important that we examine more concretely some of the ways in which the operaton of a capitalist system creates contradictions between health and profit.

First, the physical processes of commodity production itself will affect health in a variety of ways. Clearly the imperatives of capital accumulation condition the nature of the labour process, and the need for shiftwork, de-skilling, overtime or the use of dangerous chemicals, will all be reflected in the health or ill health of workers. They may suffer directly, either through industrial injuries and diseases, or in more diffuse ways with stress-related ill health, or psychosomatic problems. Yet commodity production also has more *indirect* effects on health, and the physical effects of the production process extend beyond the workplace itself. Damage to the surrounding environment and pollution of various kinds are often the by-products of industrialized production. Finally, commodity production may damage health through the nature of the commodities themselves. Capitalist production is concerned with exchange values and, as a result, concern about the quality of a product (including its effects on health) will usually arise only in the context of an assessment of its selling potential. If it will sell, then its effects on health are likely to be of little concern to the producer, so that many health-damaging products will continue to be made simply because they are profitable.

But it is also characteristic of capitalist societies that everyone is not equally affected by these illness-producing processes. Class differences in morbidity and mortality are very pronounced. Working-class people die sooner, and generally suffer more ill health than do middle-class people. We therefore need to look at other aspects of capitalist social and economic relations – especially distribution of income and patterns of work and consumption – in order to explain these differences. The most obvious cause of class differences in morbidity and mortality will be the differential health risks of specific occupations. Certain groups of workers (often the lower paid) have more dangerous and unhealthy jobs than others, but these occupational risk factors do not account for all the observed differences in mordibity and mortality. Class differences in infant mortality rates, for example, or the increased rates of morbidity and early mortality among the wives of male manual workers remain unexplained. Some of these differences derive from physical proximity to the production process. Workers 'import' dangers from the workplace into the home, and clearly this will affect working-class families more often. In addition, they are more likely to live near industrial plants and therefore to be more affected by pollution and industrial wastes. But again, this direct or indirect contact with the production process is not enough to explain all class differences in health and illness.

The distribution of ill health in capitalist societies broadly follows the distribution of income. Those with lower incomes tend to have higher rates of morbidity and mortality, for a number of reasons. In a capitalist society income is a major determinant of the standard of housing individuals and families can obtain, of where they live, of their diet, and of their ability to remain warm and well-clothed. All of these factors are significant for health. Moreover, the quality of life (and therefore of health) is increasingly influenced by access to the goods and services provided by the state. Even where these are in principle distributed on a universalistic basis, in practice they are allocated neither equally nor in terms of need. For example, children of unskilled workers are likely to receive an inferior education and therefore to go on to low paid and probably dangerous jobs themselves. Similarly, medical care is not allocated solely on the basis of need. While a more egalitarian allocation of medical resources could not remove inequalities in morbidity and mortality, it is evident that present inequalities in resource allocation serve to reinforce more fundamental class differences in health and illness.

It is, however, in underdeveloped countries that the extremes of ill health and premature death are to be found. Here, the major causes of death are not, as is often assumed, the endemic tropical diseases, but rather infectious diseases and malnutrition. These are not 'natural', but arise in large part from the particular social and economic relationships characteristic of imperialism. The incidence and severity of infectious diseases, for example, are directly related to the misery and squalor of both urban and rural poverty. Similarly, malnutrition does not simply result from too many people and too little food in any particular country. Like urban and rural poverty, it is often a direct result of the exploitative relationship between the metropolitan countries and the underdeveloped world, and the consequent uneven development and allocation of resources.

Ill health cannot, therefore, be attributed simply to capitalism in any crude sense. On the other hand, we cannot make sense of patterns of health and illness outside the context of the mode of production in which they occur. As Eyer and Stering have said, 'A large component of adult physical pathology and death must be considered neither acts of God nor of our genes, but a measure of the misery caused by our present social and economic organization' (Eyer and Sterling, 1977).

It is the medical definition, the view of the 'experts', which now forms the basis for the social definition of health and illness throughout the developed world ... between the late eighteenth century and the present day, medicine has been characterized by what Jewson calls 'a shift from a person-oriented to an object-oriented cosmology'. Ill health is now defined primarily in terms of the malfunctioning of a mechanical system, and treatment consists of surgical, chemical or even electrical intervention to restore the machine to normal working order. The 'functional' element in the definition of health means that, in practice, health is usually defined as 'fitness' to undertake whatever would be expected of someone in a particular social position. For example, people who are able to carry on with their normal activities are not likely to be regarded as really ill, even though subjectively they may be suffering from depression, anxiety, migraine, insomnia or chronic indigestion. Put another way, health is usually defined – negatively – as the absence of incapacitating and externally verifiable pathology. Anyone not showing signs of such pathology is assumed to be healthy. The defining of health and illness in a functional way is an important example of how a capitalist value system defines people primarily as producers – as forces of production. It is concerned with their 'fitness' in an instrumental sense, rather than with their own hopes, fears, anxieties, pain or suffering. In defining health and illness in this way, the medical model limits people's own expectations of what it is to be healthy and is thus significant in keeping sickness (and also the demand for medical care) under control.

But under capitalism, health is also defined in an individualistic way. It is always individuals who become sick, rather than social economic or environmental factors which cause them to be so. As Evan Stark (1977) has commented:

> Disease is understood as a failure in and of the individual, an isolatable 'thing' that attacks the physical machine more or less arbitrarily from 'outside' preventing it

from fulfilling its essential 'responsibilities'. Both bourgeois epidemiology and 'medical ecology' ... consider 'society' only as a relatively passive medium through which 'germs' pass en route to the individual.

This emphasis on the individual origin of disease is of considerable social significance, since it effectively obscures the social and economic causes of ill health. The destruction of health is potentially a vitally important political issue, and the medical emphasis on individual causation is one means of defusing this. In recent years the individualism inherent in the scientific medical model has taken a new and more powerful form. As it has become clear that curative medicine is largely ineffective against the 'diseases of affluence', it is now being widely argued that what are referred to as 'way of life' factors – diet, stress, smoking and lack of exercise – are crucial in causing this new 'disease burden'. As a consequence, it is suggested that ill health can be explained in terms of individual moral failings – by blaming the victims for what has happened to them.[1] Contemporary epidemiology has therefore incorporated environmental factors into its understanding of ill health, but it interprets them narrowly and selectively, usually emphasizing those aspects which can be seen as the individual's own responsibility. The suggestion that individuals are to blame for their own unhealthy life-styles means that moral exhortations to be healthier, as well as self-care and self-help, are stressed as important future trends in health care. People as individuals must help themselves to stay healthy through changing their *own* lives. Navarro (1976) has summarized the obvious appeal of this approach, in the following way:

> ... it strengthens the basic ethical tenets of bourgeois individualism, the ethical construct of capitalism where one has to be free to do whatever one wants, free to buy and sell, to accumulate wealth or to live in poverty, to work or not, to be healthy or to be sick. Far from being a threat to the power structure, this life-style politics complements and is easily co-optable by the controllers of the system, and it leaves the economic and political structures of our society unchanged. Moreover, the life-style approach to politics serves to channel out of existence any conflicting tendencies against those structures that may arise in our society.

This functional and individualistic definition of health forms the background against which medicine itself is defined as essentially curative. 'Curing' as the central focus of medical activity is of broad social and economic significance in at least two ways. Most importantly, the expansion of technological curative medicine has provided the basis for an expanding and extremely profitable health care industry. The medical-industrial complex in the USA where the private sector remains predominant, provides the clearest example of the direct role of medicine in the process of capital accumulation.[2] Even in countries like Britain, however, where medical care is organized by the state, it still remains an important source of profit, since equipment and drugs continue to be purchased from the private sector, while state hospitals are built by private contractors. But the medical emphasis on cure is also of wider, though more indirect, economic significance. As we have seen, capitalist production is itself a cause of ill health in a variety of ways. As a consequence, any preventive medicine which was to be substantially effective, would need to interfere with the organization of the production process itself. Insofar as curative medicine appears to deny or at least to minimize the need for such preventive measures, it serves to protect existing economic interests.

Notes

1. Berliner, H. (1977) Emerging ideologies in medicine. *Review of Radical Political Economics*, 9(1), Spring, 116–123; Ryan, W. (1972) *Blaming the Victim*, Random House, New York. The impact of these ideas on recent British health policy is discussed in chapter five.
2. For an extremely good discussion see, Ehrenreich, B. and Ehrenreich, J. (1971) *The American Health Empire: Power, Profits and Politics*, a Report from the Health Policy Advisory Centre, Vintage Books, New York; Rodberg, L. and Stevenson, G. (1977) The health care industry in advanced capitalism. *Review of Radical Political Economics*, 9(1), Spring, 104–115.

References

Eyer, J. and Sterling, P. (1977) Stress related mortality and social organisation. *Review of Radical Political Economics*, 9(1), Spring, 2

Navarro, V. (1976) *Medicine Under Capitalism*, Croom Helm, London, p. 126.

Stark, E. (1977) 'Introduction' to the special issue on health. *Review of Radical Political Economics*, 9(1), Spring, v.

Reprinted by permission of Pluto Press, London. Lesley Doyal (with Imogen Pennell) (1979) Health, illness and capitalism. In *The Political Economy of Health*, Pluto Press, London, pp. 22–27, 32–33, 36

Chapter 3

The role of medicine: dream, mirage, or nemesis?

Thomas McKeown

Doctors have always tended to overestimate the effectiveness of their intervention and to underestimate the risks, whether removing large quantities of blood, under mistaken notions of the blood volume, in the treatment of yellow fever in the eighteenth century, or exposing patients to dangerous levels of radiation, of whose effects they were unaware, when screening for breast cancer in the twentieth. There was and is still a good deal of unjustified complacency about the extent of understanding of disease and of ability to control it, for example, in the assumptions that malaria and schistosomiasis will soon be eradicated or that there is little more to fear from airborne infections. And patients have been and continue to be exposed to pain and injury from misguided attempts to do them good. Suffering is only marginally more tolerable when inflicted with the best intentions, and the death of Charles II under treatment by his doctors was much more cruel than that of his father at the hands of his executioner. Indeed the history of treatment of illness in the aristocracy,[1] who were able to obtain the 'best' medical care, suggests that Francis Galton was generous in his conclusion that there is a considerable difference between a good doctor and a bad one, but hardly any difference between a good doctor and none at all.

A second reason for reappraisal of the role of doctors is the more independent line now taken by other health professionals. In some respects this is less a result of a fresh assessment of the needs of patients than an expression of the spirit of our times, when notions of equality and freedom are applied in all circumstances, even to the relation between parents and children. But it is also true that nurses, social workers, hygienists, and others have come to believe that they can often function just as effectively without the advice, and much more happily without the supervision of the doctor.

There is also a change in public attitudes to medicine, less evident in Britain than in the United States. In that country the image of the doctor as a devoted healer has been shaken by the resistance of professional organizations to the introduction of publicly financed and administered health services, and by the unwillingness of doctors to practise in areas which they find unattractive: even, in some cases, where patients are able to meet the costs of private medical care. To many people doctors seem less concerned about the welfare of patients than about their own convenience and standard of living. In such circumstances insistence on the delicacy of the doctor–patient relationship by the physician seems an anomaly, equivalent to the suggestion that the privacy of the confessional is intended to protect, not the sinner but the priest.

If we are neither cured when we are ill nor well cared for when we are disabled, what is the role of medicine in which so much has been invested, in hope and resources?

I have put the question in the provocative form in which it may be asked, indeed in which it has already been asked by some who have lost faith in the work of doctors. But if the question is overstated so too are likely to be the answers. From the belief that medicine can do everything, opinion is in danger of swinging to the equally untenable conclusion that it can do little or nothing. It is therefore important for the public as well as for the profession itself, that the medical role should be reconsidered, fairly and objectively, taking account of both its achievements in the past and its probable contributions in the foreseeable future.

Conclusions

In the broadest terms, the medical role is in three areas: prevention of disease by personal and non-personal measures; care of the sick who provide scope, or more accurately, under existing services, while they provide scope, for investigation and treatment; and care of the sick who are not thought to require active intervention. Medical interest and resources are focused on the second area and, to a lesser extent, on personal prevention by immunization; the other responsibilities are relatively neglected.

The immediate determinant of the traditional range of interests is the patient's demand for acute care and the physician's wish to provide it. But the approach rests also on a conceptual model, on the belief that health depends primarily on personal intervention, based on understanding of the structure and function of the body and of the disease processes which affect it.

This concept is not in accord with past experience. ... The improvement of health during the past three centuries was due essentially to provision of food, protection from hazards, and limitation of numbers; medical science and services made an important contribution to the control of hazards but only a limited one through immunization and therapy.

A theoretical assessment of the determinants of human health ... suggests that the same influences are likely to be effective in future; but there is this difference, that in developed countries personal behaviour (in relation to diet, exercise, tobacco, alcohol, drugs, etc.) is now even more important than provision of food and control of hazards. According to this interpretation few diseases, except for an ill-defined group at the end of life, are determined irreversibly at fertilization; most congenital abnormalities are probably due to intra-uterine conditions operating during implantation and early embryonic development; and most other common diseases are due to post-natal influences. Prenatal determinants are likely to be difficult to identify and control; those which are post-natal vary widely, from some which are simple and tractable (as in the case of many infections) to others which are complex and difficult (for various reasons) to remove. Nevertheless it is on recognition of such post-natal influences that hopes for a solution of the problems of the common diseases, both physical and mental, chiefly rest.

Nothing in these conclusions suggests that the traditional lines of biomedical research are useless and should be brought to an end. On the contrary, they have contributed greatly, by extending the scope and precision of hygienic measures, to a more limited extent by immunization and therapy, but above all, by providing an understanding of the body and its diseases on which the security of effective measures, originally largely intuitive, now substantially rests. However there is need for a shift in the balance of effort, from laboratory research to epidemiology, in recognition that improvement in health is likely to come in future, as in the past, from modification of the conditions which lead to disease, rather than from intervention in the mechanism of disease after it has occurred.

In health services the provision of acute care will continue, needless to say, for it is a response to what the patient usually considers to be his most urgent need. But this service does not justify the predominant place it has occupied until now in medical thought and practice. It is sometimes extremely effective, particularly in treatment of conditions such as accidents which, ideally, should not occur; but often it is ineffective, or merely tides the patient over a short illness, leaving the underlying disease condition and prognosis essentially unchanged. The limitations of the traditional concept of the medical role would have been recognized much earlier, if health had not been transformed in the past three centuries by other influences.

What is needed is an adjustment in the balance of interest and resources between the three main areas of service referred to above. It is essential to give sufficient attention to the personal and non-personal influences which are the major determinants of health: to food and the environment, which will be mainly in the hands of specialists, and to personal behaviour, which should be the concern of every practising doctor. These interests should no longer be peripheral to the medical role, in the way that health education, nutrition, and environmental medicine have been peripheral hitherto. In the field of personal care, the making of a diagnosis and the provision of acute care should be regarded as no more than the beginning of a responsibility which will continue so long as the patient is unwell; and the arbitrary and largely artificial distinctions between different types of patients (acute, chronic, mental, subnormal, etc.) should end.

Note

1. Excellently recorded for the French Court in the Memoirs of Saint-Simon.

Reprinted by permission of Blackwell Publishers, Oxford, and Princeton University Press, New Jersey. Thomas McKeown (1976) *The Role of Medicine: Dream, Mirage, or Nemesis*, The Nuffield Provincial Hospitals Trust/Blackwell, Oxford, pp. 158–160, 178–180.

Chapter 4

Epidemic psychology: a model

Philip Strong

This essay is a first attempt at a general sociological statement on the
striking problems that large, fatal epidemics seem to present to social
order; on the waves of fear, panic, stigma, moralizing and calls to action
that seem to characterize the immediate reaction. Of course, severe epidemics may also present serious threats to both the economy and to welfare.
The assault on public order is, in part, moulded by the other ravages made
by the epidemic. Singling it out for separate theoretical treatment may,
however, lead to important analytic gains. Not only may public order be
challenged in a most unusual fashion, but the subjective experience of the
first social impact of such epidemics has a compelling, highly dramatic
quality (Rosenberg, 1989). Societies are caught up in an extraordinary emotional maelstrom which seems, at least for a time, to be beyond anyone's
immediate control. Moreover, since this strange state presents such an immediate threat, actual or potential, to public order, it can also powerfully
influence the size, timing and shape of the social and political response in
many other areas affected by the epidemic.

How can this initial drama be analysed? I shall argue that the early
reaction to major fatal epidemics constitutes a distinctive psycho-social
form; one which I shall term *epidemic psychology*. Its underlying micro-
sociology may well be common to all such diseases – or so I shall
hypothesize – but is manifested in its purest shape when a disease is new,
unexpected, or particularly devastating. Versions of it may also perhaps be
found, mutatis mutandis, in other distinctive but parallel types of dramatic
social crisis, in times of war and revolution as well as those of plague.
(Hobbes' *Leviathan*, published in 1651, was both the first major analysis of
social order and written in a time of civil war.)

Epidemic psychology: notes on the model

Epidemic psychology is a phrase with a double meaning. It contains within it
a reference, not just to the special micro-sociology or social psychology of

epidemics, but to the fact that that psychology has its own epidemic nature, quite separate from the epidemic of disease. Like the disease, it too can spread rapidly from person to person, thereby creating a major collective as well as individual impact. At the same time, however, its spread can take a much wider variety of forms. Epidemic psychology, indeed, seems to involve at least three types of psycho-social epidemic. The first of these is an epidemic of fear. The second is an epidemic of explanation and moralization and the third is an epidemic of action, or proposed action. Any society gripped by a florid form of epidemic psychology may, therefore, simultaneously experience waves of individual and collective panic, outbursts of interpretation as to why the disease has occurred, rashes of moral controversy, and plagues of competing control strategies, aimed either at containing the disease itself or else at controlling the further epidemics of fear and social dissolution.

———————

[A]lthough epidemic psychology has not been a conventional subject in modern medical or micro-sociology, it seems to be a clearly recognized possibility in lay thought. It may never be elaborated in the way described here but the potential reality of the phenomenon seems a fundamental given, an all too vivid danger, in human social apprehension. Even if the apocalypse is not now, who knows when the four horsemen may ride? Everyone has deep personal experience of panic. Most of us, moreover, know something of minor social crisis and most of us, more particularly, have been taught something dramatic about bubonic plague. Many commentators have criticized the tabloids' use of the phrase 'gay plague' to describe AIDS. Fewer have noted the extraordinary historical resonance of the Black Death in popular culture. Six hundred years on, it remains one of the most powerful of all European folk memories. Epidemic psychology, then, is not just an analyst's construct but an ideal-type which is in everyday use.

Some comment must also be made on the validity of the distinctions I have just introduced between the different types of psycho-social epidemic. Any sharp separation between different types of epidemic psychology is a dubious business. To distinguish fears from action and morality from strategy seems arbitrary and inaccurate. In actual life, these matters are inseparably intertwined. Different sorts of fear, for example, generate quite different sorts of action. Analytically, however, the distinction has its uses.

Finally, it is worth elaborating a little on the point that the epidemics of fear, interpretation and action seem to be much more severe when the disease is new or strikes in a new way. Once bubonic plague had returned again to Europe in the fourteenth century, major epidemics broke out roughly once every twenty years. After the first horror of the Black Death, these outbreaks were never quite as virulent, except in particular isolated locations, but there was still an overall mortality of perhaps fifteen or twenty per cent in many towns (Open University, 1985). However, although the plague was always awful, individuals, towns and cities developed routine, often rapid, ways of responding to it – at least some of the time (Cipolla, 1973). Plague, then, became normalized and institutionalized (just as AIDs has begun to become now). In these changed circumstances, plague was still appalling but it was now, at least on some occasions, a familiar condition and could be greeted in a familiar way: 'Oh God, it's plague again, we'll have to shut up the city', rather than 'Oh my God, what is this, is it the end of the world?'

By contrast, as the instance of the Black Death so vividly illustrates, new forms of fatal, epidemic disease can potentially be much more terrifying and may generate much more extreme reactions and diverse reactions. When routine social responses are unavailable, then a swarm of different theories and strategies may compete for attention.

The different psycho-social epidemics

Consider the different psycho-social epidemics in turn. The epidemic of fear seems to have several striking characteristics, or potential characteristics, all of which will be fairly obvious to the reader, since we have just lived through such an epidemic ourselves. None the less, they are worth listing systematically. First note that the epidemic of fear is also an epidemic of suspicion. There is the fear that I might catch the disease and the suspicion that you may already have it and might pass it on to me. A second characteristic of novel, fatal epidemic disease seems to be a widespread fear that the disease may be transmitted through any number of different routes, through sneezing and breathing, through dirt and through door-knobs, through touching anything and anyone. The whole environment, human, animal and inanimate, may be rendered potentially infectious. If we do not know what is happening, who knows where the disease might not spring from?

A third striking feature, closely linked to the two above, is the way that fear and suspicion may be wholly separate from the reality of the disease. Just as HIV spread silently for several years before anyone was aware of its presence, so it is possible for great waves of panic and fear to spread among a population even when almost no-one has actually been infected. Japan seems to have experienced such a reaction to just one case of AIDS in 1987 (Ohi et al., 1988). Likewise, as soon as AIDS became a public crisis in the UK (a process which began in the last week of April 1983, when mass media coverage suddenly erupted) doctors began to see a wave of patients who were obsessed with the fear that they had the disease and could not be persuaded to the contrary (Weber and Goldmeier, 1983; see also Jaeger, 1988).

Such panic and irrationality can extend even to those who are normally best informed about the disease. Experienced doctors could still turn hot and cold when they saw their first AIDS patient, or be unable to extend the normal social courtesies to AIDS campaigners. Experienced natural scientists could find themselves unable to treat HIV like any other virus. (Strong and Berridge, 1990).

Classically associated with this epidemic of irrationality, fear and suspicion, there comes close in its train an epidemic of stigmatization; the stigmatization both of those with the disease and of those who belong to what are feared to be the main carrier groups. This can begin with avoidance, segregation and abuse and end – at least potentially – in pogroms. Personal fear may be translated into collective witch-hunts. Moreover, so we should note, such avoidance, segregation and persecution can be quite separate – analytically at least – from actions aimed at containing the epidemic. Such behaviour can occur with all types of stigma, not just with that of epidemic disease. We are dealing here with magic and taboo, not just with quarantine.

Now consider the epidemics of explanation, moralization and action, epidemics which can be a response both to plague itself and to the plague of fear. Here, too there are several different dimensions. One striking feature of the early days of such epidemics seems to be an exceptionally volatile intellectual state. People may be unable to decide whether a new disease or a new outbreak is trivial or whether it is really something enormously important. They swing backwards and forwards from one state of mind to another. There is, then, a collective disorientation (Ferlie and Pettigrew, 1990, p. 203). And if individuals do finally decide that this is something very serious, further unusual psychological states may occur in some people. The process seems rather similar to that of religious conversion. Like St. Paul on the road to Damascus, some people may suddenly find their beliefs and their lives transformed. Some of those whom we have interviewed could remember the precise moment at which they had become converted about AIDS. And some of these, in turn, became messianic – from then on, they rushed out and tried to warn, educate and convert other people.

Thus, when a disease is new and there are no routine collective ways of handling it, a thousand different converts may spring up drawn from every part of society, each possibly with their own plan of action, their own strategy for containing and controlling the disease. Moreover, this epidemic of converts, actions and strategies is matched by an epidemic of interpretation. When an epidemic is novel, a hundred different theories may be produced about the origins of the disease and its potential effects. Many of these are deeply moral in nature. All major epidemics pose fundamental metaphysical questions: how could God – or the government – have allowed it? Who is to blame? What does the impact of the epidemic reveal about our society? The Black Death was a challenge to orthodox Christianity, just as AIDS challenged, at least for a time, the power of biomedical science. Likewise, while some traditionalists have seen AIDS as a terrible judgement on the state of our sexual morality, some liberals have viewed its consequences as an appalling inditement of the state of our health services, or of our attitudes to homosexuality.

The furore and hubbub of intellectual and moral controversy may, in turn, be dramatically increased by the huge rash of control measures now proposed to contain the disease. Many suggestions for limiting the contagion may cut across and threaten our conventional codes and practice. Trade and travel may be disrupted, personal privacy and liberty may be seriously invaded, health education may be enforced on matters that are normally never talked about. Even treatment may be unethical to some (Brandt's [1987] social history of STDs contains many examples of this latter tendency.)

Finally, because of the disruption and disorientation that such epidemics produce they are also fruitful grounds not just for moral debate and moral challenge but for all kinds of 'moral entrepreneur' (Becker, 1963). For anyone who already has a mission to change the world – or some part of it – an epidemic is a new opportunity for change and conversion. Thus, cholera gave a platform to both religious revivalists and to those who wished to clean up Victorian cities. Likewise, AIDS has offered new sorts of possibility for the religiously conservative, for those who wished to reform services for STDs and drug addicts, for those gay men who were unhappy with recent trends in gay sexual expression.

In conclusion, the distinctive social psychology produced by large-scale epidemic disease can potentially result in a fundamental, if short-term, collapse of conventional social order. All kinds of disparate but corrosive effects may occur: friends, family and neighbours may be feared – and strangers above all; the sick may be left uncared for; those felt to be carriers may be shunned or persecuted; those without the disease may nonetheless fear they have got it; fierce moral controversies may sweep across a society; converts may turn aside from their old daily routines to preach a new gospel of salvation; governments may panic. For a moment at least, the world may be turned upside down.

References

Becker, H. (1963) *Outsiders: Studies in the Sociology of Deviance*, Free Press, New York
Brandt, A. (1987) *No Magic Bullet*, Oxford University Press, Oxford
Cipolla, C. (1973) *Cristofano and the Plague: A Study in the History of Public Health in the Age of Galileo*, Collins, London
Ferlie, E. and Pettigrew, A. (1990) Coping with change in the NHS: a frontline district's response to AIDS. *Journal of Social Policy*, 19(2), 191–220
Jaeger, H. (ed) (1988) *AIDS Phobia: Disease Pattern and Possibilities of Treatment*, Ellis Horwood, Chichester
Ohi, G. *et al.* (1988) Cost-benefit analysis of AIDS prevention programmes: its limitation in policy-making. In *The Global Impact of AIDS* (Fleming, A. *et al.*, eds), Alan R. Liss Inc., New York, pp. 251–262
Open University (1985) *Medical Knowledge: Doubt and Certainty*, Open University Press, Milton Keynes
Rosenberg, C. (1989) What is an epidemic? AIDS in historical perspective. *Daedalus*, 118(2), 1–18
Strong, P. and Berridge, V. (1990) No one knew anything: some issues in British

AIDS policy. In *AIDS: Individual, Cultural and Policy Dimensions* (Aggleton, P., Hart, G. and Davies, P., eds), Falmer, Basingstoke

Weber, J. and Goldmeier, D. (1983) Medicine and the media. *British Medical Journal*, 287, 420

Chapter 5

The rise of surveillance medicine

David Armstrong

If there is one image that captures the nature of the machinery of observation that surrounded the child in [the] early decades of the twentieth century, it might well be the height and weight growth chart. Such charts contain a series of gently curving lines, each one representing the growth trajectory of a population of children. Each line marked the 'normal' experience of a child who started his or her development at the beginning of the line. Thus, every child could be assigned a place on the chart and, with successive plots, given a personal trajectory. But the individual trajectory only existed in a context of general population trajectories: the child was unique yet uniqueness could only be read from a composition which summed the unique features of all children. A test of normal growth assumed the possibility of abnormal growth, yet how, from knowledge of other children's growth, could the boundaries of normality be identified? When was a single point on the growth and weight chart, to which the sick child was reduced, to be interpreted as abnormal? Abnormality was a relative phenomenon. A child was abnormal with reference to other children, and even then only by degrees. In effect, the growth charts were significant for distributing the body of the child in a field delineated not by the absolute categories of physiology and pathology, but by the characteristics of the normal population.

The socio-medical survey, first introduced during World War II to assess the perceived health status of the population, represented the recruitment to medicine of an efficient technical tool that both measured and reaffirmed the extensiveness of morbidity. The survey revealed the ubiquity of illness, that health was simply a precarious state. The post-war fascination with the weakening person–patient interface – such as in the notion of the clinical iceberg which revealed that most illness lay outside of health care provision (Last, 1963), or of illness behaviour which showed that people experience symptoms most days of their lives yet very few were taken to the doctor (Mechanic and Volkart, 1960) – was evidence that the patient was inseparable from the person because all persons were becoming patients.

Dissemination of intervention

The blurring of the distinction between health and illness, between the normal and the pathological, meant that health care intervention could no longer focus almost exclusively on the body of the patient in the hospital bed. Medical surveillance would have to leave the hospital and penetrate into the wider population.

The new 'social' diseases of the early twentieth century – tuberculosis, venereal disease, problems of childhood, the neuroses, etc. – were the initial targets for novel forms of health care, but the main expansion in the techniques of monitoring occurred after World War II when an emphasis on comprehensive health care, and primary and community care, underpinned the deployment of explicit surveillance services such as screening and health promotion. But these later radiations out into the community were prefigured by two important inter-war experiments in Britain and the United States that demonstrated the practicality of monitoring precarious normality in a whole population.

The British innovation was the Pioneer Health Centre at Peckham in south London (Pearse and Crocker, 1943). The Centre offered ambulatory health care to local families that chose to register – but the care placed special emphasis on continuous observation. From the design of its buildings that permitted clear lines of sight to its social club that facilitated silent observation of patients' spontaneous activity, every development within the Peckham Centre was a conscious attempt to make visible the web of human relations. Perhaps the Peckham key summarizes the dream of this new surveillance apparatus. The key and its accompanying locks were designed (though never fully installed) to give access to the building and its facilities for each individual of every enrolled family. But as well as giving freedom of access, the key enabled a precise record of all movement within the building. 'Suppose the scientist should wish to know what individuals are using the swimming bath or consuming milk, the records made by the use of the key give him this information' (Pearse and Crocker, 1943, pp. 76–77).

Only 7 per cent of those attending the Peckham Centre were found to be truly healthy; and if everyone had pathology then everyone would need observing. An important mechanism for operationalizing this insight was the introduction of extensive screening programmes in the decades following World War II. However, screening, whether individual, population, multiphasic, or opportunistic, represented a bid by Hospital Medicine to reach out beyond its confines – with all its accompanying limitations. First, it was too focused on the body. It meant that screening still confronted the localized lesion (or, more commonly, proto-lesion) within the body and ignored the newly emerging mobile threats that were insinuated throughout the community, constantly reforming into new dangers. Second, techniques to screen the population have always had to confront points of resistance, particularly the unwillingness of many to participate in these new procedures. The solution to these difficulties had already begun to emerge earlier in the twentieth century with the development of a strategy that involved giving responsibility for surveillance to patients themselves. A strategy of health promotion could potentially circumvent the problems inherent in illness screening.

The process through which the older techniques of hygiene were transformed into the newer strategy of health promotion occurred over several decades during the twentieth century. But perhaps one of the earliest experiments that attempted the transition was the collaborative venture between the city of Fargo in North Dakota and the Commonwealth Fund in 1923. The nominal objective of the project was the incorporation of child health services into the permanent programme of the health department and public school system (Brown, 1929) and an essential component of this plan was the introduction of health education in Fargo's schools, supervised by Maud Brown. Brown's campaign was, she wrote, 'an attempt to secure the instant adoption by every child of a completely adequate program of health behaviour' (Brown, 1929, p. 19).

The Commonwealth Fund project was a two pronged strategy. While the classroom was the focus for a systematic campaign of health behaviour, a periodic medical and dental examination both justified and monitored the educational intervention. In effect 'health teaching, health supervision and their effective coordination' were linked together.

From its insistence on four hours of physical exercises a day – two of them outdoors – to its concern with the mental maturation of the child, Fargo represented the realization of a new public health dream of surveillance in which everyone is brought into the vision of the benevolent eye of medicine through the medicalization of everyday life.

After World War II this approach began to be deployed with more vigour in terms of a strategy of health promotion. Concerns with diet, exercise, stress, sex, etc., become the vehicles for encouraging the community to survey itself. The ultimate triumph of Surveillance Medicine would be its internalization by all the population.

The tactics of Hospital Medicine have been those of exile and enclosure. The lesion marked out those who were different in a great binary system of illness and health, and processed them (in the hospital) in an attempt to rejoin them to the healthy. The tactics of the new Surveillance Medicine, on the other hand, have been pathologization and vigilance. The techniques of health promotion recognize that health no longer exists in a strict binary relationship to illness, rather health and illness belong to an ordinal scale in which the healthy can become healthier, and health can co-exist with illness; there is now nothing incongruous in having cancer yet believing oneself to be essentially healthy (Kagawa-Singer, 1993). But such a trajectory towards the healthy state can only be achieved if the whole population comes within the purview of surveillance: a world in which everything is normal and at the same time precariously abnormal, and in which a future that can be transformed remains a constant possibility.

References

Brown, M. A. (1929) *Teaching Health in Fargo*, Commonwealth Fund, New York
Kagawa-Singer, M. (1993) Redefining health: living with cancer. *Social Science and Medicine*, **37**, 295–304
Last, J. M. (1963) The clinical iceberg. *Lancet*, **2**, 28–30
Mechanic, D. and Volkart, E. H. (1960) Illness behaviour and medical diagnoses. *Journal of Health and Human Behaviour*, **1**, 86–90
Pearse, I. H. and Crocker, L. H. (1943) *The Peckham Experiment: A Study in the Living Structure of Society*, George Allen and Unwin, London

Reprinted by permission of Blackwell Publishing, Oxford. David Armstrong (1995) The rise of surveillance medicine. *Sociology of Health and Illness*, **17**(3), 397–400, 404.

Chapter 6

The conceptualization of functioning, health and quality of life

Ann Bowling

Clinicians and researchers interested in health care are increasingly focusing their attention on the measurement of health outcomes, or consequences, of care. The conceptualization and measurement of outcomes are controversial. There is now recognition that meaningful measures of health-related quality of life should be used to evaluate health-care interventions. Most existing indicators reflect a 'disease' model. The 'disease' model is a medical conception of pathological abnormality which is indicated by a set of signs and symptoms. A person's 'ill health' is indicated by feelings of pain and discomfort or perceptions of change in usual functioning and feeling. Illnesses can be the result of pathological abnormality, but not necessarily so. A person can feel ill without medical science being able to detect disease. Measures of health status need to take both concepts into account. What matters in the 20th century is how the patient feels, rather than how doctors think they ought to feel on the basis of clinical measurements. Symptom response or survival rates are no longer enough; and, particularly where people are treated for chronic or life-threatening conditions, the therapy has to be evaluated in terms of whether it is more or less likely to lead to an outcome of a life worth living in social and psychological, as well as physical, terms.

Measuring health outcome

In order to measure health outcome a measure of health status is required which in turn must be based on a concept of health. The limitations of the widely used negative definition of health as the absence of disease and the World Health Organization's (WHO) 1946 definition of health as total social, psychological and physical well-being have long been recognized (WHO, 1958). In the absence of satisfactory definitions of this basic concept how should health outcome be defined? Typical indices of health status in current use in the Western world focus on disease, illness and negative concepts. They include mortality rates and biochemical data (e.g. haemo-globin levels); routinely collected statistics on health-service use; subjective indicators: self- or other-reported morbidity, disability and behavioural data (e.g. smoking, alcohol use, etc.).

Mortality and morbidity indicators used by clinicians

Clinicians ultimately tend to judge the value of a therapy in terms of the five-year-survival period. In the developed world mortality rates are routinely collected; on the other hand, mortality statistics are subject to error and also ignore the living – many health-care programmes and interventions will have little or no impact on mortality rates. Survival time needs to be inter-preted more broadly in terms of the impact and consequences of treatment.

The major outcome measures in most clinical trials are mortality and morbidity. Measures of morbidity used by clinicians in assessing outcome commonly focus on results of biochemical tests, observed symptom rates or role performance (e.g. number of days off work, bed disability days). Wilson Barnett (1981) has reviewed research attempting to measure outcome among post-operative cardiac patients. She reported that the most frequently used measures related to mortality rates (length of survival), morbidity (serious complication), physical condition (e.g. exercise testing, cardiac function, angiography), patency of grafts, symptoms (pain, dyspnoea) and return to work. Return to work is one of the most commonly used non-biological indicators of health status. This is of limited value as it is influenced by economic and social opportunities and age.

Service utilization

Another source of data to which there is relatively easy access in the USA and the UK in particular is service-use information. The USA relies heavily on health insurance data for information about service use, the UK relies on routinely collected information from the National Health Service about deaths and discharges from hospital by condition, age and sex. Some in-formation is also available from periodic morbidity surveys in general med-ical practice. Much of Europe has little tradition of data collection of this type. All routinely collected data about usage is subject to problems of inaccuracy. Also, while hospital readmission rates, length of hospital stay and other indices of service use are frequently used as outcome and mor-bidity measures, they often reflect the policies of individual clinicians and service provision, and provide no information about the impact of the treatment on the patient's life.

Subjective health indicators

More detailed information about health and illness is only available from surveys. These take the form of either community-based population surveys, which collect data about individuals' self-reports of illness and disability, or studies of clinic populations based on patient-, and sometimes physician-assessed, morbidity.

An example of a physician-assessed morbidity-rating scale is the Olsson Health Scale which was developed using New York Heart Association gradings which range from 'dead' to 'alive' with various complications, to 'alive' with I to IV grades of activity limitation (Olsson *et al.*, 1986). The classifications give no indication of the effects of the condition on specific areas of physical, economic, psychological, social and domestic functioning. This also provides an example of how, in relation to the assessment of morbidity, health is generally conceptualized as being at one extreme of a continuum, generally defined negatively as the absence of symptoms, and with death at the other. There are differing views as to the gradations that may exist between 'perfect health' and 'death'. For example, Dorn (1955) represents the health spectrum as perfect health at one end, passing through conditions predisposing to disease (e.g. obesity), latent or incipient disease, early apparent disease, far advanced disease and then to death. The problem with such frameworks is that each stage is blurred as a disease may or may not manifest itself for a period of time and may or may not be recognized by the individual or presented to, and diagnosed by, a doctor. Moreover, in passing along the continuum, the point at which a state of health no longer exists is unknown.

Routine information about illness, obtained from individuals responding to large community samples, has been collected annually by government interview surveys in the USA, since 1956, in the UK since 1971, and in Finland since 1964. There is also an increasing number of *ad hoc* surveys carried out by research organizations, university and health departments.

Routine government health surveys typically report on the incidence of acute illness and injuries requiring either medical attention or restriction of daily activity; number of days of restricted activity and activity limitation resulting from various diseases and conditions; absence from work or school; self-reported chronic diseases and impairments; and discharges from hospital. Some also include symptom check-lists. Early methodologies concentrated on the collection of morbidity data, reflecting a disease model. More recent studies also reflect this model but are also more likely to encompass a behavioural approach – e.g. the annual UK General Household Survey often includes questions on behaviour such as alcohol and tobacco use.

There are multiple influences upon patient outcome, and these require a broad model of health. The non-biological factors which can affect recovery and outcome include patient psychology, motivation and adherence to therapy, socioeconomic status, availability of health care, social support networks and individual and cultural beliefs and behaviours. Outcome should thus also be measured more comprehensively in relation to people's value systems. More recently developed 'subjective health indicators' reflect these non-biological inputs. They are also recognized in research on health behaviour, for example the health-belief model refers to people's perceptions of the severity of an illness, their susceptibility to it, and the costs and benefits incurred in following a particular course of action (Becker, 1974).

The concept of functional ability

One of the most common methods of assessing outcome of care in a broader sense is in terms of people's ability to perform tasks of daily living. Disability measures are more meaningful to people's lives than objective biochemical measures or measures of timed walking or grip strength.

The terms 'impairment', 'disability' and 'handicap' are often erroneously used interchangeably. The increasing use of the concept of functional dependency has recently added to the confusion. The distinctions between these concepts first requires clarification. The World Health Organization's (1980) *International Classification of Impairments, Disabilities and Handicaps* provides a consistent terminology and a classification system.

This defines the terms 'impairment', 'disability' and 'handicap' and links them together conceptually:

Disease or Disorder $\longrightarrow$ Impairment $\longrightarrow$ Disability $\longrightarrow$ Handicap

e.g.:

Blindness $\longrightarrow$ Vision $\longrightarrow$ Seeing $\longrightarrow$ Orientation

Rheumatism $\longrightarrow$ Skeletal $\longrightarrow$ Walking $\longrightarrow$ Mobility

Impairment is defined as: 'In the context of health experience, an impairment is any loss or abnormality of psychological, physiological or anatomical structure or function.' It represents deviation from some norm in the individual's biomedical status. While impairment is concerned with biological function, disability is concerned with activities expected of the person or the body.

Disability is defined as 'In the context of health experience, a disability is any restriction or lack (resulting from an impairment) of ability to perform an activity in the manner or within the range considered normal for a human being'.

Functional handicap represents the social consequences of impairments or disabilities. It is thus a social phenomenon and a relative concept. The attitudes and values of the non-handicapped play a major part in defining a handicap. It is defined as:

In the context of health experience, a handicap is a disadvantage for a given individual, resulting from an impairment or a disability, that limits or prevents the fulfilment of a role that is normal (depending on age, sex and social and cultural factors) for that individual.

These constitute working definitions of impairment, disability and handicap. A working definition, as distinct from an operational definition, must be precise enough to suggest the content of the indicators but must not be so precise that it cannot be generalized to a variety of contexts. Operational definitions, in contrast, are usually specific to a particular measurement instrument and even to a particular type of study. They define the specific behaviour and the ways in which they are to be classified.

These concepts lead to the concept of dependency on other people or service providers. Impairment and disability may or may not lead to dependency in the same way they lead to handicap. As with the concept of handicap, functional 'dependency' is a social consequence – societal attitudes decide on its definition and existence. Wilkin (1987) defined dependency as 'A state in which an individual is reliant upon other(s) for assistance in meeting recognized needs'.

In summary, impairment and disability may lead to dependency in the same way they lead to handicap. However, they cannot be equated with dependency, nor is there a necessary relationship.

The concept of positive health

Health is usually referred to negatively as the absence of disease, illness and sickness. All measures of health status take health as a baseline and then measure deviations away from this. They are really measuring ill health. It is easier to measure departures from health rather than to find indices of health itself. When studying severely ill populations, the best strategy may be to employ measures of negative health status. However, only approximately 15 per cent of a general population in a Western society will have chronic physical limitations, and some 10–20 per cent will have substantial psychiatric impairment (Stewart et al., 1978; Ware and Young, 1979). Thus reliance on a negative definition of health provides little information about the health of the remaining 80–90 per cent of general populations. A positive conception of health is difficult to measure because of the lack of agreement over its definition. Clinical judgements focus upon the absence of disease; lay people may hold a variety of concepts such as the ability to carry out normal everyday tasks, feeling strong, good, fit and so on. Without an operational definition it is not possible to determine if and when a state of health has been achieved by a population.

The WHO has recommended the development of measures of positive health (Scottish Health Education Group, 1984). In its 1946 constitution (WHO, 1958), the WHO specified that 'Health is a state of complete physical, mental and social wellbeing and not merely the absence of disease and infirmity'. No conceptual or operational definitions were provided. Despite the controversy provoked by this utopian definition, it has generated a new focus on a broader, more positive concept of health, rather than a narrow, negative (disease-based) focus (Seedhouse, 1986). The World Health Organization's (1985) ideal of 'Health for all by the Year 2000' and the *Ottawa Charter for Health Promotion* (1986) with its emphasis on assisting the individual to increase control over and improve health, both employ broader definitions of health than those traditionally employed. They highlight the inadequacy of existing negative concepts of health (Thuriaux, 1988).

There is now broad agreement that the concept of positive health is more than the mere absence of disease or disability and implies 'completeness' and 'full functioning' or 'efficiency' of mind and body and social adjustment. Beyond this there is no one accepted definition. Positive health could be described as the ability to cope with stressful situations, the maintenance of a strong social-support system, integration in the community, high morale and life satisfaction, psychological well-being, and even levels of physical fitness as well as physical health (Lamb *et al.*, 1988). It is composed of distinct components that must be measured and interpreted separately.

Partly confusing conceptual issues further are the other related multi-faceted concepts such as 'social well-being' or 'social health' and 'quality of life', which are components of a broad concept of positive health.

The concept of social health

Donald *et al.* (1978) have called a broader view of health than the reporting of symptoms, illness and functional ability 'social health'. Social health was viewed as a dimension of individual well-being distinct from both physical and mental health. They conceptualized social health both as a component of health-status outcomes (as a dependent variable) and, following Caplan (1974) and Cassel (1976):

> in terms of social support systems that might intervene and modify the effect of the environment and life stress events on physical and mental health (as an intervening variable). Measurement of social health focuses on the individual and is defined in terms of interpersonal interactions (e.g. visits with friends) and social participation (e.g. membership in clubs). Both objective and subjective constructs (e.g. number of friends and a rating of how well one is getting along, respectively) are included in this definition (Donald *et al.*, 1978).

The authors attempted to measure social health, or social well-being as they also sometimes called it, in the Rand health insurance study.

Other authors have also conceptualized social health as a separate component of health status, defining it in terms of the degree to which people function adequately as members of the community (Renne, 1974; Greenblatt, 1975). Lerner (1973) noted that health status may be a function of non-healthy factors external to the individual, such as the environment, the community and significant social groups. He recommended that social well-being measures focus on constructs such as role-related coping, family health and social participation. He hypothesized that socially healthy persons would be more able to cope successfully with day-to-day challenges arising from performance of major social roles; would live in families that are more stable, integrated and cohesive; would be more likely to participate in community activities; and would be more likely to conform to societal norms. In relation to psychiatric illness, Leighton (1959) has described how individual personalities can be influenced by the quality and quantity of interpersonal relationships. Lack of social integration may produce psychological stress and decrease the individual's resources for dealing with it, possibly resulting in psychiatric disorders. Lack of social support has also been implicated in poor outcome of depressive illness (George *et al.*, 1989).

Social support can thus be regarded as a key concept in theory and research on 'social health'. Kaplan (1975) outlines several areas of social support, including work achievements and position in the hierarchy; family support, social activity and friendships; financial adequacy; personal life (e.g. existence of a confidante); personal achievements and philosophy and sexual satisfaction. In sum, studies of social health tend to focus on the individual, rather than on the community, and the concept is used as a dimension of another imprecisely defined term: 'quality of life'.

The concept of quality of life

In general terms quality can be defined as a grade of 'goodness'. Quality of life is a broader concept than personal health status and also takes social well-being, as described above, into account. There is no consensus over a definition of quality of life. The literature covers a range of components: functional ability including role functioning (e.g. domestic, return to work), the degree and quality of social and community interaction, psychological well-being, somatic sensation (e.g. pain) and life satisfaction. It is becoming fashionable to equate all non-clinical data with 'quality of life' which is likely to be a source of conceptual confusion. Health and functional status are just two dimensions of health-related quality of life.

There is little empirical research attempting to define those qualities which make life and survival valuable. Mendola and Pelligrini (1979) have defined quality of life as 'the individual's achievement of a satisfactory social situation within the limits of perceived physical capacity'. This is a fairly limited definition and no more easy to operationalize than more complex definitions. Shin and Johnson (1978) have suggested that quality of life consists of 'the possession of resources necessary to the satisfaction of individual needs, wants and desires, participation in activities enabling personal development and self actualization and satisfactory comparison between oneself and others', all of which are dependent on previous experience and knowledge. Patterson (1975) approached this differently by identifying certain characteristics deemed essential to any evaluation of quality of life. These included general health, performance status, general comfort, emotional status and economic status, all of which are contributory to the proposition made by Shin and Johnson. Basically quality of life is recognized as a concept representing individual responses to the physical, mental and social effects of illness on daily living which influence the extent to which personal satisfaction with life circumstances can be achieved. It encompasses more than adequate physical well-being, it includes perceptions of well-being, a basic level of satisfaction and a general sense of self-worth. It is an abstract and complex concept comprising diverse areas, all of which contribute to the whole, personal satisfaction and self-esteem.

Quality of life as an outcome measure: whose assessment?

Existing global measurement scales of health outcome, aiming to encompass the measurement of 'quality of life', are based on either physicians' or individuals' own assessments.

Slevin *et al.* (1988) attempted to determine whether assessments of quality of life of cancer patients by health professionals are meaningful and reliable by analysing the associations between professionals' and patients' assessments. The instruments used were the Karnofsky Performance Scale, the Spitzer Quality of Life Index, the Hospital Anxiety and Depression Scale and a series of linear analogue self-assessment scales. The wide discrepancies between doctors' and patients' assessments led the authors to conclude that doctors could not adequately measure the patients' quality of life. The implication is that measures of outcome should take account of individuals' self-assessments.

References

Becker, M. (1974) The health belief model and personal health behaviour. *Health Education Monographs*, 2, 326–373

Caplan, G. (1974) *Support Systems and Community Mental Health*, Behavioral Publications, New York

Cassel, J. (1976) The contribution of the social environment to host resistance. *American Journal of Epidemiology*, 104, 107–123

Donald, C. A., Ware, J. E., Brook, R. H. *et al.* (1978) *Conceptualization and Measurement of Health for Adults in the Health Insurance Study*, Vol. IV, Social Health, Rand Corporation, Santa Monica, California, R-1987/4-HEW

Dorn, H. F. (1955) Some applications of biometry in the collection and evaluation of medical data. *Journal of Chronic Diseases*, 1, 638–664

George, L. K., Blazer, D. G., Hughes, D. C. *et al.* (1989) Social support and the outcome of major depression. *British Journal of Psychiatry*, 154, 478–485

Greenblatt, H. N. (1975) *Measurement of Social Well-being in a General Population Survey*, Berkeley, Human Population Laboratory, California State Department of Health

Kaplan, B. H. (1975) An epilogue: toward further research on family and health. In *Family and Health: An Epidemiological Approach* (Kaplan, B. H. and Cassel, J. C., eds), University of North Carolina, Institute for Research and Social Science, Chapel Hill

Kaplan, R. (1985) Social support and social health. In *Social Support Theory, Research and Application* (Saranson, I. and Saranson, B., eds), Nijhoff, The Hague

Lamb, K. L., Brodie, D. A. and Roberts, K. (1988) Physical fitness and health-related fitness as indicators of a positive health state. *Health Promotion*, 3, 171–182

Leighton, A. H. (1959) *My Name is Legion: Foundations for a Theory of Man in Relation to Culture*, Basic Books, New York

Lerner, M. (1973) Conceptualization of health and well-being. *Health Services Research*, 8, 6–12

Mendola, W. F. and Pelligrini, R. V. (1979) Quality of life and coronary artery bypass surgery patients. *Social Science and Medicine*, 13A, 457–461

Olsson, G., Lubsen, J. and Van Es, G. A. (1986) Quality of life after myocardial infarction: effect of long-term metoprolol on mortality and morbidity. *British Medical Journal*, 292, 1491–1493

Patterson, W. (1975) The quality of survival in response to treatment. *Journal of the American Medical Asociation*, 233, 280–281

Renne, K. S. (1974) Measurement of social health in a general population survey. *Social Sciences Research*, 3, 25–44

Scottish Health Education Group (1984) *European Monographs in Health Education Research*, No. 6, Scottish Health Education Group, Edinburgh

Seedhouse, D. (1986) *Health: The Foundations of Achievement*, John Wiley, Chichester

Shin, D. C. and Johnson, D. M. (1978) Avowed happiness as an overall assessment of the quality of life. *Social Indicators Research*, 5, 475–492

Slevin, M. L., Plant, H., Lynch, D. *et al.* (1988) Who should measure quality of life, the doctor or the patient? *British Journal of Cancer*, 57, 109–112

Stewart, A. L., Ware, J. E., Brook, R. H. *et al.* (1978) *Conceptualization and Measurement of Health for Adults in the Health Insurance Study*, Vol. II: *Physical Health in Terms of Functioning*, Rand Corporation, Santa Monica, R-1987/2-HEW

Thuriaux, M. C. (1988) Health promotion and indicators for health for all in the European Region. *Health Promotion*, 3, 89–99

Ware, J. E. and Young, J. (1979) Issues in the conceptualization and measurement of value placed on health. In *Health: What Is It Worth?* (Mushkin, S. J. and Dunlop, D. W., eds), Pergamon Press, New York

WHO (1958) *The First Ten Years. The Health Organization*, World Health Organization, Geneva

WHO (1980) *International Classification of Impairments, Disabilities and Handicaps*, World Health Organization, Geneva

WHO (1985) *Targets for Health for All by the Year 2000*, World Health Organization, Regional Office for Europe, Copenhagen

Wilkin, D. (1987) Conceptual problems in dependency research. *Social Science and Medicine*, 24, 867–873

Wilson Barnett, J. (1981) Assessment of recovery: with special reference to a study with post-operative cardiac patients. *Journal of Advanced Nursing*, 6, 435–445

Reprinted by permission of the Open University Press, Buckingham. Ann Bowling (1991) The conceptualization of functioning, health and quality of life. In *Measuring Health – A Review of Quality of Life Measurement Scales*, Open University Press, Buckingham, pp. 1–10.

Chapter 7

The health service consumer: a sociological misconception

Margaret Stacey

It has become fashionable in the last decade to speak of patients as health service consumers, a fashion to which I have succumbed (Stacey, 1974). More careful analysis suggests, however, that the term 'consumer' is of limited value in understanding the status and role of the patient;[1] that it is an economic term which implies a theoretical model of the health service which is quite inappropriate and which conceals as much as it illuminates. Deriving from economics it has now become a social actor's term[2] and is a political term, in the sense that it has been used by certain social actors to legitimate alterations in the power structure. 'Health service consumer' is inappropriate terminology to describe a sociological conception of the patient.

The notion of a patient as a consumer has arisen, it seems, from two sources. The first is the application of an economic industrial model to the health service; the second is from the consumer movement. The term is therefore located in two distinct developments, both with specific historical referrents.

The nub of my argument is that the health service can better be seen as a process of continuing interaction between patient and health care professionals and workers than as an industry or other predominantly economic activity. There is a sense in which the health service is an economic enterprise of course. The NHS is the largest British employer and only Shell and BP have a larger turnover.[3] Not only is the health service much more than economic enterprise, in so far as one does think of the health service as an industry, a patient can be said to be a producer as much as a consumer of that elusive and abstract good: health.

What are the alternative models? There is first of all the professional–client model, that is, in this case, the traditional doctor–patient model. This model is still clung to by many members of the medical profession but serves only an ideological purpose bearing little relation to social reality. Indeed, the model is embodied in the NHS reorganization documents (DHSS, 1972) associated with the notion that a doctor can be accountable only to his patient. However, it is clear that the complexity of modern health services has made this model largely obsolete. Few professionals work on their own and in consulting a doctor a patient is calling upon the skill of many other personnel, many of whom he never even sees. The notion of a client is one who consults a particular professional. The concept is stretched when applied to mass medicine to which patients contribute financially in an unspecified way when well as well as when ill, either through the state or through insurance schemes.

It is perhaps because of the mass nature of modern health services that the industrial model has come to be applied. But this model really fits the health service badly. A simple industrial model imagines a management which employs workers to produce a good which is then sold to customers or consumers as the economists have it. Consumers are essentially those who consume goods produced by industry. There are, of course, service industries which produce an intangible good or service. This sevice is commonly bought by customers or clients who have come to be called consumers in economic theory. Service industries as a whole are clearly distinguishable from productive industries in that a service and not a good is produced. But the important distinction in health is that this is a service industry which does things *to* people rather than *for* people. This is of course, true also to some extent of other services: education, for example, seeks to manipulate the minds of the scholars. In education of course, the pupils may well be compelled to submit to this attention. This is also true of some health service patients: child patients are presented by their parents; the very elderly, the mentally and physically handicapped, the mentally ill have often no choice but to submit to treatment, or to custodial care in the name of medicine. If there is a sense in which a patient is a consumer, it has to be said that he is at the same time a work object. A patient of the health service offers his body and his person as a work object. He is suffering and seeks relief. The service which a patient requests or buys is one which requires that his body or, in the psychiatric services, his mind, be in some way processed. The analogy of a patient as a work object is seen most clearly in operations, particularly in batch operations where large numbers of people are operated on for the same condition *seriatim* and recover together in the same ward. Thinking of a patient as work object shows one way in which the industrial model is inappropriate. It would have consumers as products of the industry.

Yet one can readily take the model of the patient as work object too far. For a patient is rarely a merely passive recipient of a service, he can never be wholly objectified. Goffman showed how, despite the tendencies to depersonalize patients in one of the situations in which they are most vulnerable, namely a mental hospital, patients used various means to retain some individuality and independence (Goffman, 1971). As Freidson also showed (1961), and as Stimson and Webb have recently shown (1975), a patient is not altogether a passive actor. Patients, in association with the professionals who are working on them and also on their own account, are decision makers. In any industry certain decisions are made on the shop floor, if only the important decision as to whether to produce the goods or not. But the importance of decisions on the 'shop floor' of the health service is particularly marked. The patients decide whether to attend, what to tell the doctor and whether to accept his advice. The doctors make decisions about the illness and the best method of treatment. The many exchanges of this kind which go on continually, together with their outcomes, largely determine the nature of the health service. It is for this reason that I argue that the health service is better thought of as a process or more or less prolonged interaction between the minds and bodies of the patients and the health care workers.

It is noticeable that management experts tend to define out the kind of decisions that are taken by patients, doctors and nurses in interaction as not being decision-making in the policy sense in which they understand it. Their analysis is the poorer for that. Whatever decisions may be taken round the board room table, in committee or at the administrator's desk depend upon many workers, professional, para-professional and other, for their execution. This is true of any industry but is particularly true of the health service as our difficulties in controlling expenditure show (Culyer, 1975). The decisions made by patients are the actions of private actors but they can be understood only in the context for collective actions and interactions in the health service. If it is inevitable that decision-making analyses shall exclude decisions made in the course of working or being worked on, then this is further evidence of the inappropriateness of the management–consumer model.

To stress the nature of the health service as an interactive process is not to say that there should not be a concern with outcomes. Indeed, Culyer (1975) is right to argue for much greater concern with outcomes. There is certainly a case for looking at the health service as an economic enterprise for costs have to be counted, outcomes measured and priorities determined. In an economic context it might be permissible to think of a patient as consumer and to ask whether he has value for money. But this is surely not essential for the economic exercise. Furthermore, the essential nature of a patient's involvement in the process must be understood to count the costs adequately. I have suggested that the concept of 'consumer' clouds this understanding.

Stelling and Bucher (1973) have argued that patients are more concerned with the outcome, while doctors are more concerned with the process. This is shown in the acquisition by medical students of a 'vocabulary of realism' which does not include the notion of mistakes measured by outcome in the way in which a layman would think of a mistake. The medics concentrate on the process and the procedure and think in terms of judgement. A patient is necessarily primarily concerned with outcome, but this outcome is not a good, independent of himself, but is integral with him and more or less vital to his life, for the outcome is something done to his body or mind.

The differences of interest between doctor and patient are, therefore, real but they do not have a producer–consumer nature. They can be said to have a worker–work object nature and at the same time some of the characteristics of a shared enterprise. In this context the concept of a partnership between professional and patient is perhaps the most appropriate.

The partnership is not an equal one, for the professionals tend always to be in the most powerful positions. This is particularly true in the NHS or any other service where the financial arrangements ensure a permanent clientele for the professionals (Johnson, 1972). In this case the dependence of health care workers on the patients is reduced. A patient also lacks choice because of a shortage of professionals and/or amenities, his own lack of knowledge, reinforced by bureaucratic complexities.[4] Many partnerships are unequal and the concept of a partnership need not necessarily be vitiated for that reason. Because of the peculiar nature of the health service, one of the partners is also the work object of the others. This juxtaposition produces many tensions. The patients are also the service objects of the professions at the same time as they are the work objects. But because they are thinking actors involved in their own treatment some of the characteristics of a partnership remain. It seems that, in order to reduce the tensions that exist in working on fellow men, many social arrangements, with their associated ideologies, have developed to reduce patients to unquestioning, non-participating work objects and to obliterate the aspects of partnership.

It was in face of these arrangements and ideologies, which tended to reduce the status of and depersonalize patients, that the notion of a patient as consumer appeared to be liberating. Here was an understandable identity and a platform from which to argue. It is noticeable that patients are very little organized and that there is no coherent shared ideology to support the role of patient as actor, decision maker or partner in the health enterprise. The ideologies that there are derive from the status of the dominant partners in the interaction and stress the value of the 'good patient' who is compliant, does what he is told, does not question, is deferential.

Consumerism offered an ideology to fill this gap. And it was à la mode. But is the consumer ideology the right one for the patients? Is it appropriate? Surely the analysis above must suggest that the concept of patient as consumer *undervalues* the patient status. In the ideal of free, perfect competition the consumer held high status: the consumer was always right. In monopoly capitalism, in the bureaucracies of the welfare state this is no longer true. In these circumstances the consumer has low status. What else are all the consumers' rights movement about? Only the disadvantaged or threatened develop movements to defend or enhance their rights.

The patient lacks status relative to the doctors and other professionals, but to redefine the patient as consumer will in no way enhance his/her status or power. On the contrary, this redefinition was used to cut patients out of 'consumers' in Community Health Councils which had watchdog functions but no executive power. The remarkable delay in getting the CHCs off the ground also suggests low priority and low status for patient affairs. This is evidence of the political nature of the redefinition of patient as consumer. As such, of course, it may be turned on its head. The latent power of the patient as citizen may be used in and through Community Health Councils in association with other citizenship statuses to shift the balance of power again. Already a Labour government has made some moves in this direction. This would be the aim of radical consumer movements. But it must also be argued that those who do not study the nature and operation of patient power, who fail to recognize the decision-making role of patients, are not only colluding with, but actively encouraging, an ideology which seeks to keep the patients quiet, docile and compliant. In short they are helping to maintain, indeed actively fostering, the present gross inequalities in the collective partnership that is the National Health Service.

The concept we need for the sociological analysis of patients begins with the notion of a patient as social actor of which his role as economic actor is an important part, but only a part; the concept also has to include the notion of a patient as one who offers himself for servicing, i.e. offers himself as a work object; the concept therefore has to allow for interaction between a patient as social actor and others, but a special kind of interaction in which the patients become work objects of the others, at least temporarily; the concept also must recognize that while the relationship may have some characteristics of a partnership, it may also be exploitive; this may happen because of the inequalities between health care professionals and patients, especially patients as work objects; it may happen because of disabilities which lead patients to be disvalued in the wider society and also by their kin and friends and the health care professionals so that they do not offer themselves as work objects, but are offered. As yet I have no one term and have to be content with an indicative phrase such as 'the patient as partner but also work object' (papwo?). Certainly not consumer: the term disvalues and oversimplifies. And it is amusing to notice in the OED that as well as meaning employer of a professional, customer, 'client' meant a plebeian under the protection of a noble in Roman times and archaically was a dependant or hanger on. Perhaps just patient will do since it derives from the Latin *pati*, to suffer.

Notes

1. Status and role here are used as defined in the glossary of Stacey, M., Batstone, E., Bell, C. and Murcott, A. (1975) *Power, Persistence and Change*, Routledge and Kegan Paul, London.
2. It was as an involved participant in health service administration, a member of the Welsh Hospital Board and the Michael Davies Committee at the time of the NHS reorganization in the early '70s, that I first came to use it. One took the available language of discourse of the dominant participants.

3. Arthur Francis, private communication.
4. This argument I have developed more fully elsewhere. (See Stacey 1974; forthcoming).

References

Culyer, A. J. (1975) Health: the social cost of doctors' discretion. *New Society*, 27 February, 517–519
DHSS (1972) *Management Arrangements for the Reorganised National Health Service*, HMSO, London, 1.18
Freidson, E. (1961) *Patients' View of Medical Practice*, Russell Sage Foundation, New York
Goffman, E. (1971) *Asylums*, Doubleday Anchor, New York
Johnson, T. (1972) *Professions and Power*, Macmillan, London
Pill, R. and Jacobs, R. (1974) *Report on a pilot study on the problems of long stay children in hospital*. Medical Sociology Research Centre, mimeo, University of Swansea
Stacey, M. (1974) Consumer complaints procedures in the British National Health Service. *Social Science and Medicine*, 8, 429–435
Stacey, M. (forthcoming) *Dilemmas of Participation. The Case of the Health Service Consumer*. Edinburgh Faculty Seminar
Stelling, J. and Bucher, R. (1973) Vocabularies of realism in professional socialization. *Social Science and Medicine*, 7, 661–675
Stimson, G. and Webb, B. (1975) *Going to see the Doctor: The Consultation Process in General Practice*, Routledge and Kegan Paul, London

Reprinted by permission of Blackwell Publishers, Oxford. Margaret Stacey (1976) The health service consumer: a sociological misconception. In *Sociological Review Monograph 22, The Sociology of the National Health Service*, Blackwell, Oxford, pp. 194–200.

Chapter 8

A model of the lay evaluation of medical care

Michael Calnan

[O]ne important area related to illness management much neglected at both the conceptual and empirical level is lay evaluation of medical care.

The intention is [here] to identify the elements that shape lay perceptions of medical care.

The model identifies three interrelated elements that might shape the way lay people evaluate medical care. These three interrelated elements are:

1. The socio-political values or ideologies upon which the particular medical care system is based.
2. The level of experience of use of medical care.
3. The goals of those seeking medical help in each specific instance.

It is suggested that, at the broadest level, the socio-political values or ideologies upon which the particular medical care system is based structures in a general way what lay people expect. It is possible to identify at least two different sets of values about medical care. The first is where medical care is provided directly by the state as a public utility. The avowed objectives are to have equity in the availability and distribution of services and to ration services and resources according to need. Decisions about the allocation of resources are usually determined by the state, which is usually the largest and the only employer of professionals and others who provide the medical service.

The second model of medical care suggests that its provision should be determined by a market economy. Medical care should be treated like any other commodity and be subject to market forces. Thus, the emphasis is on individual choice and consumer sovereignty and medical care is usually purchased on a fee-for-service basis. Thus, health care would be paid for privately, although the various schemes are supported to a greater or lesser degree by a community pool of funds or a public subsidy. Professionals act on their own or in small groups as entrepreneurs and would attempt to respond to the demands of the consumer.

These models are ideal types and are not found in pure form, although the health care system in the United States is more congruent with the ideological stance of the second model, and the Swedish health care system more congruent with the first. The NHS may have been seen to be affiliated with the first model, although in recent times with the increased emphasis in current government policy documents on the need for consumer choice (Klein, 1986) it is now moving or being pushed towards a form of the mixed health economy model where consumerism and paternalistic rationality are blurred (Hunter, 1983). However, it is not as mixed as other western European health care systems, and, with the near monopoly of the NHS, is much closer to the first model than many of its European neighbours. Prospective patients in the NHS obviously may critically discriminate between seeking and not seeking medical care, although the level of shopping around for medical care in the NHS is reduced to choosing between doctors within a group practice or between a GP and a hospital accident and emergency department. There are still structural impediments to changing family doctors, although current government policy is suggesting a need for change (HMSO, 1986). The lack of choice and the idea that providers will define patients' needs appears to have led to an acceptance of the philosophy of providers. 'Don't waste the doctor's time with trivia' or 'only use the hospital accident emergency department for "emergencies"' are examples of this philosopy which has been taken on to some degree by patients (Calnan, 1983). For example, one common finding in studies of patients' patterns of help-seeking behaviour is patients' concern not to waste the doctor's time with inappropriate conditions, that is, a fear of overutilization. It is doubtful whether such a finding would be identified in studies of the use of privately financed medical care, where supply is claimed to respond to patient demands. Professional control and influence over provision and resource use is also prevalent in the market economy model primarily because health care has special qualities that differentiate it from other consumer products (Titmuss, 1969). In the market economy there is a greater risk of overprovision to those who can pay and lack of access to those who cannot (Hunter, 1983).

The second element that, it is suggested, will influence patient perceptions of medical care will be the level and nature of the individual's (and his or her close social network) experiences of medical care. The uncertainties and unpredictabilities that surround illness, and the professional medical care provided to treat and manage it, suggest that patients only become knowledgeable when they or their network of friends and relations experience medical care. Thus, any expectations they may have will be created by their experience and those with limited experience may have to rely on general ideological beliefs. However, as was pointed out previously, the emphasis in the NHS on provider-defined need might suggest that expectations at the level of ideology may be weak.

The third element in the conceptual framework suggests that patient evaluation of medical care can be understood in terms of the specific reasons why the sufferer or his family sought medical care in each specific instance. Patients seek medical care, particularly from general practitioners, for a wide variety of complaints that are physical, psychological, and social, or a combination of these elements. In each of these instances, they will have specific wants and make specific demands they will expect to be met by those providing the service. The family doctor might be expected to play a variety of roles that include doctor as technician to treat minor cuts, doctor as diagnostician and information-giver for problematic signs and symptoms, doctor as advice-giver and reassurer for anxious parents, and doctor as counsellor for psycho-social problems. Patients will make different demands and will evaluate medical care according to whether or not their demands are met.

A clear example of this can be found in a study examining (Calnan, 1983) the illness behaviour of those with minor cuts and minor lacerations and their decision to go to a general practitioner or to a hospital accident and emergency department in England. It is evident ... that patients assessed the appropriateness of the care in terms of their specific needs.

Patients with injuries such as cuts tended to self-diagnose and to choose between medical care settings on the grounds of the presence of appropriate medical facilities. Assessments of the appropriate place for treatment were also influenced by the perceived costs to patients in terms of wasted time. There were also the costs of upsetting their doctor with a condition he might regard as a waste of his valuable time. Some patients emphasized the need to take 'trivial' complaints to the hospital as the hospital was anonymous and thus it would not have implications for the relationship with their GP. Only a small number of patients adopted the practice of routinely contacting their GP for everything. Thus, waiting at casualty is much preferred to waiting for the GP to be available. Once the process of self-diagnosis or lay diagnosis has taken place, and the decision to seek medical care is made, then the most convenient place for treatment in terms of time and accessibility is sought. In the cases involving minor cuts, lay people appear to make calculated decisions about the appropriate source of medical care. In the case of illness, self-diagnosis or lay diagnosis is more problematic and GPs are seen to be more legitimate sources of advice and care. In the cases involving illness, costs of time and accessibility are much less important than receiving satisfactory and detailed information about the diagnosis and prognosis of the condition. The person with a cut, because he or she is able to self-diagnose, appears to retain some control over his or her body and does not necessarily become dependent on medical advice. In the cases involving cuts, technological expertise is required, but only on a short-term basis. On the other hand, illness involves uncertainty among patients about what is wrong and what the implications of their problems are. Thus, in these cases, the sufferer may find it necessary to enter into a dependent position in the doctor–patient relationships so as to obtain further information about their condition. Thus, in the case of illness, satisfaction was expressed in terms of the ability of the doctor to listen to the patients' wishes and to communicate what was wrong and what treatment was required. However, in the case of cuts, medical care and the performance of professionals was evaluated in instrumental and technical terms.

These findings also have implications for the study of doctor–patient relations. Sufferers with 'illnesses' tended to be willing, at least initially, to adopt the traditional patient position and defer to what they believe to be superior medical knowledge. On the other hand, patients with traumatic conditions such as cuts tend to know what is wrong with them, have a reasonable explanation of why they are suffering from this complaint, and appear to have specific ideas about the treatment required. Such an active and knowledgeable patient seems to be the opposite of what has been traditionally portrayed in doctor–patient relations. This patient seems to fit with the consumerist approach to patienthood, which emphasizes the need to be active and critical, and seems to conflict with what doctors tend to define as a 'good' patient.

The relationship between experience and motives for seeking medical help are clearly closely related. Patients will soon learn about the best source of medical care for certain problems. For example, in the case of minor cuts that need stitching, many patients learn that the most appropriate setting for treatment is the hospital accident and emergency department rather than their general practitioner.

This then is the conceptual framework within which it is proposed that lay evaluation of medical care should be analysed. However, social inequalities are inherent in the United Kingdom and many countries in the western world and thus they have a major influence on ideologies about health care and its provision, patients' experience of health and health care, and patterns of utilization. For example, studies in the United Kingdom have shown that levels of satisfaction may vary by social class and income, although the evidence is not consistent and is difficult to interpret. While the lower social classes and those with lower incomes may have poorer quality services than their more affluent counterparts, the latter group may be more critical because they have higher expectations and greater access to information. However, the strongest or most consistent pattern of evidence points to a relationship between age and levels of satisfaction (Halpern, 1985). Once again, this might be explained by lower expectations about health care or about health associated with ageing, or may be related to differences in approaches to medical care associated with different generations. These examples provide a clear illustration of how an analysis of lay evaluation of medical care needs to take into account the likelihood of variation in perceptions by social class, age, gender, religious and political affiliation, and ethnic background. Each of these factors will possibly influence the three elements in the model independently in a number of different ways that are difficult to identify at present without further empirical research.

References

Calnan, M. (1983) Managing minor disorders: pathways to a hospital accident and emergency department. *Sociology of Health and Illness*, 5, 149–167

Halpern, S. (1985) What the public thinks of the NHS. *Health and Social Services Journal*, 6 June, 703–704

HMSO (1986) *Primary Health Care: An Agenda for Discussion*, HMSO, London

Hunter, D. (1983) The privatisation of public provision. *Lancet*, 1, 1264–1268

Klein, R. (1986) Weighing up opposing models of health care. *Health and Social Services Journal*, 8 May, 618–619

Titmuss, R. (1969) The culture of medical care and consumer behaviour. In *Medicine and Culture* (Poynter, F., ed), Wellcome, London

Reprinted by permission of Routledge (Tavistock Publications), London and New York. Michael Calnan (1987) A model of the lay evaluation of medical care. In *Health and Illness: The Lay Perspective*, Tavistock Publications, London and New York, pp. 184–188.

Chapter 9

The process of becoming ill
David Robinson

One of the perennial quests in the study of illness behaviour is for some kind of understanding of why one person with a particular illness condition legitimately occupies the status sick when another person with the same condition does not. Any achievements in the field of medical sociology will be prompted largely by the attempt to explain this problem. Problems do not arise unless those who discover them already have certain theories which lead them to problems. The sociologist's interest in the study of illness behaviour arises from the observation that a person's readiness to consider himself, or another, ill cannot adequately be explained by reference to the severity of the symptomatic person's condition.

Although there is grudging recognition that each of us will die sometime, illness is assumed to be a relatively infrequent, unusual or abnormal phenomenon. Moreover, the statistics used in the discussion of illness tend to support this assumption. Specifically diagnosed conditions, days out of work and visits to the doctor do occur for each of us relatively infrequently. Though such data represent only professionally validated illness we rarely question whether or not they give a full picture. Usually implicit, further, is the notion that people who do not consult doctors and other medical agencies, and thus do not appear in the statistics, may be regarded as healthy.

Signs clearly vary with the family status of the potentially ill person. The wife/mother and young children were most likely to be seen to be more irritable and tired than usual when they were not feeling fully fit. Husbands and older children were likely to be considered quieter than usual when they did not feel well, while for children, both young and old, going off their food was considered a sign of forthcoming illness. Signs also differed according to the class of the potentially ill person. Tiredness, for example, was never seen as a sign of illness in working-class men. Tiredness is, perhaps, for them a mere fact of everyday life. In fact, for all statuses tiredness was less likely to be seen as a sign of illness for people in working-class families.

If different people are seen to be not feeling well when they exhibit certain signs, then this is one clue to the way in which people may be differentially classified as sick. The fact that in working-class families tiredness was less likely to be considered a sign of being unwell than in middle-class families may be due to difference in tolerance to tiredness, or different beliefs about tiredness as an acceptable fact of everyday life. If so, it would not be surprising to find that people of different occupations, class or family status will have differential expectations about what signs or symptoms it is appropriate to ignore, live with, treat or consult about. These ideas will not persist unchanged over time for or about any particular person or condition, or even throughout the whole course of any one condition.

Mrs M's account of her husband's leg injury illustrates the kind of manoeuvrings which were made around the notion of being ill and the role of the doctor. Mr M, aged 28, twisted his leg playing football on the Saturday prior to the Wednesday of one of my visits. Mrs M reported that he had not consulted the doctor even though the pain in his leg had become gradually worse. By the Wednesday it prevented him from driving their old car.

> *Mrs M*: 'It wasn't too bad when he came in, just tender round the knee. It was stiff [on] Sunday and I said he'd have to go to the surgery on the Monday . . . but he wouldn't. He started his new job with X's and you can't go sick on the first day. He'd have got his note no trouble last month. Last week he was home anyway [between jobs] I could have looked after him. Just rest and he wouldn't have needed the doctor. Trust him to do it when he can't be on the sick. Next week he can make out he did it on the site. It's not that bad[1] mind.'

Mr and Mrs M obviously shared quite clear notions of when it was appropriate for Mr M to be sick and when to consult a doctor. When Mr M (the previous month) had been with his old employer as a laundry delivery-van driver it would have been quite proper for him to have taken time off from work, consult a doctor and get the necessary medical certificate to legitimize is absence. During the time between jobs Mrs M could have looked after her husband and, because rest was all that Mr M was considered to require, he 'wouldn't have needed the doctor'. However, Mr and Mrs M felt that the demands and obligations of being in his new job as a machine operator were such that it was impossible, even though the condition was worsening, for Mr M to take time off from the aluminium factory even if he had been able to obtain the official approval of the doctor (which would readily have been given).

From the M family's point of view 'being ill' would in the previous month have impaired the performance of Mr M's normal work role but would have been adequately sanctioned by the doctor. Between jobs, 'being ill' could have been Mr M's major social role and would not have needed the sanctioning of the doctor. In the new job it was felt necessary to accommodate the injury until such time as it was felt appropriate to allow Mr M to take steps to gain legitimate access to the sick role. Because of the

M family's perception of the seriousness of the injury (false, as it turned out) the doctor's role at the time of Mrs M's report was not considered in terms of healer, but solely in terms of agent of legitimization for access to the status sick. His role as healer was considered only when the injury was subsequently felt to be, and diagnosed as being, in need of specialist medical treatment.

Few families produced illness reports which so clearly highlighted a series of differential responses to one illness condition. However, several families reported on, or discussed, illness situations in such a way as to make it quite clear that the decisions taken by the M family would have been readily understood and considered appropriate by many other respondents. Mrs O, for example, kept her nine-year-old son at home from school and in bed when he had a heavy cold, but only, she said, because it was very near the end of term. If it had been 'a proper week' she would have made him go. Her stated philosophy with regard to family illness was 'to push them' to keep going. But even though the threshold of what she considered an illness condition was higher than most other respondents, she still made clear differential decisions about illness conditions in the light of the circumstances of the symptomatic person. Similarly the C and D families, like the M's, when jobs changed, readily accepted that commitment to a full and satisfactory job performance, or at least attendance at work, took primacy over 'being ill', a role which would have been considered legitimate by their doctor.

Note

1. In fact when Mr M did go to the doctor the following week, and subsequently to the hospital out-patient department, it was revealed that ligaments in his knee were damaged. He was off work for over two months and the injury almost certainly put a premature end to his football playing.

Reprinted by permission of Routledge and Kegan Paul, London. David Robinson (1971) *The Process of Becoming Ill*, Routledge and Kegan Paul, London, pp. 7, 13–16.

Chapter 10

The social character of illness: deviance or politics

Elihu M. Gerson

We may begin by noting a fundamental flaw in the traditional conceptualization of the relationship between physician and patient: the assumption, first made by Henderson in 1935 and since enshrined in the medical sociology literature, that the interests of physician and patient are harmonious if not congruent. In fact, this situation applies only in limited circumstances, and the relationship is fraught with inherent contradictions which may appear – to the detriment of physician, patient, or both – in most contemporary medical settings. The failure to recognize these contradictions is in large part responsible for both the sterility of traditional medical sociology and the ineffective public policies of the physicians who have sponsored it.

The physician–patient relationship has a dual nature, even in its simplest form. On one side, practicing medicine is the work of the physician, and he must necessarily be as concerned with the conditions of his work as with the particular medical situation of particular patients. By this, I do not mean simply the problem of fixing fees, but rather the more general problem of defining the circumstances under which he must work, circumstances which include the fixing and collection of fees, determining hours of work, the distribution of honor and prestige for exceptional accomplishment (and of opprobrium for misfeasance), the nature of working relationships with a host of colleagues and other professionals, and the character of relationships with a wide variety of complex organizations (hospitals, insurance companies, government agencies, and so on). Furthermore, physicians do not exist simply in some 'professional role' divorced from other aspects of ordinary life – they are spouses and parents, they live in complex communities. All of these make for differing assessments of work and work contingencies, and for different patterns of risk in making decisions about working conditions. Finally, physicians must handle the problem of emotional involvement with patients and emotional response to their problems, despite what their teachers and sociologists have told them. Styles, tactics and strategies for doing this vary enormously from physician to physician, although certain broad patterns can easily be identified.

From the perspective of the patient, an illness is *not* work in the sense of 'making a living': it is a grossly uncomfortable, often painful, often embarrassing, frequently terrorizing experience involving the fundamental character of the self. That is why patients approach physicians in the first place. They may approach with an attitude ranging along a broad continuum from total unreasoning trust to total unreasoning suspicion, but they approach in, and because of, a cloud of pain and fear. Along with the illness and the patient's reaction to it come a wide variety of other concerns and considerations. The patient wants, not only relief of suffering, reassurance, and information on his physical condition: he wants them at a minimum of monetary cost; he wants them in a minimum amount of time; he wants them with a minimum of disruption to his usual activities; and he wants them with a minimum of further discomfort, fear, and inconvenience. In addition, patients have families, friends, jobs, and other interests as well, and an illness impacts these settings to the degree that the patient is prevented from operating effectively in them. Such interference is as often a result of the prescribed regimen as it is of the disease proper, and patients do not often bother to distinguish too carefully between the two; indeed, it is often difficult for the physician to do so in the face of the extreme side effects of many kinds of drugs and procedures.

The physician then, must manage both his work and the disease as best he can simultaneously, while the patient must manage his disease *and the physician's work*. And therein lies the essential contradiction in the physician–patient relationship: there is an inherent conflict of interest which can rebound with enormous damage to both parties if it is not adequately managed. And here lies, in turn, the principal defect of medical sociology: for to say that the patient must adhere in his conduct to the norms of the sick role is merely to take the side of the physician; while to assert simply that illness is 'labelling' is merely to take the side of the patient. One task of medical sociology therefore, is the analysis of the processes by which the inherent contradictions in the physician–patient relationship are managed by all parties to the relationship. These include not only patient and physician, but the enormous complex of commitments and obligations which both have in their surrounding social organizations.

There are a variety of circumstances which tend to 'mask' the contradictory nature of the physician–patient relationship, while at the same time compounding the difficulties of management. Two of these have overwhelming importance: the fact that medical care is increasingly provided in very large complex settings, and the fact that many illnesses are short-term and relatively inconsequential in their 'social side effects' to the patients. Traditional medical sociology has tended to focus rather arbitrarily, on relatively short-term acute conditions, often treated by the physician in his office. Thus, the 'model' disease has been the common cold or influenza, with an occasional nod to the possibility of acute appendicitis, surgical correction of hernia, and so forth. Under such circumstances, the pain, discomfort, and fear of the patient are at a relative minimum: he can look forward to resuming a normal life in a few days, essentially 'cured' of the problem which drove him to the physician. These are however, the very procedures and problems which are most highly routinized in medical practice, which have the lowest rates of error, which are best understood by the general public, and which allow for a relatively smooth and efficient processing by the physician and the hospital, as well as 'third-party' insurance carriers and other interested bureaucracies.

Catastrophic, long-term, and chronic illnesses which require elaborate continuing management by a complex medical organization and which severely impact (if they do not eliminate) the normal activities of patients are an entirely different story. It is, in fact, from sociological studies of such diseases (Davis, 1963) that the notion of illness as politics rather than deviance clearly emerges. The process of managing such illnesses requires a different order of skills and procedures on the part of both patient and staff. The patient must become medically quite sophisticated in order to 'hold up' his end of the treatment; he must somehow reconcile himself to a lowered level and restricted range of activity; to the loss of friends, and other social consequences of his disease; and to his potential pauperization by the high costs of the treatment. He must often learn to live with some specific chronic pain or discomfort, and (certainly not least) he must learn to deal with a host of complex bureaucracies which are notably idiosyncratic in their procedures.

The physician, on the other hand, must reconcile himself to 'managing' rather than 'curing' the illness; to surrendering much of his technical autonomy to a host of specialists and consultants; to developing and managing relatively extensive and intimate relationships with patients and their associates; to suffering the endlessly repeated failure of procedures which do not work, treatments which damage more than they help, and the bitterly fought loss of patient after patient after patient. In addition, there are the compounding difficulties of ethical dilemmas: the precise definition of death, the moral burdens accompanying the use (or non-use) of heroic measures, and the management of involvement with patients. And finally, physicians must learn to deal with a host of complex bureaucracies which are notably idiosyncratic in their procedures.

In such situations, the contradictions inherent in the fact that a single organism embodies one person's work and another person's self, come rapidly to the fore and generate a host of detailed management problems for both physician and patient. These problems are inherently political – they are concerned with 'who gets what, when, where, how'. They involve extensive maneuvering on the part of all concerned to maximize advantage and minimize disadvantage under conditions in which 'advantage' and 'disadvantage' vary both across parties and over time for each part. They involve the exercise of power: sometimes subtly and indirectly; sometimes coercively, even brutally.

The balance of power is usually with the medical organization (which may or may not be *politically* separable from the attending physician) while the important outcomes and consequences are with the patient. Patients of course, come to realize this very quickly, and react in a variety of ways. Generally, the immediate effect is to increase the patient's fear and helplessness. In turn, this may make for more difficult 'management' problems for medical personnel, as they confront an ever-intensifying series of worries, complaints, and even threats. One of the most powerful strategies for handling this situation is the ability of the physician (and often nurses as well), to define the problematic conduct of the patient as 'symptomatic' rather than political, and thus react by prescribing rather than negotiating. Thus, often the consequences of the organizational defects of medical practice are passed on to the patient in doubled form: once through direct impact on patient quality of life, and again through oppressive responses to legitimate complaint. This is known in traditional sociology as 'sanctioning conformity to the norms of the sick role', and occurs precisely when the technical capacities of the medical institutions are *least able to deliver their 'normative' service*. The *reductio ad absurdum* of this situation occurs when the patient is himself a physician, or at least medically knowledgeable. The increased technical sophistication of the patient on the one hand, combined with the increased involvement of the medical staff with 'one of their own' on the other, naturally heightens both the probability and the potential damage of the general process.

Becoming 'uncooperative' however, is not the only strategy open to the patient in these situations; and defining the patient as psychologically or (what is tantamount to the same thing) morally defective is not the only strategy open to the medical staff. Indeed, the emergence of such a situation is relatively rare, and such strategies are often last resorts on the part of physicians and patients alike. Patients may in fact cultivate a studiously ignorant and deferential helplessness, which thrusts upon the medical staff the necessity of vastly more intense monitoring of the patient's condition and adherence to the prescribed regimen. Thus, such patients may effectively force the commitment of a disproportinate amount of time and emotional involvement from the medical staff; at the same time they jeopardize their own chances of success through their inability or unwillingness to manage the details of their own illness careers.

References

Davis, F. (1963) *Passage Through Crisis: Polio Victims and Their Families*, Bobbs-Merrill, Indianapolis

Henderson, L. J. (1935) Physician and patient as a social system. *New England Journal of Medicine*, **212**, 819; Parsons, T. (1951) *The Social System*, Free Press, Glencoe, Ill

Reprinted from *Social Science and Medicine*, 10, Elihu M. Gerson, The social character of illness: deviance or politics, pp. 220–222, 1976, with permission from Elsevier Science Ltd, The Boulevard, Langford Lane, Kidlington OX5 1GB, UK.

Chapter 11

A view of the patient

Gerry Stimson and Barbara Webb

... the ideal consultation. The doctor's attention is devoted exclusively for a short period of time to the life and problems of another human being. He is there to listen and to help. His training will have made him receptive to a wide range of distress signals and given him the means, or knowledge of the means, to answer them. The occasion will be unhurried and something will be gained by both participants; a good consultation brings satisfaction to the doctor as well as to the patient.

> *The Future General Practitioner*, by a
> Working Party of the Royal College of
> General Practitioners, 1972, p. 13.

When I'm walking in my doctor's, he just finds out first of all if I've got the children with me, which I've come for, or whether I've come for myself, and once he's found that out he's writing the name and address on the prescription while I'm talking to him. He doesn't know what I want, you know. I say, 'One of these days' – I went into him and I said, 'One of these days you'll write the prescription out before I even tell you what's wrong!' You know he's in the middle of doing it as I'm talking to him, you know.

> Woman talking about her doctor.

[Here] we look at the process of consultation with the general practitioner. Nearly everybody goes to see the doctor at some time and nearly everybody is at some time a patient to a doctor. What we have attempted to do is to write about the contact between patient and doctor from the point of view of the patient.

While something is known about the shape of the consultation in terms of where it takes place, how long it lasts, how many patients a doctor sees each day, and how many times a year a patient sees a doctor, there is no adequate account of consulting behaviour.

Consultation we see as a special type of social encounter in which one person seeks information or advice from another. It is akin to a focused interaction (Goffman, 1961, p. 7) in so far as both parties sustain for a time a single focus of attention. Consultation with the doctor is distinguished from everyday conversational social acts in that (1) it is geographically and temporally inflexible: consultation usually takes place at a certain place and at a certain time; (2) there is specificity: the advice will be the reason for the interaction – other topics may be raised but only incidentally; and (3) as Waitzkin and Stoeckle (1972) point out, there is a competence gap between advice seeker and advice giver.

In looking at the consultation *process* we are extending the social activity of consultation temporally and consequently spatially. We include actions outside the face-to-face contact of patient and doctor, but with reference to that contact. Analytically, we have divided the process into three stages: the stage *prior to the consultation* which includes the expectations of the consultation, and the rehearsal for the consultation (these pre-consultation elements have been called 'anticipations' by Kuhn, 1962); second, the *face-to-face interaction* of patient and doctor when the consulting action takes place, which includes the performance of the patient in presenting his self and his problems, the strategies of interaction used by patients and doctors, and the expressive and communicative aspects of the consultation; and third, there is the period *after the consultation*, during which the patient makes sense of what happened, reassesses the consultation and the doctor's action, and makes his treatment decisions.

The ways in which people present themselves in the surgery may be viewed as strategies influencing the course of the consultation. We do not claim that the patient or the doctor always consciously adopt strategies to influence each other. The desire to influence may only be implicit in the presentation. The way in which the facts are presented to the doctor is an expression of a certain approach on the part of the patient, whether this approach is a request for a sickness certificate, a desire that the doctor should give his attention to symptoms that are seen to be a problem, or simply a desire that the doctor makes all the decisions. Verbal and non-verbal control strategies are attempts to put across and reinforce that approach. Likewise, the doctor attempts to influence the interaction along his own desired course. The doctor may have repeated his actions so often that they are generally performed at the level of routine and are not consciously invoked except when that routine is disrupted. For both, the strategies are part of a repertoire, to be invoked when the situation permits. The efforts made by each to influence the interaction give the consultation its bargaining quality.

In the following example from a surgery consultation, a patient is trying to persuade the doctor that her problem merits medical attention. The woman patient presents her symptoms to the doctor. He can find no explanation for them in the examination he makes or from the medical history on the patient's record card. As a position of stalemate is reached, the patient herself finally offers a proposed course of action in the light of the doctor's seeming inaction. She persists in offering the symptoms as a matter of concern and succeeds, by proposing a solution of her own, in gaining the doctor's recognition that some action should be taken. The consultation began with the woman describing 'odd pains' and giddiness and complaining that she had put on weight. We begin the dialogue with her speaking whilst the doctor examines her:

> Patient: 'I've taken tablets. I thought I could fight it off.'
> Doctor: 'Mmm. Uh-huh.'
> Patient: 'This morning I couldn't even drink my cup of tea so I knew something was wrong.'
> Examination ends.
> Doctor: 'Well, that's normal, there's nothing wrong there.'
> Patient: 'Well, I don't know what causes it, I'm sure.'
> Doctor: 'Your blood pressure's all right, there's nothing the matter there.'
> Patient: 'Nothing to worry about? Oh well, there you are then.'
> Doctor: 'Are you sure you've put on half a stone?'
> Patient: 'Definitely.'
> Pause in dialogue.
> Patient: 'Is there something I could stop eating? I can't wear my clothes now.'
> Doctor: 'Cut out sugar in your tea and flour products, take them only in moderation. Try that and see how you go on. It'll take some time mind.'
> Patient (laughing): 'Oh I know that!'
> Both begin to joke about eating and weight problems.

There is rarely open conflict in the negotiation in the consultation. Both parties generally recognize and retain some semblance of formality and exercise restraint to prevent the encounter from completely 'breaking down'. A patient seldom makes accusations to a general practitioner's face about what are considered to be inefficiencies and inadequacies; similarly, a doctor rarely loses his temper with a patient. If it appears that this point is being approached, one actor seems to step down and attempts to avoid the issue or heal the breach. A patient who failed to keep her hospital appointment evoked the doctor's annoyance. During the consultation he said to her: 'Well I'm sorry Betty. What do you expect me to do? I've done as much as I can. ... What's the use if you don't do anything I say?' Betty remained silent throughout, muttering her apologies just before leaving. Verbal and non-verbal control strategies are often covert and rarely obvious or explicit. On the part of the patient particularly they appear to operate beneath a façade of compliance and acquiescence. The thoughts of the patient which are not articulated during tense or difficult exchanges such as that above, may form the basis for 'stories' told about doctors when the patient is well away from the surgery.

There are three ways in which patients can exert control over doctors and thus over the medical care that they receive. First, patients can exert control by choosing which, if any, doctor to consult. [P]eople may choose between doctors in a practice, a choice often based upon the doctor's reputation for certain preferred types of action, which enables the patient to fit the doctor to the problem. In such cases, the patient will have clearly-defined expectations of the encounter.

Following from this ... patients can exert control by influencing the interaction in the face-to-face consultation with the doctor. The way in which the patient presents himself, what he chooses to tell or not to tell the doctor, what he emphasizes and so on, are all ways of attempting to exert control.

Third, decisions made by the patient concerning the utilization of the treatment which the doctor has prescribed are also a means of exerting control. The patient may make his own decisions about taking a medicine when, for example, the patient's own experience of a particular drug overrides, in his estimation, the importance of the instructions given by the doctor. Again, where the patient's expectations were not met in the consultation and the doctor failed to persuade the patient to accept his perspective of the problem, then the patient may not use the prescribed treatment as directed. Yet as a means of exerting control over doctors, not using the treatment is a rather negative sanction.

Limits to patient control

Apart from the interactive strategies that doctors use to maintain control in their dealings with patients, there are several limits to what the patient can do in the way of exerting control over doctors. These limits are the professional ideology of doctors, legal controls, and the structural limitations imposed by the organisation of medical care.

Professional ideology as a limit to patient control

The impact of client choice on the behaviour of the doctor comes out in the work of Freidson. He stresses the ability of the patient to affect the practice of medicine, an ability that rests on the assumption that 'the physician does not have the power to force the layman to use his services' (1961, p. 167), an assumption similar to Goode's. How far is the person independent of the profession in this way? It appears to us that it is sometimes difficult for people to decide not to consult a doctor, when doctors have been fairly successful at defining what people need in the way of medical services, and in the way of what constitutes illness.

Doctors have not, of course, been entirely successful in providing these definitions for they still perceive the complementary problems of trivial consultations on the one hand, and reluctance to consult on the other. Yet the fact that some doctors do define various complaints as trivia and can define the reluctant consulter, shows their claim to decide what constitutes the nature of illness and its treatment.

We use the term 'professional ideology' to describe the system of beliefs and ideas that doctors collectively hold about the nature of man, disease, and the treatment of disease. The ideology is reflected in the work orientation of the doctor and his orientation to patients. The doctor feels that he is the person who defines, with his colleagues, what an illness is. He does this right down to the level of his day-to-day interaction with patients when he is concerned to make it clear, as we have shown, 'who the doctor is'. Furthermore, not only does the doctor provide the definitions regarding illness and treatment but he also attempts to define the way in which the patient, his client, should behave, determining the basis upon which relations between them are to proceed. Balint (1971) terms this the doctor's 'apostolic function', and notes that the effect of this is often to induce patients to adopt the doctor's standards and thereby accept his orientation towards their problem.

> It was almost as if every doctor had revealed knowledge of what was right and what was wrong for patients to expect and to endure, and further, as if he had a sacred duty to convert to his faith all the ignorant and unbelieving among his patients (p. 216).

The patient's defence is often to hold the doctor in person in disrespect and to adopt an attitude of healthy scepticism towards the knowledge of the profession. An individual patient may contest the doctor's opinions and judgments upon the basis of his own common sense and intuition and so 'defy' the expert. [...T]his defiance usually occurs away from the vicinity of the doctor, rather than in his presence.

Legal controls as limits to patient control

Doctors have been so successful in their claims to be the only holders of certain knowledge and skills that their claimed monopoly is recognized by the State and is often embodied in statutes. The medical profession has a legal monopoly over access to, and the distribution of, certain resources, and this limits the freedom of choice of the person to use or not to use the doctor for his problem. There is little alternative but to consult the doctor if, for example, it is certain controlled drugs which are desired. The doctor does not only give advice for the patient to act upon, but acts as a gatekeeper in making resources available. Because these resources are only available through the doctor the patient's freedom to choose whether or not to consult, and thus his control over the doctor, is limited.

The organization of the National Health Service and patient control

The organization of the National Health Service also puts constraints on the possible courses of action open to the patient and thus affects the interaction between patient and doctor. It is difficult for patients to choose between doctors in the United Kingdom, except within one practice, because of the way in which the NHS is organized with the emphasis on personal primary medical care. Each patient has only one doctor of first contact. The patient has to apply to be on the 'list' of the doctor, and there are various administrative procedures for dealing with such applications, and for remunerating doctors partly in terms of the number of patients that they have on their list. Whilst there are arrangements for the treatment of patients in emergency or temporary situations, a patient who is a permanent resident must register with a doctor in order to be able to get ongoing access to the doctor when treatment is needed. It is difficult to 'shop around' among different doctors or to choose a particular doctor for a particular illness. Access to hospital care, and thus specialist doctors, is available only through general practitioners. (We are ignoring in this argument the use of private practice at the general practice level because it is rare and effectively unavailable to most people.)

———————

Changing doctors is seen to be difficult by patients. The patient often has little option open to him, and 'choice' is hardly an appropriate term to describe the paucity of alternatives. Very few people in fact change doctors because of dissatisfaction. Cartwright (1967) reports 3 per cent in five years changing because of dissatisfaction, and Klein (1973) suggests a similar rate of about four for every thousand patients each year. If it is difficult to change doctors, it is equally difficult for the patient to push disagreement or dissatisfaction with what the doctor does to the level of open conflict. The patient is very often in a position of 'take it or leave it'.

———————

Thus, the organization of the NHS effectively limits client choice and thus client control. The consultation process which we have described must be seen in this broader context. The structure in which medical care is provided affects what is possible in the contact between patient and doctor.

References

Balint, M. (1971) *The Doctor, His Patient and the Illness*, Pitman Medical, London. First published, 1957
Cartwright, A. (1967) *Patients and their Doctors*, Routledge and Kegan Paul, London
Freidson, E. (1961) *Patients' Views of Medical Practice*, Russell Sage Foundation, New York
Goffman, E. (1961) *Encounters*, Bobbs-Merrill, Indianapolis
Klein, R. (1973) *Complaints Against Doctors*, Charles Knight, London
Kuhn, M. H. (1962) The interview and the professional relationship. In *Human Behaviour and Social Processes* (A. M. Rose, ed.), ch. 10, Routledge and Kegan Paul, London
Royal College of General Practitioners Working Party (1972) *The Future General Practitioner*, Royal College of General Practitioners, London
Waitzkin, H. and Stoeckle, J. D. (1972) The communication of information about illness. *Advances in Psychosomatic Medicine*, 8, 180–215

Reprinted by permission of Routledge and Kegan Paul, London. Gerry Stimson and Barbara Webb (1975) A view of the patient. In *Going to See the Doctor: The Consultation Process in General Practice*, Routledge and Kegan Paul, London, pp. 1, 2, 7, 8, 48–50, 135–138.

Chapter 12

Women, health and medicine

Lesley Doyal and Mary Ann Elston

Women as consumers of medical care

Women constitute the majority of NHS patients and use general practitioner, psychiatric, geriatric and most preventive services more frequently than men. This is often seen as a paradox because, on average, women live longer than men and therefore one might conclude that they are healthier than men and use medical services less. In 1981 a woman's life expectancy at birth was 76.2 years compared with 70.2 years for a man. At the age of 60, life expectancy was 20.4 and 15.9 respectively.

The practical result of these differences is that women need more medical care rather than less. Women now form a significant majority of the elderly in the population: among those over 75, there are now two women for every man. Since the very elderly always have great need of medical services, the longevity of women in obviously important in explaining their predominance among patients in NHS hospitals.

Another reason for women's greater use of health services is their reproductive capacity, which brings them into the medical orbit in a variety of different ways. Women are obviously the only users of maternity services, and they come into frequent contact with the health-care system during the processes of pregnancy and childbirth. They are also the most frequent users of services connected with fertility control, since women are increasingly taking responsibility for contraception, and most female contraception techniques involve some degree of medical intervention, whether in the prescribing of a pill or the fitting of an intra-uterine device (IUD). Finally, since women bear the major responsibility for childcare, they frequently accompany children on visits to the doctor.

Because women are often using medical services in connection with reproduction, they may well visit their doctors when they are perfectly healthy. They are not then 'patients' in the classic sense of the term, yet doctors and health workers often treat them as though they were sick and dependent and in need of medical intervention. [...T]his problem of the healthy woman being treated as ill is perhaps at its most acute in the context of childbirth.

Generally speaking, women are treated for psychiatric problems rather more often than men, whether we compare GP consultation rates for 'emotional' problems, outpatient psychiatric visits or admittance to a psychiatric hospital. In 1970 it was calculated that one woman in six in England and Wales would enter hospital because of mental illness at some time in her life, compared with one man in nine. Psychiatric admissions have fallen considerably since then, largely because of changes in treatment policy (more people are treated as outpatients), but the difference between the proportions of women and men still remains.

The most obvious conclusion that could be drawn from these figures would be that women suffer from mental illness more often than men and this is reflected in a straightforward way in their greater use of psychiatric services. However, we cannot assume simple relationship between the use of medical services and the level of physical or psychological ill-health in a community. A great deal of illness is never brought before a doctor, so official consultation rates only represent the tip of an iceberg, with most illness remaining invisible.

On the other hand, many medical consultations do not arise directly from physical or psychological illness but are actually a response to a social or economic problem for which there appears to be no alternative source of help. Tranquilizer advertisements aimed at doctors show that this is well recognized by the drug industry. The companies that manufacture tranquilizers have realized that many women's unhappiness or 'depression' is caused by the circumstances in which they live, since women are pictured in advertisements in bad housing conditions, surrounded by piles of washing-up and screaming children. However, the answer shown is not to change the situation, but to prescribe a pill to dull the pain. Not surprisingly, problems presented to a doctor – whatever their origin – will usually be interpreted only in medical terms. This can lead to an overemphasis on the rate of illness in a community and an underestimate of other social and economic problems.

These difficulties of definition and measurement are particularly acute when we are trying to compare the frequency with which women and men consult doctors. This is because studies have shown that there are differences between sexes in what sociologists call 'illness behaviour', that is, the way people behave when they are ill. These are likely to lead to an overestimation of the amount of ill-health among women compared with that of men. First, it appears that women are more likely than men to express their problems through anxiety, depression or other symptoms of illness. In general, it is more socially acceptable for women to admit weakness and to seek help, particularly when their problems are emotional. Therefore, women may find it easier than men to take problems of this kind to a doctor. Moreover, the fact that psychological weakness is not only more readily tolerated but may even be expected in women, will affect the perceptions that doctors have of their patients. Hence doctors often interpret a woman's symptoms as psychosomatic (psychological in origin) when they might consider similar symptoms in a man to be physical in origin (Lennane and Lennane, 1973).

It seems then, that some of the greater use made of medical services, and psychiatric services in particular, by women can be explained by sex differences in attitudes towards illness and towards the seeking of medical care. However, it also seems likely that we cannot explain the entire difference in this way. If we cannot explain away the greater female use of psychiatric services, then we have to look at alternative explanations for why women should exhibit higher rates of certain kinds of mental illness than men.

Some of the excess, particularly in admission to hospital for senile dementia (a form of mental confusion that sometimes accompanies ageing), is again accounted for by the number of elderly women in the population. However, far more women than men are also treated for anxiety and depression, and despite the problems in interpreting the statistics, this does seem to reflect real differences between the sexes.

One argument that is frequently used to explain – implicitly or explicitly – is the suggestion that women are genetically (biologically) more prone to certain kinds of mental illness than men. That is to say, they are inherently more excitable and emotionally unstable, and are therefore more likely to go 'over the top' or 'off the rails' and find themselves in a doctor's surgery. The most important argument against this idea that all women have a genetic predisposition to mental illness is that it ignores all the social and environmental factors that also influence women's lives and inevitably affect their experiences of sickness and health. A more appropriate starting point for understanding female mental illness would not be women's genes but an analysis of the role of women in our society in order to ascertain whether or not it is liable to make them more likely than men to suffer from anxiety and depression.

Feminists have also pointed out that the role of a woman in our society is in many ways a 'sick' one – that femininity itself is somehow equated with sickness. Thus there is a sense in which to be a 'normal' woman is often to be a neurotic human being. Another suggestion is that the behaviour and attitudes expected of a woman may sometimes be so intolerable or contradictory that anxiety or depression become a reasonable response. The hysteria sometimes exhibited by middle-class women in the nineteenth century, for instance, has been described as an entirely understandable response to their sheltered lives – and possibly even as a form of protest. Finally, it is argued that the lives many women lead – the nature of their living and working conditions and the quality of their relationships with other people – will often be conducive to depression and or anxiety. One example of this might be the middle-aged woman who is depressed because her children have left home, and who now has little sense of her own identity or worth. Another illustration would be the prevalence of depression among working-class housewives at home with small children. Obviously, the reasons behind this phenomenon are complex, but among the most important must be the social isolation of these women combined with the very low value placed on their work (Brown and Harris, 1978).

Women as producers of medical care

Although medicine is usually thought of as a male sphere of activity, it is women who make up the majority of health workers. Over 70 per cent of people working for the NHS are female. But women are by no means evenly distributed within the health labour force. Only about 25 per cent of NHS doctors are women, and most female health workers are found low down in the occupational hierarchy, particularly in nursing and ancillary work. These involve the traditionally female task of caring for the intimate needs of the sick and the domestic duties of cooking, cleaning and laundering; thus the sexual division of labour in health care reflects that of the wider society. If we look at the relationship between doctors and nurses, for instance, we find that it often mirrors the relationship traditionally found between the sexes. That is to say, the (usually) male doctor makes the 'hard' intellectual decisions while the (usually) female nurse carries them out and provides 'tender loving care' for the patient. Most NHS work is therefore 'women's work' and this is reflected in the inferior status, low pay and often unpleasant conditions that characterize many jobs in the health service as well as women's work in other sectors of the economy.

But women's role in caring for the sick is by no means confined to the NHS. Women also provide a vast and largely invisible reservoir of care for those people who are in need but who are not deemed to be the responsibility of the healthcare system. In practice, most of the chronically sick and disabled, the mentally handicapped and the elderly are not cared for by paid workers either in institutions or in the community, but by individual women who feel morally bound to do so – usually by ties of kinship or marriage.

Women are also held responsible for maintaining the health of their families. This idea that women should look after the health of others is not a new one. If we go back to the nineteenth and early twentieth centuries we find that it was often mothers who were blamed for the high infant mortality rate. Rather than paying any serious attention to the problems of poverty, insanitary housing, and lack of medical attention during labour, most reformers blamed mothers themselves for their 'ignorant' and 'feckless' behaviour. In later years the content of this criticism of mothers has changed, but the logic remains the same. Thus the immediate post-war period was dominated by the notion of 'maternal deprivation' which was said to cause a wide variety of psychological problems in children whose mothers went out to work.

References

Brown, G. W. and Harris, T. (1978) *The Social Origins of Depression*, Tavistock, New York

Lennane, K. J. and Lennane, R. J. (1973) Alleged psychogenic disorders in women: a possible manifestation of sexual prejudice. *New England Journal of Medicine*, **288**, 288–292

Reprinted by permission of the Open University Press, Buckingham. Lesley Doyal and Mary Ann Elston (1986) Women, health and medicine. In *Women in Britain Today* (Beechey, V. and Whitelegg, E., eds), Open University Press, Buckingham, pp. 174–177, 207.

Chapter 13

You are dangerous to your health: the ideology and politics of victim blaming

Robert Crawford

The victim blaming ideology as applied to health is emerging alongside the limits of medicine argument. Indeed, that argument is its first premise. Basing itself on the irrefutable and increasingly obvious fact that medicine has been oversold, the new ideology argues that individuals, if they take appropriate actions, if they, in other words, adopt life-styles which avoid unhealthy behavior, may prevent most diseases. 'Living a long life is essentially a do-it-yourself proposition', as it was put by one pundit. Policy, it is argued, must be redirected away from the extension of social programs which characterized the 1960s toward a health promotion strategy which calls upon the individual to become more responsible for his or her own health rather than to rely on ineffective medical services.

At a time when people seem to want medicine most, its continuing availability and expansion threaten powerful economic and political interests. Further, much to the concern of industry, medicine is clearly inadequate in dealing with the contemporary social production of disease, and is therefore increasingly unable to perform its traditional role of resolving societal tensions which emerge when people identify the social causes of their individual pathologies. In the face of these trends, it is fascinating and revealing that we are witnessing the proliferation of messages about our own personal responsibility for health and an attack on individual life-styles and at-risk behaviors.

The politics of diversion

Social causation of disease has several dimensions. The complexities are only beginning to be explored. The victim blaming ideology, however, inhibits that understanding and substitutes instead an unrealistic behavioral model. It both ignores what is known about human behavior and minimizes the importance of evidence about the environmental assault on health. It instructs people to be individually responsible at a time when they are becoming less capable as individuals of controlling their health environment (Eyer, 1977; Anon., 1977a). Although environmental dangers are often recognized, the implication is that little can be done about an ineluctable, modern, technological, and industrial society. Life-style and environmental factors are thrown together to communicate that individuals are the primary agents in shaping or modifying the effects of their environment. Victor Fuchs, for example, while recognizing environmental factors as 'also relevant', asserts that 'the greatest potential for reducing coronary disease, cancer, and other major killers still lies in altering personal behavior' (Fuchs, 1974, p. 46). 'Emphasizing social responsibility', he philosophizes, 'can increase security, but it may be the security of the "zoo" – purchased at the expense of freedom' (p. 26). Or as Whalen (1977) writes:

> Many of our most difficult contemporary health problems, such as cancer, heart disease and accidental injury, have a built-in behavioral component.... *If they are to be solved at all*, we must change our style of living [emphasis added].

The diffusion of a psychological world view often reinforces the masking of social causation. Even though the psychiatric model substitutes social for natural explanations, problems still tend to be seen as amenable to change through personal transformation – with or without therapy. And with or without therapy, individuals are ultimately held responsible for their own psychological well-being. Usually, no one has to blame us for some psychological failure; we blame ourselves. Thus, psychological impairment can be just as effective as moral failing or genetic inferiority in blaming the victim and reinforcing dominant social relations (Edelman, 1974). People are alienated, unhappy, dropouts, criminals, angry, and activists, after all, because of maladjustment to one or another psychological norm.

The ideology of individual responsibility for health lends itself to this form of psychological social control. Susceptibility to at-risk behaviors, if not a moral failing, is at least a psychological failing. New evidence relating psychological state to resistance or susceptibility to diseases and accidents can and will be used to shift more responsibility to the individual. Industrial psychologists have long been employed with the intention that the best way to reduce plant accidents in lieu of costly production changes is to intervene at the individual level (Anon., 1977b). The implication is that people make themselves sick, not only mentally but physically. If job satisfaction is important to health, people should seek more rewarding employment. Cancer is a state of mind.

In another vein, many accounts of the current disease structure in the United States link disease with affluence. The affluent society and the life-styles it has wrought, it is suggested, are the sources of the individual's degeneration and adoption of at-risk behaviors. Halberstam, for example, writes that 'most Americans die of excess rather than neglect or poverty' (quoted in Somers, 1971, p. 22).

Thus, even though some may complain about environmental hazards, people are really suffering from over-indulgence of the good society. It is that over-indulgence which must be checked. Further, by pointing to life-styles, which are usually presented as if they reflect the problems of a homogenized, affluent society, this aspect of the ideology tends to obscure the reality of class and the impact of social inequality on health. It is compatible with the conception that people are free agents. Social structure and constraints recede amidst the abundance.

Of course, several diseases do stem from the life-styles of the more affluent.

But are the well-established relationships between low income and high infant mortality, diseases related to poor diet and malnutrition, stress, cancer, mental illness, traumas of various kinds, and other pathologies (Hurley, 1971; Anon., 1972; Kitagawa and Hauser, 1973; Anon., 1975; Sherer, 1977) now to be ignored or relegated to a residual factor? While long-term inequality in morbidity and mortality is declining (Antonovsky, 1967), for almost every disease and for every indicator of morbidity incidence increases as income falls (Anon., 1976, pp. 620–621). In some specific cases, the health gap appears to be widening (Jenkins, 1976; Eyer and Sterling, forthcoming).

Finally, by focusing on the individual instead of the economic system, the ideology performs its classical role of obscuring the class structure of work. The failure to maintain health in the workplace is attributed to some personal flaw. The more than 2.5 million people disabled by occupational accidents and diseases each year and the additional 114,000 killed (Page and O'Brien, 1973; Brodeur, 1974) are not explained by the hazards or pace of work as much as by the lack of sufficient caution by workers, laziness about wearing respirators or the like, psychological maladjustment, and even by the worker's genetic susceptibility. Correspondingly, the overworked, overstressed worker is offered TM, biofeedback, psychological counseling, or some other 'holistic' approach to healthy behavior change, leaving intact the structure of incentives and sanctions of employers which reward the retention of health-denying behavior.

Corporate management appears to be increasingly integrating victim blaming themes into personnel policies. Physical and especially psychological health have acquired more importance for management faced with declining productivity and expanding absenteeism.

Holding individual workers responsible for their susceptibility to illness, or for an 'unproductive' psychological state, reinforces management attempts to control absenteeism and enhance productivity. Job dissatisfaction and job-induced stress (in both their psychological and physical manifestations), principal sources of absenteeism and low productivity, will become identified as life-style problems of the worker. Programs are now being expanded to screen workers for susceptibility to job hazards. Not only genetic susceptibility but also other at-risk health behaviors, such as smoking, use of alcohol, or improper diet, help legitimize screening programs. But while alerting individual workers to their susceptibility, these programs do not address the hazardous conditions which to some degree affect all workers. Thus, all workers may be penalized *to the extent* that such programs function to divert attention from causative conditions. To the degree that the causative agent remains, the more susceptible workers are also penalized in that they must shoulder the burden of the hazardous conditions either by looking for another, perhaps nonexistent job, or, if it is permitted, by taking a risk in remaining. It is worth noting in this regard that some women of childbearing age barred from working in plants using lead are reported to be obtaining sterilizations in order to regain their jobs.

The ideology of individual responsibility promotes a concept of wise living which views the individual as essentially independent of his or her surroundings, unconstrained by social events and processes. When such pressures are recognized, it is still the individual who is called upon to resist them. Nevertheless, an alternate political understanding, directed not toward individuals, but toward relations among individuals, will profoundly influence the politics of health in the coming period. The commercial and industrial assault on health is becoming too grave to be ignored. A crisis characterized by an increasing involvement of unions, consumer groups, and environmental activists in confrontation with the 'manufacturers of illness' threatens to extend far beyond the normal boundaries of health politics.

This politicization of environmental and occupational health issues suggests an erosion of the power of medicine to function as a diversion from social causation. This may be occurring even though overall utilization of medical services continues to rise and the hope for medical deliverance remains intense. The failure of medicine to contain the new epidemics is a partial explanation for that erosion. The cost crisis also leads to an ideological shift away from medicine. Given people's expectations and political pressures for protection and extension of entitlements, a justification for retrenchment must be offered. Thus, people are told that they rely too much on ineffective medical services, and they must think instead about prevention. However, to the extent that medicine is delegitimized, its traditional social control function of individualizing disease through the biological model, and of providing a 'technological fix' as a substitute for social change, is also weakened. As people come to understand the limitations of medicine and technology as a means to better health, there is increasing potential for the development of a movement willing to confront dominant interests over the systematic denial of health.

The ideology of individual responsibility poses an alternate social control formulation. It replaces reliance on therapeutic intervention with a behavioral model which only requires good living. Like medicine, the new ideology continues to 'atomize both causation and solution to illness' (Ziem, 1977), although now that ideological function is performed outside the therapeutic structure.

The success of such an approach, however, is problematic. A deinstitutionalized individualism cannot perform as an effective social control device in a technological age. For this reason it is important not to overemphasize the abandonment of medicine.

=====

The continuing utility of medicine will come not so much from a newly found effectiveness, but from its potent redemptive and other social control qualities. Although medicine is not the only institution capable of performing such critical functions, the therapeutic ideology will remain the 'paradigm for modernized domination' (McKnight, undated, p. 8). Through masking political relations by calling them medical (Edelman, 1974), and through the technical definition of social problems, medicine provides an institutionalized form of control that the concept of individual responsibility cannot.

Finally, although the victim blaming ideology is linked with the attack on medicine, there is no inherent reason why the celebration of a 'reformed' medicine and notions of individual responsibility cannot coexist. Each counterbalances the weakness of the other. Even as the attack on medicine gains popularity, a reintegration may be under way. After all, victim blaming may let medicine off the hook as well.

References

Anon. (1972) *Infant Mortality Rates: Socioeconomic Factors*, Series 22, No. 14, U.S. Public Health Service, Washington, D.C.

Anon. (1975) *Selected Vital and Health Statistics in Poverty and Nonpoverty Areas of 19 Large Cities, United States, 1969–71*, Series 21, No. 26, U.S. Public Health Service, Washington, D.C.

Anon. (1976) *Preventive Medicine USA*, Prodist, New York

Anon. (1977a) The social etiology of disease (part I). *HMO–A Network for Marxist Studies in Health*, No. 2, January

Anon. (1977b) *New York Times*, April 3

Antonovsky, A. (1967) Social class, life expectancy, and overall mortality. *Millbank Memorial Fund Quarterly*, 45 (2, part I) , 31–73.

Brodeur, P. (1974) *Expendable Americans*, Viking Press, New York

Edelman, M. (1974) The political language of the helping professions. *Politics and Society*, 4(3), 295–310

Eyer, J. (ed.) (1977) Special Issue on the Economy, Medicine, and Health. *International Journal of Health Services*, 7(1), 1–150

Eyer, J. and Sterling, P. Stress related mortality and social organization. *Review of Radical Political Economy*, forthcoming

Fuchs, V. (1974) *Who Shall Live? Health, Economics, and Social Choice*, Basic Books, New York

Hurley, R. (1971) The health crisis of the poor. In *The Social Organization of Health* (Dreitzel, H. P., ed.), Macmillan, New York

Jenkins, C. D. (1976) Recent evidence supporting psychologic and social risk factors for coronary heart diseases. *New England Journal of Medicine*, 294(18), 987–994; 294(19), 1033–1038

Kitagawa, E. and Hauser, P. (1973) *Differential Mortality in the United States: A Study in Socioeconomic Epidemiology*, Harvard University Press, Cambridge

McKnight, J. The medicalization of politics. Northwestern University, unpublished paper (undated)

Page, J. A. and O'Brien, M. (1973) *Bitter Wages*, Grossman, New York

Sherer, H. (1977) Hypertension. *HMO – A Network for Marxist Studies in Health*, No. 2, January 1977

Somers, A. (1971) *Health Care in Transition: Directions for the Future*, Hospital Research and Educational Trust, Chicago

Whalen (1977) *New York Times*, April 3

Ziem, G. (1977) Ideology, the state, and victim blaming: a discussion paper for the East Coast Health Discussion Group. Johns Hopkins University, unpublished paper

Chapter 14

Health and lifestyles

Mildred Blaxter

One important finding of this study has been that, in fact, few people's lifestyles are totally healthy or unhealthy: most are mixed. Only about 15 per cent of the sample were found to have 'healthy' habits in all the four areas of life examined, and only about 5 per cent had totally 'unhealthy' lives in these respects. Thus the effect of any one good or bad habit has to be considered in context, not in isolation. It is true that the minority whose lifestyles, judging from the limited criteria available here, are totally healthy, are likely to demonstrate health much better than the norm, and unhealthy habits will depress health markedly, even in favourable living circumstances. It is true that those who behave in totally unhealthy ways, and at the same time are subject to economic or social stress, were found to have the very worst health. The avoidance of behavioural risk factors was found, however, to be protective to only a small degree when involuntary lifestyles were unhealthy.

This is, of course, an over-simplified summary.

There are several firm conclusions, however: firstly, it has been shown that health is – as lay people clearly believe – multi-dimensional. Different groups or individuals can lay emphasis on different aspects or be unhealthy and healthy in different ways: circumstances and health-related habits can affect one dimension of health rather than another. In considering whether there are any practical or policy implications, therefore, this first point must be made: receipes for a healthier society must be clear about what they mean by 'health', and what aspect of health they are directed at.

A second conclusion is that there is clear evidence for social differentiation in everyday experience of health. It is not only in mortality rates, or in the distribution of specific disease conditions, that social classes differ. Indeed, variation in health more widely defined is probably greater. Differences in subjectively-experienced aspects of health – in the prevalence of common symptoms, in feelings of positive healthiness, in psycho-social well-being – are certainly greater than differences in objectively-measured physical fitness or the prevalence of diagnosed disease.

It has also been clearly shown that almost all the associations between social circumstances and health are strongest, especially for men, in the middle years of life. Some differences were apparent among even the youngest adults studied here, but commonly they were not great. Amongst older men and women, health became more 'equal' amongst those who survived to any given age. But in the 40s, 50s and 60s the accumulated effects of disadvantaged lives showed themselves most strongly.

Other important findings to which attention must be drawn relate to differences between men and women. Commonly, in health statistics women show less variation by social class than men (e.g. in mortality figures). It is possible that this is due to the use of 'husband's occupation' for the classification of married women, which – since their 'own' class may not be the same as their husbands's – may thus smooth out some of the variation between classes.

———

[I]t was certain relationships between social circumstances or behaviour and health which appeared to differ for women and men. Exercise appeared to be more protective for the fitness of male manual smokers than non-manual, and a good diet was not associated with less illness among non-manual men with otherwise unhealthy habits. For women, these class relationships were reversed: exercise was not protective for manual smokers, and diet had more effect among non-manual than manual women. Area of residence impinged on health in different ways and behavioural patterns were not necessarily associated with area in the same manner.

One of the more important conclusions of this analysis relates more generally to the effects of area of residence. In general, certain types of 'small area' (cities, industrial areas) were likely to demonstrate both worse health and less healthy behaviour than others (rural areas, high status areas): this is not surprising. Within small areas, however, class differences in health or in behaviour could be more or less marked: they were usually small in rural areas, for instance, and considerable in cities. They might even reverse: alcohol consumption was higher among non-manual than manual men in high status areas, but the reverse was true in industrial areas. The 'North/South divide' was shown to have limited significance of itself, and to be less important than type of area wherever geographically situated. This is the more notable, given the rather crude categories of area necessarily used here.

A conclusion must be that although broad statements about the effects of class or income or area of residence, or the relationship of behaviour to health, may seem to offer simple implications for policy, they can never be assumed to be universally applicable.

Reprinted by permission of Routledge (Tavistock Publications), London and New York. Mildred Blaxter (1990) *Health and Lifestyles*, Routledge/Tavistock, London and New York, pp. 234–236.

Chapter 15

The effects of unemployment on family life

Leonard Fagin and Martin Little

The causal link between unemployment and health

We want to consider the question of whether the health histories of these families can be linked in any way to the event of unemployment. Looking at the descriptive accounts of the families, one has to conclude that health problems played an important part in their adjustment to unemployed life and even in re-employment. In such a small sample of families, without any other control than themselves through time, it is impossible to arrive at firm conclusions and predictable generalizations, but especially in those families where health difficulties followed unemployment, these changes appeared to be associated more closely to job loss than to any other significant event occurring in the family's life at the time. But that still leaves us with the questions, 'Does unemployment cause ill health?' and 'If so, how?'

The evidence reviewed ... strongly suggests that there is an association between health and unemployment. The link, however, is far from straightforward, and the possibility is that they are connected through many pathways which increase or decrease the possibility that health may be affected. First of all one must accept that the majority of individuals are not likely to express their problems in terms of health, and that those that do suffer fall into clearly demarcated vulnerable groups – unfortunately that sector of society which always responds less well to adverse social conditions and can rarely avoid bearing the brunt of them: the frail and sick, the elderly, the ethnic minorities, the unskilled, the young and the poor.

The fact that most of the families considered unemployment to be an extremely unpleasant experience leads us to think that stress could be a mechanism, or a mediator, by which unemployment may lead to illness. It must be emphasized, however, that stress can also be the mediator towards successful adjustment. Figure [1] is a model which takes into account the major contributory factors.

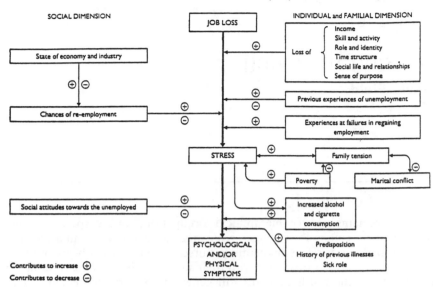

Figure [1]   Possible pathways from unemployment to ill health

All of the factors mentioned in Figure [1] appeared in the families we interviewed, in each one carrying a different weight and exercising different influences. It may well be that some of these factors are more deleterious than others, and this will only be ascertained if further research is able to isolate them and study them in larger numbers. If we are to intervene and try to prevent some of the most harmful consequences of unemployment, we shall only be able to be effective if we know where and when to act.

Reprinted by permission of Penguin Books, Harmondsworth. Leonard Fagin and Martin Little (1984) The effects of unemployment on family life. In *The Forsaken Families*, Penguin Books, Harmondsworth, pp. 204–207.

Chapter 16

Nursing the dying

David Field

Nursing remains a very hierarchical occupation, and despite the new 'professional' emphasis in nurse education to encourage initiative and decision making, it seems that trainee nurses are not normally encouraged to question or discuss treatment with their superiors during their training on the wards. In the wards they are still generally expected to remain silent, accept orders, and respond to commands. Where work is organized on a basis of task allocation their capacity to develop expert knowledge of their patients is diminished, and they are unlikely to be able to exercise autonomy in their care of patients. One can see that in such situations nurses are unlikely to develop or be allowed to practise the types of decision-making and communication skills necessary for the good nursing care of the terminally ill. By contrast, where nurses have a high degree of autonomy and where individualized patient care is the norm, as on the medical ward and the CCU, the organization of work seems to encourage – even demand – greater initiative, self-sufficiency, and decision making from the nurses, and serves to support caring attitudes. In such situations the nurse can develop expert knowledge of patients which others will lack, and can therefore contribute meaningfully to the planning and delivery of good patient care.

Changing attitudes towards the care of the dying

In the more than two decades since Glaser and Strauss published their seminal work, *Awareness of Dying* (1965), there has been a shift in the attitudes of health care professionals towards the care of dying people. The debates generated by the work of Glaser and Strauss, Saunders, Kubler-Ross, and others about *whether* to disclose a terminal prognosis to a dying patient have been largely superseded by questions about *how* to disclose such a prognosis. True, the situation described by Duff and Hollingshead (1968, p. 303) where 'Each member of the group functioned within a framework of ambiguous definitions of what *might* be done, what *should* be done, what *must* be done' (emphasis in the original) has not altered significantly, but the way of responding to such ambiguity seems to have shifted towards openness with patients and away from the evasion which Duff and Hollingshead and so many other researchers have found. While not all doctors and nurses believe that dying people should be informed of their impending death, 'expert opinion' is certainly to do so. Why has this change occurred?

In large part the change has been consequent upon, or at the very least closely linked with, changes in the practical care of people who are dying. The management of pain and other distressing physical symptoms which dying people experience are now much better understood and are more likely to be successfully treated, and so doctors and nurses can now feel that they can offer something positive to their dying patients. Research reported by Parkes (1985) and Wilkes (1984) suggests that at least some British hospitals are achieving levels of pain relief found in the hospices. This is not to deny that there are still major deficits, or that too many people die in unnecessary pain and unrelieved suffering, especially those dying at home. Still, the possibility exists, and is *known* to exist, for the relief of physical distress. It is also recognized that the control and relief of such physical symptoms as pain and breathlessness contribute significantly to the alleviation and reduction of anxiety, depression, and psychological distress among those who are dying. These changes in technology and in knowledge, by providing the means for better physical care of dying patients and a better understanding of how to manage the process of dying, have been important factors leading to greater openness with the terminally ill. Equally important is that many doctors and nurses are no longer seeing death as a failure (Wilkes, 1986). The development and dissemination of such attitudes, expertise, and knowledge have been largely a product of the hospice movement which has demonstrated the possibility of holistic patient-centred care, which treats dying people with dignity and involves both them and all those caring for them in the decisions which are made about their care.

Changes in medical and nurse education may also have been consequential in the changing attitudes towards the care of dying patients. In Britain one of the results of the Royal Commission on Medical Education (1968) was the introduction of behavioural science teaching into most British medical schools. In nursing schools such teaching has a longer, better established, and more accepted role. Thus, the present generation of doctors and nurses is more firmly grounded in basic human sciences than previous generations were. They are likely to be exposed to teaching about communication skills, the effect of cultural differences on healthy and illness behaviour, practitioner–client relationships, and other topics which are relevant to the practice and appreciation of 'whole person' care. In particular nurse education incorporates such an approach as a core feature of nursing practice. They are also likely to receive direct teaching about death, dying, and bereavement, and about their role in caring for those who are dying and their relatives. Despite the acknowledged deficiencies, not least the discrepancy between what is taught in the nursing school and what the trainee experiences and observes on the wards, it seems likely that such changes have led to some changes in attitudes among health professionals and to a greater likelihood of the disclosure of a terminal prognosis to the dying person with probable improvements in care as a result.

The impact of AIDS

The importance of nurses' attitudes towards those they care for is clearly shown by the current concerns and fears among nurses about the treatment of patients with Acquired Immune Deficiency Syndrome (AIDS). The rapid rise in the number of people suffering from AIDS poses particular problems for nurses, who are the group of health care workers most closely involved in their care. People with AIDS tend to be young adults – a category of terminally ill patients whom nurses find particularly distressing to care for. They are also likely to be members of two stigmatized groups in our society: homosexuals and drug addicts. There is currently no known cure for or immunization against AIDS, and the death rate of AIDS patients is very high. AIDS patients are thus likely to constitute a particularly problematic category of terminally ill patients whom nurses are likely to perceive as difficult, dangerous, and unrewarding to care for.

Geiss and Fuller (1985) in a study of the reaction of hospice staff to their first (homosexual) AIDS patients report that contacts with AIDS patients caused problems for the staff by threatening the non-judgemental stance which many of them adopted towards the values and beliefs of their patients, and by challenging their professional and caring roles. One solution to such problems adopted by the staff was avoidance of the AIDS patients even though this ran counter to the hospice philosophy. Geiss and Fuller identify three issues, which run throughout the literature reviewed: fear of contagion, unresolved feelings about homosexuality (homophobia), and embarrassment by staff about their irrational responses to the patient.

The nursing care of terminally ill AIDS patients thus poses additional challenges and difficulties for nurses. In particular, the fear of death may assume the status of a very real and direct threat for the nurse caring for an AIDS patient. Thus clear procedures to prevent contagion, and in-service and nursing school training about the actual threat of contagion and ways to minimize it, are necessary to alleviate such fears. Given the high level of stress associated with nursing AIDS patients, homophobia and other negative attitudes towards AIDS patients, and the moral dilemmas surrounding their care, staff support and counselling also seem to be high priorities (Geiss and Fuller, 1985). In contrast to the United States, nursing guidelines for the care of AIDS patients have been slow to emerge in Britain. A survey of British nursing schools found that while all of the responding schools provided AIDS-related information in the RGN courses there was a 'low level of commitment to skills training' with 62 per cent of the responding schools reporting no such training (Baldwin and Vidler, 1988, p. 38). Half of the schools had no policy regarding the management of AIDS. It is imperative that such guidelines are developed and disseminated speedily.

Powerless patients

An enduring aspect of doctor–nurse, nurse–patient, and doctor–patient relationships in each case is the control of the information given to the latter by the former. Many writers have noted that control of information and communication is an important way in which people control others. Sharing knowledge is equivalent to sharing power. Controlling the information they give to nurses is an important way in which doctors maintain their authority and control over them. Game and Pringle (1983) argue that in a similar way nurses maintain control over patients. Withholding information from patients denies them autonomy and makes it impossible for them to break down the hierarchical relations which are the normal pattern within hospitals, and so contributes to the depersonalization of patient care.

An endemic feature of hospital care is the neglect of the patient as a person. Patients are treated as passive receivers of what the experts (i.e. doctors) deem is best for them. Medical expertise is typically focused upon intervention and cure of pathological disease processes and conditions. The experts concentrate on the sub-individual features of symptoms, pathological processes and bodily signs, and apply their sophisticated medical and surgical technology to the treatment of these. Such treatment may often be inappropriate for the care of chronically ill and dying patients, where palliative care is more appropriate. In all this medically defined activity the needs of the patient as a person are often overlooked. Nurses usually accept doctors' definitions of treatment and care and so support this depersonalization of patients. They are more likely to act as advocates and interpreters of the doctor to the patient than vice versa. The widespread failure of hospital staff to provide patients with information about their condition seems firmly rooted in these attitudes towards treatment, despite the evidence suggesting that clinical outcomes can be improved by giving patients routine and simple information about their condition and its treatment (Egbert et al., 1964; Korsch and Negrette, 1972; Skipper and Leonard, 1968). Further, dying patients in hospitals are often denied knowledge about their condition while their relatives are told. Not only may this have negative consequences for their symptom management and psychological state and place strains on family relations and communication, but this is also a breach of confidence. There are strong ethical grounds for disclosure of information about their prognosis to people who are dying.

Although the majority of deaths in Britain occur in hospitals, most of the care of dying people occurs in their own homes where they are looked after by their relatives, with admission to hospital coming towards the end of their terminal illness. A number of studies report that the quality of life for terminally ill people being cared for at home is often poor (Bowling and Cartwright, 1982; Cartwright *et al.*, 1973; Parkes, 1985; Wilkes, 1984). Admission to hospital usually occurs because the main carer cannot cope with care and/or because of problems of symptom control. Despite the emphasis on encouraging community care in place of hospital care for a whole range of conditions the growth of community nursing services which bear the brunt of expert care of the sick and dying in the community is not keeping pace with the increased demand for services (DHSS, 1983). An immediate question, then, is to ask why the care of those who are dying in their own homes – where it seems most people would want to die – cannot be improved. Why should hospitals have become the place where people go to die, particularly as the wards are often too busy to be suitable places for dying patients? Is the poor quality of care at home at least partly a result of patients not being adequately informed about their terminal prognosis, and hence not being fully involved in the decisions which are being made about their care?

The realization of nursing care for the whole person and the derivation of satisfaction and reward from such caring nursing can flow from the types of structural arrangements identified in this work. In particular they seem to be closely associated with individualized methods of allocating patient care. Far from being detrimental to the nurse a certain level of emotional involvement with patients seems to be to the mutual benefit of nurse and patient, and can pertain ... even in such an apparently negative situation as nursing dying patients.

======

The current pressures in the NHS combined with persisting patterns of nursing organization and work seem to make the provision of such healthy work environments within British hospitals unlikely. Unless nurses can work in a humane system which gives them respect and rewards them for humane and holistic patient care, it is unrealistic to expect them consistently to provide such care. If current trends continue the prospects are that their caring labour will become less caring and more laborious, to the detriment of all those concerned.

References

Baldwin, S. and Vidler, K. (1988) AIDS and general nursing training curricula: a survey of UK schools of nursing. *Nurse Education Today*, 8, 36–38
Bowling, A. and Cartwright, A. (1982) *Life after a Death. A Study of the Elderly Widowed*, Tavistock, London and New York
Cartwright, A., Hockey, L. and Anderson, J.C. (1973) *Life Before Death*, Routledge and Kegan Paul, London
Department of Health and Social Security (1983) *Health Care and Its Costs. The Development of the National Health Service in England*, HMSO, London

Duff, R. S. and Hollingshead, A. B. (1968) *Sickness and Society*, Evanston, New York, Harper and Row, London

Egbert, L. D., Battit, G. E., Welch, C. E. and Bartlett, M. K. (1964) Reduction of post-operative pain by encouragement and instruction of patients. *New England Journal of Medicine*, 270, 825–827

Game, A. and Pringle, R. (1983) *Gender at Work*, Allen and Unwin, London

Geiss, S. and Fuller, R. L. (1985) The impact of the first gay AIDS patients on hospice staff. *Hospice Journal*, 1(3), 17–36

Glaser, B. G. and Strauss, A. L. (1965) *Awareness of Dying*, Aldine, Chicago, IL

Korsch, B. M. and Negrette, V. F. (1972) Doctor–patient communication. *Scientific American*, 227, 66–72

Parkes, C. M. (1985) Terminal care: home, hospital, or hospice? *The Lancet*, 1, 155–157

Royal Commission on Medical Education (1968) *Report of the Royal Commission on Medical Education 1965–68* (Todd Report), HMSO, London

Skipper, J. and Leonard, R. (1968) Children, stress and hospitalization: a field experiment. *Journal of Health and Social Behaviour*, 9, 257–287

Wilkes, E. (1984) Dying now. *The Lancet*, 28 April, 950–952

Wilkes, E. (1986) Terminal care: how can we do better? *Journal of the Royal College of Physicians of London*, 20, 216–218

Reprinted by permission of Routledge (Tavistock Publications), London and New York. David Field (1989) *Nursing the Dying*, Tavistock Publications, London and New York, pp. 137–143, 147–149.

Chapter 17

Asylums

Erving Goffman

Introduction

Every institution captures something of the time and interest of its members and provides something of a world for them; in brief, every institution has encompassing tendencies. When we review the different institutions in our Western society, we find some that are encompassing to a degree discontinuously greater than the ones next in line. Their encompassing or total character is symbolized by the barrier to social intercourse with the outside and to departure that is often built right into the physical plant, such as locked doors, high walls, barbed wire, cliffs, water, forests, or moors. These establishments I am calling *total institutions*, and it is their general characteristics I want to explore.

The total institutions of our society can be listed in five rough groupings. First, there are institutions established to care for persons felt to be both incapable and harmless; these are the homes for the blind, the aged, the orphaned, and the indigent. Second, there are places established to care for persons felt to be both incapable of looking after themselves and a threat to the community, albeit an unintended one: TB sanitaria, mental hospitals, and leprosaria. A third type of total institution is organized to protect the community against what are felt to be intentional dangers to it, with the welfare of the persons thus sequestered not the immediate issue: jails, penitentiaries, POW camps, and concentration camps. Fourth, there are institutions purportedly established the better to pursue some worklike task and justifying themselves only on these instrumental grounds: army barracks, ships, boarding schools, work camps, colonial compounds, and large mansions from the point of view of those who live in the servants' quarters. Finally, there are those establishments designed as retreats from the world even while often serving also as training stations for the religious; examples are abbeys, monasteries, convents, and other cloisters. This classification of total institutions is not neat, exhaustive, nor of immediate analytical use, but it does provide a purely denotative definition of the category as a concrete starting point. By anchoring the initial definition of total institutions in this way, I hope to be able to discuss the general characteristics of the type without becoming tautological.

Before I attempt to extract a general profile from this list of establishments, I would like to mention one conceptual problem: none of the elements I will describe seems peculiar to total institutions, and none seems to be shared by every one of them; what is distinctive about total institutions is that each exhibits to an intense degree many items in this family of attributes. In speaking of 'common characteristics', I will be using this phrase in a way that is restricted but I think logically defensible. At the same time this permits using the method of ideal types, establishing common features with the hope of highlighting significant differences later.

A basic social arrangement in modern society is that the individual tends to sleep, play, and work in different places, with different co-participants, under different authorities, and without an overall rational plan. The central feature of total institutions can be described as a breakdown of the barriers ordinarily separating these three spheres of life. First, all aspects of life are conducted in the same place and under the same single authority. Second, each phase of the member's daily activity is carried on in the immediate company of a large batch of others, all of whom are treated alike and required to do the same thing together. Third, all phases of the day's activities are tightly scheduled, with one activity leading at a prearranged time into the next, the whole sequence of activities being imposed from above by a system of explicit formal rulings and a body of officials. Finally, the various enforced activities are brought together into a single rational plan purportedly designed to fulfil the official aims of the institution.

Individually, these features are found in places other than total institutions. For example, our large commercial, industrial, and educational establishments are increasingly providing cafeterias and free-time recreation for their members; use of these extended facilities remains voluntary in many particulars, however, and special care is taken to see that the ordinary line of authority does not extend to them. Similarly, housewives or farm families may have all their major spheres of life within the same fenced-in area, but these persons are not collectively regimented and do not march through the day's activities in the immediate company of a batch of similar others.

The handling of many human needs by the bureaucratic organization of whole blocks of people – whether or not this is a necessary or effective means of social organization in the circumstances – is the key fact of total institutions. From this follow certain important implications.

When persons are moved in blocks, they can be supervised by personnel whose chief activity is not guidance or periodic inspection (as in many employer–employee relations) but rather surveillance – a seeing to it that everyone does what he has been clearly told is required of him, under conditions where one person's infraction is likely to stand out in relief against the visible, constantly examined compliance of the others. Which comes first, the large blocks of managed people, or the small supervisory staff, is not here at issue; the point is that each is made for the other.

In total institutions there is a basic split between a large managed group, conveniently called inmates, and a small supervisory staff. Inmates typically live in the institution and have restricted contact with the world outside the walls; staff often operate on an eight-hour day and are socially integrated into the outside world.[1] Each grouping tends to conceive of the other in terms of narrow hostile stereotypes, staff often seeing inmates as bitter, secretive, and untrustworthy, while inmates often see staff as condescending, highhanded, and mean. Staff tends to feel superior and righteous; inmates tend, in some ways at least, to feel inferior, weak, blameworthy, and guilty.[2]

Social mobility between the two strata is grossly restricted; social distance is typically great and often formally prescribed. Even talk across the boundaries may be conducted in a special tone of voice, as illustrated in a fictionalized record of an actual sojourn in a mental hospital:

'I tell you what,' said Miss Hart when they were crossing the day-room. 'You do everything Miss Davis says, Don't you think about it, just do it. You'll get along all right.'

As soon as she heard the name Virginia knew what was terrible about Ward One. Miss Davis. 'Is she the head nurse?'

'And how,' muttered Miss Hart. And then she raised her voice. The nurses had a way of acting as if the patients were unable to hear anything that was not shouted. Frequently they said things in normal voices that the ladies were not supposed to hear; if they had not been nurses you would have said they frequently talked to themselves. 'A most competent and efficient person, Miss Davis,' announced Miss Hart. (Ward, 1955.)

Although some communication between inmates and the staff guarding them is necessary, one of the guard's functions is the control of communication from inmates to higher staff levels. A student of mental hospitals provides an illustration:

Since many of the patients are anxious to see the doctor on his rounds, the attendants must act as mediators between the patients and the physician if the latter is not to be swamped. On Ward 30, it seemed to be generally true that patients without physical symptoms who fell into the two lower privilege groups were almost never permitted to talk to the physician unless Dr Baker himself asked for them. The persevering, nagging delusional group – who were termed 'worry warts', 'nuisances', 'bird dogs', in the attendants' slang – often tried to break through the attendant-mediator but were always quite summarily dealt with when they tried. (Belknap, 1956.)

Just as talk across the boundary is restricted, so, too, is the passage of information, especially information about the staff's plans for inmates. Characteristically, the inmate is excluded from knowledge of the decisions taken regarding his fate. Whether the official grounds are military, as in concealing travel destination from enlisted men, or medical, as in concealing diagnosis, plan of treatment, and approximate length of stay from tuberculosis patients,[3] such exclusion gives staff a special basis of distance from and control over inmates.

All these restrictions of contact presumably help to maintain the antagonistic stereotypes.[4] Two different social and cultural worlds develop, jogging alongside each other with points of official contact but little mutual penetration. Significantly, the institutional plant and name come to be identified by both staff and inmates as somehow belonging to staff, so that when either grouping refers to the views or interests of 'the institution', by implication they are referring (as I shall also) to the views and concerns of the staff.

The staff-inmate split is one major implication of the bureaucratic management of large blocks of persons; a second pertains to work.

In the ordinary arrangements of living in our society, the authority of the work place stops with the worker's receipt of a money payment; the spending of this in a domestic and recreational setting is the worker's private affair and constitutes a mechanism through which the authority of the work place is kept within strict bounds. But to say that inmates of total institutions have their full day scheduled for them is to say that all their essential needs will have to be planned for. Whatever the incentive given for work, then, this incentive will not have the structural significance it has on the outside. There will have to be different motives for work and different attitudes towards it. This is a basic adjustment required of the inmates and of those who must induce them to work.

Sometimes so little work is required that inmates, often untrained in leisurely pursuits, suffer extremes of boredom. Work that is required may be carried on at a very slow pace and may be geared into a system of minor, often ceremonial payments, such as the weekly tobacco ration and the Christmas presents that lead some mental patients to stay on their jobs. In other cases, of course, more than a full day's hard labour is required, induced not by reward but by threat of physical punishment. In some total institutions, such as logging camps and merchant ships, the practice of forced saving postpones the usual relation to the world that money can buy; all needs are organized by the institution and payment is given only when a work season is over and the men leave the premises. In some institutions there is a kind of slavery, with the inmate's full time placed at the convenience of staff; here the inmate's sense of self and sense of possession can become alienated from his work capacity. T. E. Lawrence (1955) gives an illustration in his record of service in an RAF training depot:

> The six-weeks men we meet on fatigue shock our moral sense by their easy-going. 'You're silly —, you rookies, to sweat yourselves' they say. Is it our new keenness, or a relic of civility in us? For by the R.A.F. we shall be paid all the twenty-four hours a day, at three halfpence an hour; paid to work, paid to eat, paid to sleep: always those halfpence are adding up. Impossible, therefore, to dignify a job by doing it well. It must take as much time as it can for afterwards there is not a fireside waiting, but another job.

Whether there is too much work or too little, the individual who was work-oriented on the outside tends to become demoralized by the work system of the total institution. An example of such demoralization is the practice in state mental hospitals of 'bumming' or 'working someone for' a nickel or dime to spend in the canteen. Persons do this – often with some defiance – who on the outside would consider such actions beneath their self-respect. (Staff members, interpreting this begging pattern in terms of their own civilian orientation to earning, tend to see it as a symptom of mental illness and one further bit of evidence that inmates really are unwell.)

There is an incompatibility, then, between total institutions and the basic work-payment structure of our society. Total institutions are also incompatible with another crucial element of our society, the family. Family life is sometimes contrasted with solitary living, but in fact the more pertinent contrast is with batch living, for those who eat and sleep at work, with a group of fellow workers, can hardly sustain a meaningful domestic existence.[5] Conversely, maintaining families off the grounds often permits staff members to remain integrated with the outside community and to escape the encompassing tendency of the total institution.

Notes

1. The binary character of total institutions was pointed out to me by Gregory Bateson, and has been noted in the literature. See, for example, Ohlin, Lloyd E. (1956) *Sociology and the Field of Corrections*, Russell Sage Foundation, New York, pp. 14, 20. In those situations where staff are also required to live in, we may expect staff to feel they are suffering special hardships and to have brought home to them a status dependency on life on the inside which they did not expect. See Record, Jane Cassels (1957) The marine radioman's struggle for status, *American Journal of Sociology*, LXII, 359.
2. For the prison version, see Weinberg, S. Kirson (1942) Aspects of the prison's social structure, *American Journal of Sociology*, XLVII, 717–726.
3. A very full case report on this matter is provided in a chapter titled 'Information and the control of treatment', in Julius A. Roth's forthcoming monograph on the tuberculosis hospital. His work promises to be a model study of a total institution. Preliminary statements may be found in his articles, What is an activity? *Etc.*, XIV (Autumn 1956), pp. 54–56, and Ritual and magic in the control of contagion, *American Sociological Review*, XXII (1957), 310–314.
4. Suggested in Ohlin, op. cit., p. 20.
5. An interesting marginal case here is the Israeli *kibbutz*. See Spiro, Melford E. (1956) *Kibbutz, Venture in Utopia*, Harvard University Press, Cambridge, Mass., and Etzioni, A. (1957) The organizational structure of 'closed' educational institutions in Israel. *Harvard Educational Review*, XXVII, 115.

References

Belknap, I. (1956) *Human Problems of a State Mental Hospital*, McGraw-Hill, New York, p. 177
Lawrence, T. E. (1955) *The Mint*, Jonathan Cape, London, p. 40
Ward, M. J. (1955) *The Snake Pit*, New American Library, New York, p. 72

Reprinted by permission of Penguin Books, Harmondsworth. Erving Goffman (1961, reprinted 1976) *Asylums: Essays on the Social Situation of Mental Patients and Other Inmates*, Penguin Books, Harmondsworth, pp. 14–22.

Chapter 18

Normal rubbish: deviant patients in casualty departments

Roger Jeffery

The material on which this [extract] is based was gathered at three Casualty departments in an English City. The largest was in the city centre, the other two were suburban; of the seven months of field work, $4\frac{1}{2}$ were in the city centre.

====

In general, two broad categories were used to evaluate patients: good or interesting, and bad or rubbish. They were sometimes used as if they were an exhaustive dichotomy, but more generally appeared as opposite ends of a continuum.

(CO to medical students) If there's anything interesting we'll stop, but there's a lot of rubbish this morning.

We have the usual rubbish, but also a subdural haemorrhage.

On nights you get some drunken dross in, but also some good cases.

====

Good patients

Good patients were described almost entirely in terms of their medical characteristics, either in terms of the symptoms or the causes of the injury. Good cases were head injuries, or cardiac arrests, or a stove-in chest; or they were RTA's (Road Traffic Accidents). There were three broad criteria by which patients were seen to be good, and each related to medical considerations.

(i) If they allowed the CO to practise skills necessary for passing professional examinations

In order to pass the FRCS examinations doctors need to be able to diagnose and describe unusual conditions and symptoms. Casualty was not a good place to discover these sorts of cases, and if they did turn up a great fuss was made of them. As one CO said, the way to get excellent treatment was to turn up at a slack period with an unusual condition. The most extreme example of this I witnessed was a young man with a severe head injury from a car accident. A major symptom of his head injury was the condition of his eyes, and by the time he was transferred to another hospital for neurological treatment, twelve medical personnel had looked into his eyes with an ophthalmoscope, and an *ad hoc* teaching session was held on him. The case was a talking point for several days, and the second hospital was phoned several times for a progress report.[1] Similar interest was shown in a man with gout, and in a woman with an abnormally slow heart beat. The general response to cases like this can be summed up in the comments of a CO on a patient with bilateral bruising of the abdomen:

> This is fascinating. It's really great. I've never seen this before.

(ii) If they allowed sta to practise their chosen speciality

For the doctors, the specific characteristics of good patients of this sort were fairly closely defined, because most doctors saw themselves as future specialists – predominantly surgeons. They tended to accept, or conform to, the model of the surgeon as a man of action who can achieve fairly rapid results. Patients who provided the opportunity to use and act out this model were welcomed. One CO gave a particularly graphic description of this:

> But I like doing surgical procedures. These are great fun. It just lets your imagination run riot really (laughs) you know, you forget for a moment you are just a very small cog incising a very small abscess, and you pick up your scalpel like anyone else (laughs). It's quite mad when you think about it but it's very satisfying. And you can see the glee with which most people leap on patients with abscesses because you know that here's an opportunity to do something.

Another one put it like this:

> Anything which involves, sort of, a bit of action ... I enjoy anything which involves bone-setting, plastering, stitching, draining pus.

For some CO's, Casualty work had some advantages over other jobs because the clientele was basically healthy, and it was possible to carry out procedures which showed quick success in terms of returning people to a healthy state.

In two of the hospitals much of this practical action was carried out by the senior nurses, and the doctors left them the more minor surgical work. These nurses too were very pleased to be able to fulfil, even if in only a minor way, the role of surgeon, and found it very rewarding.

(iii) If they tested the general competence and maturity of the sta

The patients who were most prized were those who stretched the resources of the department in doing the task they saw themselves designed to carry out – the rapid early treatment of acutely ill patients. Many of the CO's saw their Casualty job as the first in which they were expected to make decisions without the safety net of ready advice from more senior staff. The ability to cope, the ability to make the decisions which might have a crucial bearing on whether a patient lived or died, this was something which most staff were worried about in advance. However, they were very pleased with patients who gave them this experience. The most articulate expression of this was from a CO who said:

> I really do enjoy doing anything where I am a little out of my depth, where I really have to think about what I am doing. Something like a bad road traffic accident, where they ring up and give you a few minutes warning and perhaps give you an idea of what's happening. ... And when the guy finally does arrive you've got a rough idea of what you are going to do, and sorting it all out and getting him into the right speciality, this kind of thing is very satisfying, even though you don't do very much except perhaps put up a drip, but you've managed it well. And I find that very pleasing. It might be a bit sordid, the fact that I like mangled up bodies and things like this, but the job satisfaction is good.

Good patients, then, make demands which fall squarely within the boundaries of what the staff define as appropriate to their job. It is the medical characteristics of these patients which are most predominant in the discussions, and the typifications are not very well developed. Indeed, unpredictability was often stressed as one of the very few virtues of the Casualty job, and this covered not only the variability in pressure – sometimes rushed off their feet, sometimes lounging around – but also the variability between patients, even if they had superficial similarities. This is in marked contrast to 'rubbish'.

Rubbish

While the category of the good patient is one I have in part constructed from comments about 'patients I like dealing with' or 'the sort of work I like to do', 'rubbish' is a category generated by the staff themselves. It was commonly used in discussions of the work, as in the following quotes:

> It's a thankless task, seeing all the rubbish, as we call it, coming through.

> We get our share of rubbish, in inverted commas, but I think compared with other Casualty departments you might find we get less rubbish.

> I wouldn't be making the same fuss in another job – it's only because it's mostly bloody crumble like women with insect bites.

> I think the (city centre hospital) gets more of the rubbish – the drunks and that.

> He'll be tied up with bloody dross down there.

Rubbish appeared to be a mutually comprehensive term, even though some staff members used other words, like dross, dregs, crumble or grot.

===

...[T]o get a better idea of what patients would be included in the category of rubbish I asked staff what sorts of patients they did not like having to deal with, which sorts of patients made them annoyed, and why. The answers they gave suggested that staff had developed characterisations of 'normal' rubbish – the normal suicide attempt, the normal drunk, and so on – which they were thinking of when they talked about rubbish.[2] In other words, staff felt able to predict a whole range of features related not only to his medical condition but also to his past life, to his likely behaviour inside the casualty department, and to his future behaviour. These expected features of the patient could thus be used to guide the treatment (both socially and medically) that the staff decided to give the patient. Thus patients placed in these categories would tend to follow standard careers, as far as the staff were concerned, in part because of their common characteristics and in part because they were treated as if they had such common characteristics. The following were the major categories of rubbish mentioned by the staff.

(i) Trivia

The recurring problem of casualty departments, in the eyes of the doctors, has been the 'casual' attender. In the 19th century the infirmaries welcomed casual attenders as a way of avoiding the control of the subscribers, but since before the inauguration of the NHS there have been frequent complaints about the patients who arrive without a letter from their GP and with a condition which is neither due to trauma nor urgent.[3]

For the staff of the casualty departments I studied, normal trivia banged their heads, their hands or their ankles, carried on working as usual, and several days later looked into Casualty to see if it was all right. Normal trivia drops in when it is passing, or if it happens to be visiting a relative in the hospital. Trivia 'didn't want to bother my doctor'. Normal trivia treats Casualty like a perfunctory service,[4] on a par with a garage, rather than as an expert emergency service, which is how the staff like to see themselves.

> They come in and say 'I did an injury half an hour ago, or half a day ago, or two days ago. I'm perfectly all right, I've just come for a check-up.'
>
> (Trivia) comes up with a pain that he's had for three weeks, and gets you out of bed at 3 in the morning.

Trivia stretches the boundaries of reasonable behaviour too far, by bringing for advice something which a reasonable person could make up his own mind about. Trivia must find Casualty a nice place to be in, else why would they come? For trivia, Casualty is a bit of a social centre: they think 'It's a nice day, I might as well go down to Casualty'. By bringing to Casualty conditions which should be taken to the GP, trivia trivializes the service Casualty is offering, and lowers its status to that of the GP.

(ii) Drunks[5]

Normal drunks are abusive and threatening. They come in shouting and singing after a fight and they are sick all over the place, or they are brought in unconscious, having been found in the street. They come in the small hours of the night, and they often have to be kept in until morning because you never know if they have been knocked out in a fight (with the possibility of a head injury) or whether they were just sleeping it off. They come in weekend after weekend with the same injuries, and they are always unpleasant and awkward.

> They keep you up all hours of the night, and you see them next day, or in out-patients, and they complain bitterly that 'the scar doesn't look nice' and they don't realize that under there you've sewn tendons and nerves, that they're bloody lucky to have a hand at all.

> The person who comes along seeking admission to a hospital bed at 2 o'clock in the morning and he's rolling around and is incomprehensible, and one's got other much more serious cases to deal with but they make such a row you've got to go to them.

(iii) Overdoses[6]

The normal overdose is female, and is seen as a case of self-injury rather than of attempted suicide. She comes because her boy-friend/husband/parents have been unkind, and she is likely to be a regular visitor. She only wants attention, she was not seriously trying to kill herself, but she uses the overdose as moral blackmail. She makes sure she does not succeed by taking a less-than-lethal dose, or by ensuring that she is discovered fairly rapidly.

> In the majority of overdoses, you know, these symbolic overdoses, the sort of '5 aspirins and 5 valiums and I'm ill doctor, I've taken an overdose'.

> By and large they are people who have done it time and time again, who are up, who have had treatment, who haven't responded to treatment.

> Lots of the attempts are very half-hearted. They don't really mean it, they just want to make a bit of a fuss, so that husband starts loving them again and stops going drinking.

> Most of the people I've met, they've either told someone or they have done it in such a way that someone has found them. I think there's very few that really wanted to, you know.

(iv) Tramps

Normal tramps can be recognized by the many layers of rotten clothing they wear, and by their smell. They are a feature of the cold winter nights and they only come to Casualty to try to wheedle a bed in the warm for the night. Tramps can never be trusted: they will usually sham their symptoms. New COs and young staff nurses should be warned, for if one is let in one night, then dozens will turn up the next night. They are abusive if they don't get their way: they should be shouted at to make sure they understand, or left in the hope that they will go away.

> (Tramps are) nuisance visitors, frequent visitors, who won't go, who refuse to leave when you want them to.
>
> (Tramps are) just trying to get a bed for the night.

These four types covered most of the patients included in rubbish, or described as unpleasant or annoying. There were some other characterizations mentioned less frequently, or which seemed to be generated by individual patients, or which seemed to be specific to particular members of staff. 'Nutcases' were in this uncertain position: there were few 'typical' features of psychiatric patients, and these were very diffuse. Nutcases might be drug addicts trying to blackmail the CO into prescribing more of their drug by threatening to attempt suicide if they do not get what they want; but in general they are just 'irrational' and present everyone with insoluble problems. Since Casualty staff tended to be primarily surgical in orientation they had little faith in the ability of the psychiatrists to achieve anything except to remove a problem from the hands of Casualty. 'Smelly', 'dirty' and 'obese' patients were also in this limbo. Patients with these characteristics were objected to, but there was no typical career expected for these patients: apart from the one common characteristic they were expected to be different.

As Sudnow (1965) suggests, staff found it easier to create typical descriptions if they had to deal with many cases of that sort. However, it was not necessary for any one member of staff to have dealt with these cases, since the experiences of others would be shared. 'Rubbish' was a common topic of general conversations, and in this way staff could find out not only about patients who had come in while they were off duty, but also about notable cases in the past history of the department. The register of patients would also contain clues about the classification of patients this way – staff frequently vented their feelings by sarcastic comments both on the patient's record card and on the register. Again, the receptionists tended to be a repository for information of this kind, partly because they and the senior nurses had worked longest in the departments. In the departments I studied this common fund of knowledge about patients was sufficient to recognize regular visitors and tramps; other departments were reputed to keep 'black books' to achieve the same purpose.

The departments thus varied in the categories of patients typified under rubbish. The city centre hospital had all types, but only one of the suburban hospitals had tramps in any number, and neither of them had many drunks. Overdoses and trivia were, it seems, unavoidable. Comments on drunks and tramps in the suburban hospitals tended to stress their infrequency and staff had difficulty in typing them. As one CO at a suburban hospital said about drunks,

> Some are dirty, but so are some ordinary people. Some are clean. Some are

aggressive, some are quiet. Some are obnoxious. It's the same with ordinary people.

The features of rubbish which are attended to are not the strictly medical ones – they are left as understood. These non-medical features were not essential parts of any diagnosis, since it is not necessary to know that a man is a drunk or a tramp to see that he has cut his head. Similarly, the medical treatment of an overdose does not depend on the intentions of the patient, nor on the number of previous occasions when an overdose has been taken. The features which were attended to were more concerned with the ascription of responsibility or reasonableness. However, the staff could find out these features of patients in the course of the routine questions asked in order to establish a diagnosis (Strong and Davis, 1978). Thus the questions 'when did this happen?' and 'how did this happen?' provide information not only relevant to the physical signs and symptoms which can be expected, but also to the possibility that this is trivia. 'How many pills did you take?' establishes not only the medical diagnosis but also the typicality of the overdose. Similarly, questions designed to find out whether or not the patient will follow the doctor's orders (to change the dressing, or to return to the outpatients clinic) will affect not only the orders the doctor will give but will also provide evidence about the typicality of the tramp or drunk.

Notes

1. This case, while not as spectacular as one reported by Sudnow, does suggest a general level of depersonalization in British teaching hospitals rather higher than in American hospitals. See Sudnow, D. (1968) *Passing On*, Prentice-Hall, New York.
2. I am using normal in the sense that Sudnow uses, in Sudnow, D. (1965) Normal crimes, *Social Problems*, 12.
3. This topic recurs in the reports referenced in note 7 below, and in most of the research reports on casualty case-loads in the medical press. In an attempt to discourage casual attenders the Ministry of Health changed the title of the departments from 'Casualty' to 'Accident and Emergency' during the 1960s. However, most of the staff continued to call it Casualty (and I have followed their usage) and there is no evidence that the change of name has altered the nature of the case-load.
4. See Goffman, E. (1968) *Asylums*, Harmondsworth, Penguin, especially the section 'Notes on the Vicissitudes of the Tinkering Trades'.
5. Gibson op. cit. note 7 below, pp.164–186, discusses the ways in which 'drunk' fails as medical category since a wide variety of careers and treatments are associated with drunk patients, which tends to support the argument that this is essentially a moral category.
6. Godse, A.H. (1978) The attitudes of Casualty staff and ambulancemen towards patients who take drug overdoses, *Social Science and Medicine*, 12(5A), 341–346, suggests that there is generalized hostility towards all drug overdoses, but he elaborates his discussion with respect to three types. One of these – deliberate suicide attempts or gestures – fails to distinguish between what I call 'normal' overdoses and those believed by the staff to be serious suicide attempts. Gibson (op. cit. note 7 below, pp.186–194, also reports that staff presumed that most, if not all, cases of self-poisoning were seen as acts of self-injury, wilfully and directly caused, rather than as attempts to commit suicide.
7. See, for example, the British Orthopaedic Association (1959) Memorandum on accident services, *Journal of Bone and Joint Surgery*, 41B(3), 457–463; Nuffield Provincial Hospitals Trust (1960) *Casualty Services and their Setting*, Oxford University Press, London; and

House of Commons Expenditure Committee (1974), 4th Report, *Accident and Emergency Services*, HMSO, London. A fuller survey of this literature can be found in Gibson, H. (1977) *Rules, routines and records*. PhD thesis, Aberdeen University.

References

Strong, P. and Davis, A. (1978) Who's who in paediatric encounters: morality, expertise and the generation of identity and action in medical settings. In *Relationships Between Doctors and Patients* (Davis, A., ed.), Westmead, Teakfield, pp. 51–52
Sudnow, D. (1965) Normal crimes. *Social Problems*, **12**.

Reprinted by permission of Blackwell Publishers Ltd/The Editorial Board, Oxford. Roger Jeffery (1979) Normal rubbish: deviant patients in casualty departments. *Sociology of Health and Illness*, **1**(1), 91–98, 106–107.

Chapter 19

Chancers, pests and poor wee souls: problems of legitimation in psychiatric nursing
David May and Michael P. Kelly

There has been considerable discussion in both the sociological and nursing literature of the range of patient typifications employed by health care personnel and of the processes underlying their construction and use. It is extremely difficult to characterize satisfactorily (or fairly) so large and diverse a body of work. We will here only single out three common-enough features that bear directly on our argument.[1]

First much of the literature – and this is especially true of that written for and by nurses – sounds a high moral and prescriptive tone. Where the existence of 'problem' patients is acknowledged, it is taken in the final analysis as a manifestation of unfortunate and certainly unprofessional attitudes on the part of nursing staff to be rooted out essentially by means of educational measures. Few seem to consider the possibility that the reason why some patients are defined as 'problems' is precisely because they do in fact make nurses' lives difficult and undermine their claims to professional status.

Second, what is missing from so many accounts of nursing (and medical) typifications of patients is some recognition of the interactional and developmental nature of the process. Instead, it is portrayed as overly deterministic, and nursing and medical staff as neutral enforcers of rules in whose composition and application they have little influence, and even less interest. Whereas the truth of the matter is that in categorizing some patients as 'bad', nurses not only pronounce on patient performance, they reaffirm their own professional and personal values, and reinforce the functional solidarity of their group. In other words, it is from their dealings with patients, in part at least, that a sense of professional identity emerges.

Third, is the general failure in the literature (which in this respect only mirrors practice) to confront the special problems raised by psychiatric nursing. A recent study of general nurses' attitudes to their patients is a case in point (Rosenthal *et al.*, 1980). For these nurses 'problem' patients were defined in relation to their ideal of the 'good' patient:

> Ideally, from the nurse's perspective, all patients should be sick when they enter the hospital, should follow eagerly and exactly the therapeutic programme set up by the staff, should be pleasant, uncomplaining, fit into the hospital routine, and should leave the hospital 'cured'. Good patients handle their illnesses well, are co-operative, as cheerful as possible, comply with treatment, provide the staff with all the relevant information, follow the rules, and do not disrupt the ward or demand special privileges and excessive attention (p.27).

What is immediately striking about this description is how singularly inappropriate it seems to the situation of the psychiatric nurse. And indeed Rosenthal *et al.* observed a strong association between 'problem' patients and the failure to establish an organic basis to the illness. They also noted that a significant proportion of patients with subsequently diagnosed psychiatric illnesses fell into the problem patient category. These findings are very much in line with work reported by Roth (1972), Becker *et al.* (1961), Jeffery (1979), Strong (1980) and Hughes (1981). Indeed Jeffery suggests that for his casualty doctors the terms 'problem patient' and 'psychiatric patient' were virtually synonymous.

By treating psychiatry as a residual category that substitutes for explanation we are deceived into thinking that all that is at issue is the threat to nursing routines. This is not only unfair to nurses, but glosses over a much more complex relationship whose study promises to further our understanding of nursing generally.

––––––––

[W]e have argued that 'problem' patients for psychiatric nurses are those who in one way or another deny nurses' claims to therapeutic competence. Therapeutic aspirations are a central feature of psychiatric nurses' self-image precisely because of the difficulties inherent in identifying the skills peculiar to the profession. Because the organizational structure in which they operate tends not fully to acknowledge these aspirations, psychiatric nurses are particularly dependent on their claims being legitimated by patients.

If our argument is correct, then the question arises as to why the issues of nursing subordination and therapeutic frustration ... do not feature more prominently in the day-to-day working lives of psychiatric nurses. For assuredly nurses for the most part go about their daily tasks without the enduring sense of frustration and resentment that we have implied, and apparently too, without being embroiled in endemic conflict with either patient or doctors. The reasons for this are complex and worthy of investigation in their own right. We can here only outline some possible explanations.

First, any sense of dissatisfaction may well find expression in more indirect ways, e.g. in greater pressure towards unionization, or in absenteeism. In this respect it would be interesting to know if absenteeism rates are associated with areas of service where nurses' therapeutic aspirations are (or are felt to be) particularly frustrated.

Second, despite the relatively high proportion of male nurses in its ranks, psychiatric nursing, like nursing in general, remains a predominantly female occupation, and its subordination on this count no more than a reflection of wider sexual divisions in society. Moreover, we would argue, along with Freidson, that this position of subordination has been historically legitimated.

Third, patients rarely challenge nursing authority, nor openly reject the help that is offered to them. As Erikson (1957) has pointed out, the mentally ill are not wholly absolved from the rules governing normal social behaviour, and a regard for politeness and the feelings of others are among the most important of these.

Fourth, while ... it is misleading to draw too sharp a distinction in the management of the mentally ill between treatment and care, nevertheless it is undoubtedly the case that much of what is done for and to a patient during his time in hospital has little in the way of therapeutic content. Nor would anyone claim otherwise – least of all the nurse. So for the most part, doctors are content to allow nurses to get on with their nursing tasks, exercising only minimal, and often indirect, supervision. Even when and where nurses take it upon themselves to engage in explicitly therapeutic activities, this rarely constitutes a threat to ultimate medical authority since such activity will always remain conditional upon the therapeutic programme of the doctor, and therefore ultimately controllable by him (see e.g. Baruch and Treacher, 1978, pp.107–142).

And finally it would be idle to pretend that nurses themselves are not highly ambivalent on the issue of therapeutic responsibility, not surprisingly, since there are certain distinct psychological (and possibly, material) advantages that follow from its denial. This may well in the end present nurses with a conflict between their professional and personal interests. Doctors' authority derives in good measure from their willingness to accept ultimate therapeutic responsibility for groups. The advancement of nursing as a profession may well turn on its willingness to seize a greater share of this burden. This, however, is unlikely to be achieved without substantially increasing the pressure on individual nurses.

Note

1. We would emphasize that our strictures do not apply equally to all work in this area. Roth (1972) and Hughes (1981) are particularly important exceptions. For a critical review of the literature see Kelly and May (1982).

References

Baruch, G. and Treacher, A. (1978) *Psychiatry Observed*, Routledge and Kegan Paul, London

Becker, H. S., Geer, B. G., Hughes, E. C. and Strauss, A. L. (1961) *Boys in White*, University of Chicago Press, Chicago

Erikson, K. T. (1957) Patient role and social uncertainty: a dilemma of the mentally ill. *Psychiatry*, **20**, 263–274

Hughes, D. (1981) *Lay assessment of clinical seriousness: practical decision-making by non-medical staff in a hospital casualty department*. PhD thesis, University of Wales, unpublished

Jeffery, R. (1979) Normal rubbish: deviant patients in casualty departments. *Sociology of Health and Illness*, **1**(1), 90–107

Kelly, M. P. and May, D. (1982) Good and bad patients: a review of the literature and a theoretical critique. *Journal of Advanced Nursing*, **7**(2), 147–156

Rosenthal, C. J., Marshall, V. W., MacPherson, A. S. and French, S. (1980) *Nurses, Patients and Families*, Croom Helm, London

Roth, J. (1972) Some contingencies of the moral evaluation and control of clientele: the case of the hospital emergency service. *American Journal of Sociology*, **77**(5), 839–856

Strong, P. M. (1980) Doctors and dirty work: the case of alcoholism. *Sociology of Health and Illness*, **2**, 24–47

Reprinted by permission of Blackwell Publishers Ltd/The Editorial Board, Oxford. David May and Michael P. Kelly (1982) Chancers, pests and poor wee souls: problems of legitimation in psychiatric nursing. *Sociology of Health and Illness*, **4**(3), 280–281, 295–296.

Chapter 20

Old folks and dirty work: the social conditions for patient abuse in a nursing home

Charles Stannard

Personnel problems: marginality, turnover and absenteeism

The greatest problem the nursing home faced was securing and maintaining an adequate staff. The people who worked there reflected the unattractiveness of this type of work and the low wages the home paid, problems that appear common to nursing homes (U.S. Department of Labor, 1969; Kansas State Department of Health, 1964). Most of the people who worked in the nursing home occupied marginal positions in the labour market. Most non-supervisory employees were from the urban lower class. Of these, the bulk were black women who were divorced or widowed. Whites working in the home were often migrants from the rural South. With the exception of a few middle-class high school girls who worked as aides during the summer, the employees had little in the way of education, training or skills.

Several of the people who worked in the home had 'spoiled identities' (Goffman, 1963). These included former mental patients, several men who had criminal records (one was on probation while working at the home), a former alcoholic, several men who appeared to be homosexuals, several people whose bizarre behaviour seemed to indicate mental illness, and several men who appeared to be drifters in need of temporary employment.

Non-supervisory personnel did not develop strong commitments to their jobs or to the home. This is suggested by the turnover and absenteeism among employees. The nursing home had a very difficult time maintaining a numerically adequate staff.

The social conditions for patient abuse

Most people who worked in the nursing home regarded patient abuse as wrong and evil. The nurses felt especially strongly about this. They claimed that such activities happened infrequently in the home and that when they discovered an instance of abuse, they fired the person responsible for it right on the spot. The head nurse claimed that she had come across such behaviour only a few times during her 3-year tenure at the home, and each time she did, the person perpetrating it was fired immediately. During the research this happened only once, when a LPN [Licensed Practical Nurse] observed an aide kicking a patient and fired her. Because of its purported infrequency, the nurses did not regard patient abuse as a problem.

The aides felt the same way as the nurses, that in view of their deteriorated physical and mental conditions, the patients should be humoured and helped, not hurt. Yet patient abuse did occur in the home.[1] This happened when a patient assaulted an aide or was perceived as deliberately making her job more difficult than it had to be. Kicking, biting, punching or spitting at an aide, were, in in the aides' minds, inexcusable and punishable behaviour. Likewise, a patient who defaecated on the floor or in a waste basket when, according to the aide, she was perfectly able to use the toilet, was liable to receive abusive treatment. The fact that the patient violated institutionalized expectations of proper patient behaviour temporarily neutralized or suspended the norm prohibiting abuse of patients (Sykes and Matza, 1975; Matza, 1966). In so doing, it momentarily freed the aide from the restraining power of the norm and allowed her to use illicit force in dealing with the patient.

Why were the nurses unaware that aides and orderlies occasionally abused patients? There are several reasons for this. First, the way work was organized left the aides physically isolated with patients. Second, the nurses' hostility toward and suspicion of the other employees reduced the amount of interaction and communication between these two groups. Three, the character of the patients and personnel of the home provided the nurses with ready 'accounts'[2] for allegations of abuse. These accounts worked by denying the claim of abuse and imputing malice or ignorance to the person making the claim.

Work in the home was organized so that aides, for the most part, had a set group of patients for whom they alone provided care. The aides received very little direct supervision from the nurses, who were occupied with administrative duties at the nurses' station. As a result, much of what went on between the aide and the patient was not observable to the other aides or to the nurses. The patient's room, the toilets, the tub rooms, were areas where important interaction occurred between aides and patients that were also 'private' or could be made so by closing the door (Schwartz, 1968) to suit the aide's or the patient's needs. This isolation reduced the chances that the aide would be detected acting improperly with a patient.

Of course, this isolation of aide–patient interaction could be effective only to the extent that the patients did not verbalize their mistreatment to other aides, nurses, relatives or doctors. Thus, this factor was important especially with those patients who were unable or unwilling to communicate with people about their experiences in the home.

However, this isolation did not prevent abuse from being observed occasionally. Once in a while an aide observed another aide abusing a patient. In some instances the aide was sympathetic to the other aide, feeling that her actions were justified by the patient's actions. In those instances where the aide felt that the other aide acted improperly with a patient, she either did nothing at all or told the other aides about it. When the latter happened, the aides spoke about the personal attributes ('meanness') or objective conditions (widowed and living alone, or too old for this type of work) of the aide which they regarded as responsible for the aide's actions.

The aides rarely reported such actions to the nurses. One reason was the solidarity and cohesiveness that obtained among the small group of regular and steady employees, who did not want to harm another aide and be responsible for someone losing a job. Among the less well integrated employees, it can be that their lack of integration into the core group of aides left them uncertain about how they were to act and vulnerable to sanctions from the more experienced aides, primarily in the form of lack of co-operation and information about their jobs, and thus unlikely to report abuse to the nurses.

Equally important in restricting information about abuse were the hostility and suspicion that separated the nurses from the other employees, especially the aides. The nurses publicly communicated their dislike, distrust, and low opinion of the lower level employees, particularly the aides, to these people as they griped about their unreliability, inferiority, immorality and low intelligence at the nurses' station and other places where the nurses gathered. They literally treated these employees as 'non-persons', derogating their characters openly and in their presence, thus minimizing communication and interaction between them and other employees.

Finally, sometimes patients, their relatives, or an employee complained to the nurses about mistreatment. The usual response of the nurses to such claims was to deny the occurrence of abuse. They did this by making a counter-claim about the person making the complaint, denied the legitimacy and validity of the contentions, and accounted for them by referring to discrediting attributes of the person making the allegation. Thus, the nurses argued that the patients who made such complaints were trouble-makers or crazy and did not have to be taken seriously. Similarly, they felt that relatives who took up a patient's case were ignorant of the situation in the home, dupes of a crazy patient, or crazy themselves, and did not have to be taken seriously. When an employee made such an allegation, the nurses and owner imputed ulterior motives to him and in so doing debunked his claim; or they received it sceptically and did nothing.

The various accounts that the nurses offered to deny such claims of maltreatment were based on their definitions of reality in the home. They formed a common 'vocabulary of motives' (Mills, 1941) that stemmed from the basic characteristics of the work force and patients in the home. From the nurses' perspective, both the employees and patients had in common the fact that they were likely to have discrediting attributes or characteristics which made them untrustworthy and unreliable, character-istics which were responsible for their being in the nursing home in the first place. Furthermore, both groups manifested these attributes daily and in so doing made life miserable for the nurses. The employees did not come to work; when they did, they did not perform well; many had elements in their pasts, such as criminal arrests, a history of drunkenness, illegitimate children, etc. that were shocking and stigmatizing in terms of the nurses' conventional standards. The patients were unreliable by definition, since one of the reasons for their incarceration was the fact that they could not care for themselves in the outside world (Goffman, 1961) and exhibited their incapacities and incompetence daily by their helplessness and frequently bizarre behaviour.

The people who work in these institutions, including the professionals, tend to occupy marginal positions in the labour market. The occupants of the lowest positions, the aides and orderlies, who have the greatest contact with inmates share a latent culture (Becker and Geer, 1960) due to their lower social-class origins, which regards the use of force and aggression as legitimate means of resolving conflicts (Blumenthal et al., 1971). Because of their social class and low levels of education, these people do not entertain sophisticated and complex notions about human motivation and mental illness. Their interpretations of patients' actions are likely to be based on lay rather than medical ideologies (Strauss et al., 1964). This increases their likelihood of using already established and familiar means of handling difficulties with patients, namely force.

Conflicts between staff and patients are likely because these organizations cannot rely on rewards or the internalization by patients of their goals or norms to generate a commitment to their rules (Etzioni, 1961). As a result, those people who work most closely with patients find control of the patients to be their greatest problem and abuse to be one way of coping with it.

The professionals and semi-professionals who work in these institutions are the less successful members of their professions. Work in custodial mental hospitals and nursing homes does not bring professional recognition and is regarded as a step down by their professions in general. Once in these institutions, they find themselves with patients they cannot help, confronted by staff problems which make it difficult or impossible to achieve the goals expounded by their professions. The lofty goals of help and service learned during their professional training give way to more realistic goals of custody and order maintenance.[3] Rather than taking active leadership in caring for patients, they withdraw from this aspect of their role, become cynical, and concentrate their attention and energy on activities which reduce their contact with patients and lower level employees. Patient care becomes the almost exclusive province of the lower level employees to whom the professionals delegate a great deal of discretionary power. This insulates the lay perspectives of the lower level employees from the more sophisticated and potentially ameliorative ideas of the professionals.

In such a context, the supervisory and professional staff will seldom see abusive behaviour on the part of the other employees. Furthermore, they will probably develop a culture of accounts to deal with reputed cases of abuse which will enable them to deny the routine nature of abuse. In fact, these organizations may necessitate such a culture of accounts.[4] The professionals who stay on in such organizations will be those who have been successfully socialized to this culture. Those who do not accept the definitions and premises of such a culture are forced to leave the organization because of the dissonance created by the discrepancy between their self-images as professionals and the acknowledgement of what is really going on in the organization. The end result of these processes is the continuance of abuse.

Notes

1. Abuse refers to behaviour which would lead to negative sanctions if it were observed by a nurse. This definition is similar to the definition of deviance of Black and Reiss, Jr. (1970) Police control of juveniles. *American Sociological Review*, 35, 63–77. Pulling a patient's hair, slapping, hitting, kicking, pinching, or violently shaking a patient, throwing water or food on a patient, tightening restraining belts so that they cause a patient pain, and terrorizing a patient by gesture or word are examples of abusive behaviour. During the research, I occasionally witnessed aides abusing patients in one or another of these manners. Most of the data on abuse comes from discussions with aides about the way they and their fellow workers dealt with the patients.
2. 'An account is a linguistic device employed whenever an action is subject to valuative enquiry. Such devices are a crucial element in the social order since they prevent conflicts from arising by verbally bridging the gap between action and expectation. Moreover, accounts are "situated" according to the statuses of the interactants, and are standardized within cultures so that certain accounts are terminologically stabilized and routinely expected when an activity falls outside the domain of expectations.' (Scott and Lyman, Accounts. *American Sociological Review*, 33, 46–52.
3. Powelson and Bendix (1951) Psychiatry in prison. *Psychiatry*, 14, 73–86, find this is the case for psychiatrists who work in prisons. The situation also seems analogous to that of lawyers. Carlin (1966) found that the less successful lawyers often found themselves in situations where the corruption of their professional ethics and goals was possible and reasonable.
4. Suggested by Merton Kahne in a personal communication.

References

Becker, H. S. and Geer, B. (1960) Latent culture: a note on the theory of latent social roles. *Administrative Science Quarterly*, 5, 305–313

Blumenthal, M. D., Kahn, R. L., Andrews, F. M. and Head, K. B. (1971) *Justifying Violence*, Institute for Social Research, University of Michigan, Ann Arbor, Michigan

Carlin, J. E. (1966) *Lawyer's Ethics*, Russell Sage Foundation, New York

Etzioni, A. (1961) *Complex Organisations*, The Free Press, New York

Goffman, E. (1961) On the characteristics of total institutions: staff-inmate relations. In *The Prison* (Cressey, D. R., ed.), Holt, Rinehart and Winston, New York

Goffman, E. (1963) *Stigma*, Prentice-Hall, Englewood Cliffs, N. J.

Kansas State Department of Health (1964) *Kansas Long Term Care Study*, Topeka, Kansas

Matza, D. (1966) *Delinquency and Drift*, Wiley, New York

Mills, C. W. (1941) Situated actions and vocabularies of motives. *American Sociological Review*, 5, 904–913

Schwartz, B. (1968) The social psychology of privacy. *American Journal of Sociology*, 73, 741–752

Strauss, A. L., Schatzman, L., Bucher, R., Ehrlich, D. and Sabshin, M. (1964) *Psychiatric Ideologies and Institutions*, The Free Press, New York

Sykes, G. M. and Matza, D. (1975) Techniques of neutralisation: a theory of delinquency. *American Sociological Review*, 22, 664–670

United States Department of Labor (1969) *Industry Wage Survey: Nursing Homes and Related Facilities*, October 1967 and April 1968, Government Printing Office, Washington D.C.

Chapter 21

Dead on arrival

David Sudnow

In County Hospital's emergency ward, the most frequent variety of death is what is known as the 'DOA' type. Approximately 40 such cases are processed through this division of the hospital each month. The designation 'DOA' is somewhat ambiguous insofar as many persons are not physiologically *dead on arrival*, but are nonetheless classified as having been such.

===

When an ambulance driver suspects that the person he is carrying is dead, he signals the emergency ward with a special siren alarm as he approaches the entrance driveway. As he wheels his stretcher past the clerk's desk, he restates his suspicion with the remark, 'possible', a shorthand reference for 'possible DOA'. (The use of the term *possible* is required by law, which insists, primarily for insurance purposes, that any diagnosis unless made by a certified physician be so qualified.) The clerk records the arrival in a log book and pages a physician, informing him in code of the arrival. Often a page is not needed, as physicians on duty hear the siren alarm, expect the arrival, and wait at the entranceway. The patient is rapidly wheeled to the far end of the ward corridor and into the nearest available foyer or room, supposedly out of sight of other patients and possible onlookers from the waiting room. The physician arrives, makes his examination, and pronounces the patient dead or not. If the patient is dead, a nurse phones the coroner's office, which is legally responsible for the removal and investigation of all DOA cases.

Neither the hospital nor the physician has medical responsibility in such cases. In any instances of clear death, ambulance drivers use the hospital as a depository because it has the advantages of being both closer and less bureaucratically complicated a place than the downtown coroner's office for disposing of a body. Here, the hospital stands as a temporary holding station, rendering the community service of legitimate and free pronouncements of death for any comers. In circumstances of near-death, it functions more traditionally as a medical institution, mobilizing life-saving procedures for those for whom they are still of potential value, at least as judged by the emergency room's staff of residents and interns. The boundaries between near-death and sure death are not, however, as we shall shortly see, altogether clearly defined.

In nearly all DOA cases the pronouncing physician (commonly that physician who is the first to answer the clerk's page or spot the incoming ambulance) shows in his general demeanour and approach to the task little more than passing interest in the event's possible occurrence and the patient's biographical and medical circumstances. He responds to the clerk's call, conducts his examination, and leaves the room once he has made the necessary official gesture to an attending nurse. (The term 'kaput', murmured in differing degrees of audibility depending upon the hour and his state of awakeness, is a frequently employed announcement.) It happened on numerous occasions, especially during the midnight-to-eight shift, that a physician was interrupted during a coffee break to pronounce a DOA and returned to his colleagues in the canteen with, as an account of his absence, some version of 'Oh, it was nothing but a DOA'.

It is interesting to note that, while the special siren alarm is intended to mobilize quick response on the part of the emergency room staff, it occasionally operates in the opposite fashion. Some emergency room staff came to regard the fact of a DOA as decided in advance; they exhibited a degree of nonchalance in answering the siren or page, taking it that the 'possible DOA' most likely is 'D'. In so doing they in effect gave authorization to the ambulance driver to make such assessments. Given that time lapse which sometimes occurs between that point at which the doctor knows of the arrival and the time he gets to the patient's side, it is not inconceivable that in several instances patients who might have been revived died during this interim. This is particularly likely in that, apparently, a matter of moments may differentiate the revivable state from the irreversible one.

Two persons in similar physical condition may be differentially designated dead or not. For example, a young child was brought into the emergency room with no registering heartbeat, respirations, or pulse – the standard 'signs of death' – and was, through a rather dramatic stimulation procedure involving the coordinated work of a large team of doctors and nurses, revived for a period of eleven hours. On the same evening, shortly after the child's arrival, an elderly person who presented the same physical signs, with – as one physician later stated in conversation – no discernible differences from the child in skin color, warmth, etc., arrived in the emergency room and was almost immediately pronounced dead, with no attempts at stimulation instituted. A nurse remarked, later in the evening: 'They (the doctors) would never have done that to the old lady (attempt heart stimulation) even though I've seen it work on them too'. During the period when emergency resuscitation equipment was being readied for the child, an intern instituted mouth-to-mouth resuscitation. This same intern was shortly relieved by oxygen machinery, and when the woman arrived, he was the one who pronounced her dead. He reported shortly afterwards that he could never bring himself to put his mouth to 'an old lady's like that'.

It is therefore important to note that the category DOA is not totally homogeneous with respect to actual physiological condition. The same is generally true of all deaths, the determination of *death* involving, as it does, a critical decision, at least in its earlier stages.

———

Currently at County there seems to be a rather strong relationship between the age, social background, and the perceived moral character of patients and the amount of effort that is made to attempt revival when 'clinical death signs' are detected (and, for that matter, the amount of effort given to forestalling their appearance in the first place). As one compares practices in this regard at different hospitals, the general relationship seems to hold; although at the private, wealthier institutions like Cohen the overall amount of attention given to 'initially dead' patients is greater. At County efforts at revival are admittedly superficial, with the exception of the very young or occasionally wealthier patient who by some accident ends up at County's emergency room. No instances have been witnessed at County where, for example, external heart massage was given a patient whose heart was stethoscopically inaudible, if that patient was over 40 years of age. At Cohen Hospital, on the other hand, heart massage is a normal routine at that point, and more drastic measures, such as the injection of Adrenalin directly into the heart, are not uncommon. While these practices are undertaken for many patients at Cohen if 'tentative death' is discovered early (and it typically is because of the attention 'dying' patients are given), at County they are reserved for a very special class of cases.

Generally speaking, the older the patient the more likely is his tentative death taken to constitute pronounceable death. Suppose a 20-year-old arrives in the emergency room and is presumed to be dead because of the ambulance driver's assessment. Before that patient will be pronounced dead by a physician, extended listening to his heartbeat will occur, occasionally efforts at stimulation will be made, oxygen administered, and often stimulative medication given. Less time will elapse between initial detection of an inaudible heartbeat and nonpalpitating pulse and the pronouncement of death if the person is 40 years old, and still less if he is 70.

———

When a young person is brought in as a 'possible', the driver tries to convey some more alarming sense to his arrival by turning the siren up very loud and keeping it going after he has already stopped, so that by the time he has actually entered the wing, personnel, expecting 'something special', act quickly and accordingly. When it is a younger person that the driver is delivering, his general manner is more frantic. The speed with which he wheels his stretcher in and the degree of excitement in his voice as he describes his charge to the desk clerk are generally more heightened than with the typical elderly DOA. One can observe a direct relationship between the loudness and length of the siren alarm and the considered 'social value' of the person being transported.

The older the person, the less thorough is the examination he is given; frequently, elderly people are pronounced dead on the basis of only a stethoscopic examination of the heart. The younger the person, the more likely will an examination preceding an announcement of death entail an inspection of the eyes, attempt to find a pulse, touching of the body for coldness, etc. When a younger person is brought to the hospital and announced by the driver as a 'possible' but is nonetheless observed to be breathing slightly, or have an audible heartbeat, there is a fast mobilization of effort to stimulate increased breathing and a more rapid heartbeat. If an older person is brought in in a similar condition there will be a rapid mobilization of similar efforts; however, the time which will elapse between that point at which breathing noticeably ceases and the heart audibly stops beating and when the pronouncement of death is made will differ according to his age.

One's location in the age structure of the society is not the only factor that will influence the degree of care he gets when his death is considered possibly to have occurred. At County Hospital a notable additional set of considerations relating to the patient's presumed 'moral character' is made to apply.

The smell of alcohol on the breath of a 'possible' is nearly always noticed by the examining physician, who announces to his fellow workers that the person is a drunk. This seems to constitute a feature he regards as warranting less than strenuous effort to attempt revival.

Among other categories of persons whose deaths will be more quickly adjudged, and whose 'dying' more readily noticed and used as a rationale for apathetic care, are the suicide victim, the dope addict, the known prostitute, the assailant in a crime of violence, the vagrant, the known wife-beater, and, generally, those persons whose moral characters are considered reproachable.

Within a limited temporal perspective at least, but one which is not necessarily to be regarded as trivial, the likelihood of 'dying' and even of being 'dead' can be said to be partially a function of one's place in the social structure, and not simply in the sense that the wealthier get better care, or at least not in the usual sense of that fact. If one anticipates having a critical heart attack, he had best keep himself well-dressed and his breath clean if there is a likelihood he will be brought into County as a 'possible'.

Further reading

Feifel, H. (1959) *The Meaning of Death*, McGraw Hill, New York
Glaser, B. and Strauss, A. (1965) *Awareness of Dying*, Aldine Press, Chicago
Goody, J. (1962) *Death, Property and the Ancestors*, Stanford University Press, Stanford

Part II   Professions

The playwright and social critic, George Bernard Shaw, maintained that 'all professions are conspiracies against the laity'. Such a pessimistic view can certainly be challenged, but it usefully provides a warning that analysis of the work of health professionals may not be quite so straightforward as one might expect. In fact, many questions can be raised about the professions and these various questions tend to come into focus at different times. However, the issues of how one distinguishes the professions from other occupations, how members of the professions are recruited, educated and socialized always remain important.

After the emergence of a professional class in the nineteenth century and increasing attempts of other occupational groups to seek professional status, it is perhaps not surprising that early work focused on the problematic issue of definition. In other words, what distinguished a profession from other occupations. The first classic study of the professions was undertaken by Carr Saunders and Wilson (1933) who sought to identify the characteristics of those occupations which could be termed profession. This work set a trend whereby writers took what has come to be known as the trait or attribute approach to the study of professions. This identification of core or essential characteristics in a profession was criticized on the grounds that the characteristics were accepted uncritically and this meant that the question of power was overlooked. The functionalist approach to the study of professions followed Parsons' (1951) lead and views society as a social system in which, just as in biological systems, various parts depend upon each other for the overall smooth functioning of the system.

Sociologists in the late 1960s and 1970s were particularly exercised with the idea of the power of the professions, their usefulness and the consequences for society. In turn this led to an emphasis on the socialization of professional trainees. These classic studies of socialization into the professions focused on medicine. **Hughes** produced some of the seminal work and in a classic paper described medical education as 'a series of processes by which medical culture is kept alive'.

Merton and colleagues looked at the medical school as a socializing agency in which the students were seen as passive recipients of the knowledge that was on offer. On this essentially functionalist view it is the institution – the profession of medicine and the medical school which nurtures them – which keeps the professional culture alive. In this approach, the students are viewed as potential occupants of the role of doctor and it is the role and the expectations that go with it that are being conveyed in medical school. **Becker** and colleagues, in contrast, using an interactionist model, focused attention on the student's behaviour rather than on the professional role. In other words, they started from the view that students will react to the education process and negotiate a role for themselves accordingly.

A similar line of study was followed by **Olesen** and **Whittaker** in a study of the socialization of nurses. In the UK **Atkinson** studied the socialization of British medical students and looks at the way in which professional communities reproduce themselves. An interactionist study of the occupational socialization of nurses by **Melia** develops **Bucher** and **Strauss'** theme of 'segmentation'. Melia examines the 'differences between the idealized version of work as it is presented to new recruits and the work as it is practised daily by members of the occupation'.

Bucher and Strauss examine conflict within a professional group – medicine. They describe the various segments that exist within professions, each reflecting different identities, different values and interest. Issues surrounding professional knowledge are addressed by **Schön**. The practice disciplines, especially nursing, have become interested in Schön's ideas about 'knowing in action' and 'reflection in practice'. It is worth noting, given the amount of attention which Schön's work has attracted, that he only makes one, passing, reference to nursing.

One thing that becomes clear on reading these different approaches to the study of profession is that the term itself is problematic and difficult to define. **Freidson**, a seminal author in the sociology of the professions, looked at the question of power and occupations (as did Johnson, 1971). In his classic study *Profession of Medicine*, Freidson concluded that 'A profession is an occupation which has assumed a dominant position in the division of labour so that it gains control over the determination of the substance of its own work. Unlike most occupations it is autonomous and self-directing'.

Etzioni, on the other hand, examines occupational groups which do not quite attain the professional status of medicine. Included in these semi-professions as he calls them are teachers, nurses and social workers.

Power and status relationships between the occupational groups are important themes in the sociology of professions in health care. **Carpenter**, in an important paper, describes what he calls the 'new professionalism' in nursing developed, he argues, as a response to the 'new managerialism' brought about through the Salmon (DHSS, 1966) reforms in the occupational structure on nursing.

Gender has clearly shaped the content and nature of nursing. The whole gender issue has recently been taken up and developed at length by Davies

(1995) in what will surely become a classic text. **Gamarnikow** offers a gender analysis of nursing and its relationship with the profession of medicine. She looks at 'the structural determinants of the sexual division of labour', beginning her analysis in 1860, the year in which Florence Nightingale opened the Nightingale Fund School of Nursing at St. Thomas's Hospital in London.

In a sharp, if sometimes over-simplistic, analysis **Oakley** argues that professionalization may not be the only answer to what she sees as 'the crisis of confidence in medical care'. Returning to the theme of Florence Nightingale, **Whittaker** and **Olesen** discuss the ideological causes to which the Nightingale image can be lent. The context of their paper is the USA, but the idea is not culture specific. They suggest that the popular image from the Crimea is offered to the traditional school of nursing studies, whereas the university-based nursing students are offered the image of Florence Nightingale as liberally educated and a politically skilful woman with a knowledge of statistics who influenced public health policy. Lewis Carroll's witty, if a little cruel, anagram of Florence Nightingale's name was 'Flit on, cheering angel'. Whittaker and Olesen's analysis of the different faces of Nightingale might have changed his view!

Health care is a stressful and emotionally charged business. **Menzies** offers an insight into the long-standing mechanisms through which nurses manage the experience of working in that environment. She describes the defence mechanisms which are designed to allow nurses to manage the anxiety produced by the nurse–patient relationship. Menzies' work stands in stark contrast to the current prevailing view that the nurse–patient relationship is central to nursing care. **Armstrong** points out that it was only in the late 1950s and early 1960s that medical writers recognized that the patient's personality was important in the response to treatment. Around this time that interest in the doctor–patient relationship started to develop. Armstrong argues that, until the early 1970s, nursing like medicine was more concerned with the biological rather than the psycho-social patient. He traces this shift in his discussion of the 'fabrication of nurse–patient relationships'.

Menzies' view, while still widely cited, has been largely superseded by the idea of 'emotional labour' as being a part of health care work. It was Hochschild (1983) with her work on flight attendants who provided insight into this labour which she says 'calls for a co-ordination of mind and feeling and it sometimes draws on a self that we honour as deep and integral to our individuality'. The theme of emotional labour is taken up by **James** who argues that it is carried out both in the public domain of the workforce as well as in the privacy of the home. James goes on to argue that emotional labour in both domains is 'unrecognised, unrecorded and unrewarded'. Again, taking the theme of emotional labour in nursing, **Smith** discusses it in relation to the concept of care, asking if it is the same thing.

Emotional labour as a concept fitted in with the ideas behind the nursing process, which, as **de la Cuesta** points out, gained rapid acceptance in both the USA and the UK. The appeal of the nursing process, argues de la Cuesta, lay in its promise to reform the practice of nurses. Many attempts have been made to systematize the work of nurses, to provide a framework for their work so that it can be more clearly defined in professional terms.

The theme of power in the relationships between medicine and nursing is a recurring one. **Zola** has characterized medicine as an institution of social control, 'nudging aside' he says 'the more traditional institutions of religion and law'. **Witz** looks at the 'twin processes of professionalisation and masculinisation', illustrating the way in which gender has been an important historical element in the exclusionary tactics within the medical profession. The power of the professions within health care is examined further by **Strauss** and colleagues. In a study of the 'negotiated order' they describe the hospital as a 'professionalized locale' where the ambitions of professionals are played out and where non-professionals and patients have to learn how to negotiate life around them. The concept of managed professionalized locales resonates with the arrival of NHS Trusts in which the patients and the professions have to contend with the management and its bureaucracy in order to receive and provide treatment and care.

An interesting new slant on the professional status debate can be seen in the move of the old Colleges of Nursing into the Higher Education sector. There is often a mismatch between salary and academic qualifications, which in some ways parallels the professional status distinction which **Freidson** sought to make between medicine and the para-professions. He argued that medicine had true professional status which was determined by its place in a hierarchy of professions in society. These semi-professions have what Freidson called 'professionalism' – a kind of look-alike with many of the attributes of a true profession, but lacking standing in the hierarchy, and importantly for his analysis, also lacking in autonomy.

The debates surrounding the professions have taken on new dimensions. It is now not so much professions versus para-professions, but more managers versus professions. This has come with Griffiths (1983), the creation of internal markets, contracting out and the notion of a price for the job. (The impact of Griffiths on the professions and management within the health service has been well presented in the work by Cox, 1991, and Elston, 1991.)

Nursing is dependent upon medicine for the creation of patients, as the definition of 'sick' and the status of 'patient' depends upon medical sanction, as was seen in Part I. The emergence of the nurse practitioner and the working patterns of many practice nurses may in time leave this analysis behind. In twenty-first century health care it may not matter that one profession can be said to be independent, or another dominant, because general management will step into any power vacuum created as the professionals slug it out for place and prestige.

Concern with the professionals' relationships with patients has become more evident in recent years. Again, power is manifest in the ways in which specialist knowledge of the professions is used. **Davis**, in a paper concerned with the doctor–patient relationship, describes the concept and utility of 'uncertainty' in medical prognosis. He describes how, when a clinical uncertainly no longer obtains, doctors can carry on the idea of uncertainty in order to manage the doctor–patient relationship.

Stein's doctor–nurse game describes the way in which nurse offers advice surreptitiously to the doctor, ensuring that the status of the doctor, in the eyes of the patient, is always maintained. In a fascinating analysis of nurse–doctor interaction in a casualty department, the idea of the doctor–nurse game is developed by **Hughes**. In these games the diagnostic role played by nurses is often obscured as is the inexperience of junior doctors. It is open to question as to whether or not patients notice or are concerned about the games that these professionals play, but the games are played with patients in mind.

References

Carr Saunders, A.M. and Wilson, P.A. (1933) *The Professions*, Clarendon Press, Oxford

Cox, D. (1991) Health Service Management – a sociological view: Griffiths and the non-negotiated order of the hospital. In *The Sociology of the Health Service* (Gabe, J., Calnan, M. and Bury, M., eds), Routledge, London

Davies, C. (1995) *Gender and the Professional Predicament of Nursing*, Open University Press, Buckingham

Department of Health and Social Security (1966) *Committee on Senior Nursing Staff Structure* (Chairman Brian Salmon), HMSO, London

Elston, M.A. (1991) The politics of professional power: medicine in a changing health service. In *The Sociology of the Health Service* (Gabe, J., Calnan, S. and Bury, M., eds), Routledge, London

Griffiths, E.R. (1983) *NHS Management Enquiry*, DHSS, London

Hochschild, A.R. (1983) *The Managed Heart: Commercialization of Human Feeling*, University of California Press, Berkeley

Johnson, T.J. (1971) *Professions and Power*, Macmillan, London

Parsons, T. (1951) *The Social System*, Routledge and Kegan Paul, London

Chapter 22

The making of a physician – general statement of ideas and problems

Everett C. Hughes

Medical education

Medical education is the whole series of processes by which the medical culture is kept alive (which means more than merely imparted) through time and generations, by which it is extended to new populations or elements of the population, and by which it is added to through new learning and experiment. The education of the medical profession is part of it. For our immediate purposes we will use the phrase medical education only for the training and initiation of physicians, although there is a certain danger of distortion in using it in so limited a way. The education of the members of the medical profession is a set of planned and unplanned experiences by which laymen, usually young and acquainted with the prevailing lay medical culture, become possessed of some part of the technical and scientific medical culture of the professionals. The starting point is the lay medical culture; the end point varies, although the learning experiences are somewhat standardized and although all must take standard examinations to be licensed. But the end point is not there, for in varying ways and degrees the professionals must bring what they have learned into effective interaction with the lay medical culture again. But with a difference – for they themselves are in a new role.

Part of the medical culture of the lay world is some set of conceptions about the proper role of the physician and a set of beliefs about the extent to which he lives up to the role so conceived, and the extent to which and the ways in which he falls short. Initiation into a new role is as much a part of medical training as is the learning of techniques; indeed, part of it is to learn the techniques of playing the role well. A role is always a part in some system of interaction of human beings; it is always played opposite other roles. To play one is not to play another. One might say that the learning of the medical role consists of a separation, almost an alienation, of the student from the lay medical world; a passing through the mirror so that one looks out on the world from behind it, and sees things as in mirror writing. In all of the more esoteric occupations we have studied we find the sense of seeing the world in reverse.

The period of initiation into the role appears to be one wherein the two cultures, lay and professional, interact within the individual. Such interaction undoubtedly goes on all through life, but it seems to be more lively – more exciting and uncomfortable, more self-conscious and yet perhaps more deeply unconscious – in the period of learning and initiation. To take one example, the layman has to learn to live with the uncertainty if not of ignorance, at least of lack of technical knowledge of his own illnesses; the physician has to live and act in spite of the more closely calculated uncertainty that comes with knowing the limits of medical knowledge and his own skill.

In the process of change from one role to another there are occasions when other people expect one to play the new role before one feels completely identified with it or competent to carry it out; there are others in which one overidentifies oneself with the role, but is not accepted in it by others. These and other possible positions between roles make of an individual what is called a marginal man; either he or other people or both do not quite know to what role (identity, reference group) to refer him. We need studies which will discover the course of passage from the layman's estate to that of the professional, with attention to the crises and the dilemmas of role which arise.

Stereotype and reality

We assume that anyone embarking upon the road to medicine has some set of ideas about what the work (skills and tasks) of the physician is, about what the role is, what the various medical careers are, and about himself as a person who may learn the skills, play the role, and follow one of the possible career lines. We assume also that except in cases of extraordinary early contact with the profession, the medical aspirant's conceptions of all these things are somewhat simpler than the reality, that they may be somewhat distorted and stereotyped among lay people. Medical education becomes, then, the learning of the more complicated reality on all these fronts. It may turn out that it makes a good deal of difference whether the steps toward a more penetrating and sophisticated reality on one of these points come early or late, and whether the reality is learned from supporting teachers and colleagues or rubbed in by punishing cynics or stubborn and uncomprehending patients. It may be that the more complicated reality is in some circumstances traumatic, in others, exciting and even inspiring. Perhaps some aspects of reality can be learned in an early phase of technical training and experience, while others can be effectively learned only at some later point. There has always been considerable talk in educational institutions about what kinds of things are prerequisites for others; only in a few cases does it appear really to be known what should come first, what later – there are those who say that geometry should come before algebra, not after.

Some question the time-honored custom of having students learn anatomy from cadavers rather than from demonstrations with living persons. In the study of professional education, we have suggested a distinction between various kinds of prerequisites: conventional and symbolic, technical and role-learning. Learning the realities of medical skills, roles and careers may move *pari passu*; or it may be that some of the roles can be really learned only when a certain level of skill has been attained and certain career corners turned. The realities about career problems might at some points put a damper on the student's eagerness to learn skills and roles; at another point, a new knowledge of career realities might be a stimulus to work on the other fronts.

In professional, as in other lines of work, there grows up both inside and outside some conception of what the essential work of the occupation is or should be. In any occupation, people perform a variety of tasks, some of them approaching more closely the ideal or symbolic work of the profession than others. Some tasks are considered nuisances and impositions, or even dirty work – physically, socially or morally beneath the dignity of the profession. Part of what goes on with respect to a major aspect of life at whose center is a profession, such as the medical, is a constant sorting and re-sorting of the tasks involved among many kinds of people – inside the professions, in related professions, and clear outside professional ranks. The preparation of drugs, the taking of blood pressures, the giving of anaesthetics, the keeping of medical records, the collection of bills, the cleaning up of operating rooms, the administration of hospitals – these are but a few of the tasks which have been allocated and reallocated within the medical division of labor in fairly recent years. There is constant discussion of what is whose work in medicine and what part of it all is the physician's work, privilege and duty. We assume that the medical student is inducted into the discussion of these problems, and that it has some effect upon his motivation and his sense of mission. We may suppose that the essential, symbolically-valued part of the physician's work is diagnosis and treatment of the ailments of people, and that the other activities are – in theory at least – tolerated only as they appear necessary to it. What then, are considered essential auxiliary or peripheral activities, and what attitudes do physicians hold toward them and the people who perform them. Hospitals must be administered, and there are some who believe that physicians alone should do it. Yet, physicians do not ordinarily gain great prestige by becoming administrators – indeed, some who are say they are scarcely cor.sidered medical colleagues any longer. On the other hand, there is some tendency for auxiliary activities to become valued ends in themselves, sometimes even getting in the way of the presumed basic activity (as discipline becomes an end in itself in schools and, some say, in nursing).

The increasing variety of the central and, symbolically, most valued of medical activities themselves is reflected in the number of medical specialities. Some of the specialities are rated above others both by laymen and the profession, although these ratings are not necessarily the same. We may assume that as the student learns various skills and sees at closer hand the actual tasks of his future trade, he will undergo changes of attitude toward them as components of medical work.

Just as certain tasks and skills of medical work are rated above others, so also are the men who perform them. But we must remember that the various medical tasks differ from each other not merely in the knowledge and technical skill required, but in the social relations and social roles involved. The model member of the profession is a man of certain skills and knowledge, one who keeps proper balance between the more and the less valued activities of the profession, and who plays his role well in relation to himself, his colleagues, other personnel in medical work, and toward his patients and the public. As in other professions, we may find that some models are – like the saints – considered a little too good for ordinary men to be expected to imitate in daily practice, although they are admired as embodiments of the highest values of the profession. A study of medical education should discover not merely the saintly models, but also those the student regards as more practically (even a bit cynically) attainable by himself, the mold being as it is, and he being who he is. The shift in choice of models by the student, his definite steps or his drifting into the path that leads to one model rather than others, is a significant part of his medical education. This is, of course, not merely choice of speciality, but of various ways of practicing medicine: practice, teaching, research; practice in one social environment rather than another: rural or urban, well-off or poor, where the health standard of living is high or is low, among his own or among other kinds of people; alone or in association with others; for salary or for fees; where competition is keen or where there is more security, etc. These matters may all enter as components into models to be admired or followed, which is to say that, as suggested above, a model in effect embodies the whole professional ideology of those who choose it.

Reproduced by permission of the Society for Applied Anthropology from *Human Organization*, Winter, 1956. Everett C. Hughes (1956) The making of a physician – general statement of ideas and problems. *Human Organization*, Winter, pp.22–23.

Chapter 23

Some preliminaries to a sociology of medical education

Robert K. Merton, George G. Reader and Patricia L. Kendall

...The mores of medicine require continued scrutiny in the light of changing needs and opportunities.

Oddly enough, the capacity for such functionally appropriate changes in medicine and medical education can be greatly reinforced by a great emphasis upon the *traditions* of medicine. Ordinarily, tradition is that part of a culture which is resistant to change, persisting for a time even when it is out of sorts with the newly emerging requirements of the society. But this is a wholly formal view, not a substantive one. The social function of tradition depends upon its content. And in medicine, the great tradition is typically that associated with celebrated physicians of the past, with those who have shown a capacity to move forward when most of their colleagues were satisfied to let things remain as they were. The great tradition in medicine is in large part a tradition of commitment to the search for improved, and therefore changing, ways of coping with the problems of the sick. It is in this sense that respect for medical tradition is an enduring part of the culture of medical education. Frequent ceremonies serve to keep alive a sense of the core-values of medicine as these are exemplified in the achievements of those who have gone before. It is in this sense, also, that every truly outstanding physician is in some degree a historian of medicine, taking pride and finding precedent in the values and accomplishments of the great physicians of the past. This helps perpetuate the long-term values of medicine and provides the basis for continuing to put these into practice through newly-appropriate means. Medical schools thus become the guardians of the values basic to the effective practice of medicine.

It is within this broad institutional setting that the medical schools find their place. It is their function to transmit the culture of medicine and to advance that culture. It is their task to shape the novice into the effective practitioner of medicine, to give him the best available knowledge and skills, and to provide him with a professional identity so that he comes to think, act, and feel like a physician. It is their problem to enable the medical man to live up to the expectations of the professional role long after he has left the sustaining value-environment provided by the medical school. This is the context within which psychological and sociological inquiry into medical schools can identify the extent to which this comes about and the ways in which it comes about.

The process of socialization

Social scientists have long had an enduring interest in studying the process of 'socialization'.[1] By this is meant the process through which individuals are inducted into their culture. It involves the acquisition of attitudes and values, of skills and behavior patterns making up social roles established in the social structure. For a considerable time, studies of socialization were largely confined to the early years in the life cycle of the individual; more recently, increasing attention has been directed to the process as it continues, at varying rates, throughout the life cycle. This has given rise to theoretical and empirical analyses of 'adult socialization'.[2]

From this standpoint, medical students are engaged in learning the professional role of the physician by so combining its component knowledge and skills, attitudes, and values, as to be motivated and able to perform this role in a professionally and socially acceptable fashion. Adult socialization includes more than what is ordinarily described as education and training. Most conspicuous in the process of medical learning is, of course, the acquisition of a considerable store of knowledge and skills which to some extent occurs even among the least of these students. Beyond this, it is useful to think of the processes of role acquisition in two broad classes: direct learning through didactic teaching of one kind or another, and indirect learning, in which attitudes, values, and behavior patterns are acquired as by-products of contact with instructors and peers, with patients, and with members of the health team. It would seem particularly useful to attend systematically to the less conspicuous and more easily neglected processes of indirect learning. For as with all educational institutions, it is natural for those far removed from the details of life and work in the medical school to assume that the great bulk, and the most significant part, of what the student carries away with him is learned through formal instruction – an assumption which many members of medical faculties reject as remote from the actual facts of the case. It is clear that not all which is taught in medical school is actually learned by students and that not all which is learned is taught there, if by teaching is meant didactic forms of instruction. Students learn not only from precept, or even from deliberate example; they also learn – and it may often be, most enduringly learn – from sustained involvement in that society of medical staff, fellow-students, and patients which makes up the medical school as a social organization.

In our ongoing studies,[3] therefore, we include more than a sidelong glance at the informal and unpremeditated ways in which students come to acquire the attitudes and values by which some of them will presumably live as medical men. We have provisionally assumed that in the course of their social interaction with others in the school, of exchanging experiences and ideas with peers, and of observing and evaluating the behavior of their instructors (rather than merely listening to their precepts), students acquire the values which will be basic to their professional way of life. The ways in which these students are shaped, both by intent and by unplanned circumstances of their school environment, constitute a major part of the process of socialization.

It should be parenthetically said that although the technical skills and knowledge of medicine are, of course, central to the role of the physician, these are not considered, except incidentally, in this first set of research reports. Instead, the focus here is temporarily upon the attitude and value components of the physician's role.

Notes

1. As was implied earlier in this paper, it is advisable to acknowledge the historical fact that the word 'socialization' has quite a different and long-standing connotation in medical circles. This fact cannot be exorcized; it must, instead, be taken into account if we are not to become needlessly involved in semantic confusions and controversies. With this in mind, I have prepared a detailed terminological note on the concept of socialization in the hope of forestalling such bootless conflicts of meaning. This note will be found in Appendix A [which can be found in the original text].

2. Parsons, T. (1951) *The Social System*, The Free Press, Glencoe, Ill, Chapter VI and, in particular, the remarks on adult socialization on pp.207–208; Dollard, J. (1939) Culture, society, impulse, and socialization, *American Journal of Sociology*, 45, 50–63; Child, I. L. (1954) Socialization. In *Handbook of Social Psychology* (Lindzey, G., ed), Addison-Wesley, Cambridge, Mass., which includes an extensive bibliography.

3. A series of monographs on selected problems of this kind is now in process. These are briefly described in Appendix B [which can be found in the original text].

Chapter 24

Boys in white: student culture in medical school

Howard S. Becker, Blanche Geer, Everett C. Hughes and Anselm L. Strauss

The chooser of a professional occupation makes his first steps toward it on the basis of second-hand images, not of immediate experience; before him is a long blind flight. What happens to him between commitment and final acceptance into professional colleagueship is an important part of his life and a process which a society dependent on professions should understand. Medicine is, in many respects, the crucial case. It should be added that the signs of some reaction against an over-long professional adolescence are also turning up first in medicine; medicine may lead the reaction as it did the trend.

We have mentioned two aspects of the professional trend – the increase in the number of professions and the increase in length of training for each. A third, of equal importance, is a trend toward the practice of the professions in organizations more complex than the old-fashioned doctor's or lawyer's office. Some of the newer professions – again, note the tender of electronic computers – are bound to machines which in turn can be run only by an organization; others – again, note the hospital administrator – are themselves by-products of new trends in organization. Medicine and law themselves, the two occupations most often taken as models of the very concept of profession, are not exempt from the trend. Indeed, the more renowned members of these professions are less likely to be found practicing alone or outside larger organisations than are the less renowned. There is some evidence that a man who wishes to choose his style of practice must either found an organization (group, clinic, hospital firm, etc.) or attach himself to one. Furthermore, the trend toward practice in larger and more complicated organizations seems to occur quite independently of the degree of governmental control of the professions. It is rather a function of technology and of social organization itself.

A modern medical school, associated generally with a university and always with one or several large hospitals, with clinics and laboratories, is a far cry from clerkship in its original sense. The student is not an apprentice working with a master; he has many masters. Some are physicians; some are not. In a sense, the expensive plant, with its millions of dollars' worth of precious equipment is his master. The technicians, the nurses, and the patients are all his masters insofar as their presence affects his own behavior and his own fate. Finally, those who are most clearly and avowedly his masters, the teachers of clinical medicine, are usually removed in some measure from the nonacademic practice of medicine. Even if they are in private practice, they are likely to have had careers that are largely academic and to work under conditions somewhat different from those of nonacademic physicians. The separation of academic from nonacademic careers appears in increasing measure in professions generally. It is accompanied by some strain between professional schools and the practicing professions out in the world.

Two sets of ideas characteristic of medical students seem particularly cynical to other people. As a result of their experience in school students acquire a point of view and terminology of a technical kind, which allow them to talk and think about patients and diseases in a way quite different from the layman. They look upon death and disabling disease, not with the horror and sense of tragedy the layman finds appropriate, but as problems in medical responsibility. The technical attitude which prevents the student from becoming emotionally involved in the tragedy of patients' diseases seems to the layman cruel, heartless, and cynical.

In a more sophisticated way, some observers (in this case not only laymen, but also members of the medical faculty) think students cynical because they set for themselves some standard of a reasonable and proper level of effort. When, for instance, members of the faculty complain about the 'eight to five' student, they are complaining that students do not make as complete an effort as might be made. Similarly, our finding that freshmen decide it is necessary to select some of the material they are presented with for intensive study while ignoring other material will seem to some people an unjustifiably cynical approach to the study of medicine.

Where the immediate situation of the student dictates the development of a perspective of the kind we analyzed in our consideration of student culture, the layman is likely to see the development of ingrained, long-lasting cynicism. While this would be a misreading of our analysis, the problem warrants our making a more differentiated analysis, using a dimension of which cynicism and idealism are end-points, of what happens to students as they move through medical school. We shall point out both the ways in which students become 'cynical' in the layman's view and the ways in which, looked at from other vantage points, students may be said to be continuingly idealistic.

We believe that medical students enter medical school openly idealistic about the practice of medicine and the medical profession. They do not lose this idealistic long-range perspective but realistically develop a 'cynical' concern with the day-to-day details of getting through medical school. As they approach the end of school they again openly exhibit an idealistic concern with problems of practice. In other words, the students simultaneously maintain an idealistic view of the broader problems of medical practice, a view which has its roots in lay culture, and a narrower view which sees the only important problems as those posed by the daily exigencies of school itself. This relation between what we might refer to as extra and intramural interests occupies our attention for the rest of this chapter. The process we describe may be easily generalized to other kinds of institutions and thus have a sociological significance beyond the case under consideration.

We have already seen that medical students enter school with broad and idealistic concerns. They are not interested in medicine as a way of getting rich; this may be because they feel so sure of doing well financially in medicine. In any case, income is not a major concern of students when they enter school. They come in with a complement of ideas about healing the sick and rendering service to mankind. They resent any hints that they may have crasser motives. They are determined to learn all the facts that the medical school will give them, in order that they may do the best possible job of caring for the patients they will later have. They work long hours and are willing to work even longer ones.

These idealistic notions have little relevance to the students' activities in medical school. The work they do in the first year appears to them far removed from anything having to do with sick patients and besides, there is so much of it that they cannot possibly learn everything as they had expected to do. No matter how hard they work, they are told by the faculty, and believe, they will not be able to learn it all. This being the case, they must decide which of the many facts they are brought into contact with they will try to remember and make use of. For awhile, some students try to make this choice by thinking ahead to their prospective medical practices and seeing what will be most needed there. But they really know nothing of what will be needed in medical practice so that this is not a workable criterion.

What is much more pressing is their discovery that they must first of all pass the examinations set for them by the faculty; if they do not they will not practice medicine at all. Though the examinations sometimes appear unrelated to the problems of medical practice and arbitrary, they are still facts of life with which the students must deal. So the students, some quickly and others more reluctantly, take the view that the way to get through the first year of school is to find out what the faculty wants them to know and learn it. This concerns them deeply, for it seems to them a violation of the idealistic notions with which they entered their training. But they find it absolutely necessary to concentrate on learning in order to get through school and to give up their idealistic concern with learning in order to alleviate suffering. In the course of the upsets caused by the examinations of the first year, the students engage in increased communication across lines that formerly divided them, so that by the end of the year the entire class is united on the basic proposition that the important thing is to get through school.

It is this immediate concern with getting through school that appears cynical to many outside observers. Students do not worry much about the fact of death; they are not very much bothered by the fact that the cadavers they now dissect were once living human beings. A cadaver is primarily a device for acquiring certain facts they may be asked for on an examination. They have little time for concern with what kind of a person the cadaver once was. Successful students put such questions aside.

With the advent of the clinical years, students' concerns become more closely entangled with the fate of living patients. But here again, the pressures of school are so great that they take first place in the students' minds. Students become engrossed with the problem of 'working' faculty and house staff for as many nuggets of clinical experience and as many opportunities to exercise medical responsibility as possible. They worry about always presenting a good front to their superiors and never making a bad impression. They organize to share their collective work more equitably and to prevent situations in which one student will make the others look bad by working too hard. Students do these things because they are so earnest about using their time in school to acquire the knowledge and experience they think they will need in practice, and because they want so much to graduate and be licensed to practice. They see many of the requirements faculty make as interfering with their pursuit of knowledge by encumbering them with 'busy work'; students' dislike of doing admission laboratory work on patients, for instance, falls in this category.

We have shown that the students collectively set the level and direction of their efforts to learn. There is nothing unusual about such a finding. What is significant – as we insist throughout – is that these levels and directions are not the result of some conscious cabal, but that they are the working-out in practice of the perspectives from which the students view their day-to-day problems in relation to their long-term goals. The perspectives, themselves collectively developed, are organizations of ideas and actions. The actions derive their rationale from the ideas; the ideas are sustained by success in action. The whole becomes a complex of mutual expectations.

To these perspectives, we give the name *student culture*. In so doing we follow the essence of anthropological practice; for culture is commonly defined as a body of ideas and practices considered to support each other and expected of each other by members of some group of people. Such a group forms a *community of fate*, for however individualistic their motives, they share goals, a body of crucial experiences, and exposure to the same perils. We do not follow that accidental part of anthropological usage, which attributes the persistence of culture solely to the initiation of each generation by its predecessor to tradition. In fact, our evidence suggests that if the perspectives – the student culture – we describe go on from generation to generation of students, it is because each class enters medical school with the same ideas and objectives and finds itself faced with the same combination of short-run and long-term problems.

A perspective, to be more precise, contains several elements: a definition of the situation in which the actors are involved, a statement of the goals they are trying to achieve, a set of ideas specifying what kinds of activities are expedient and proper, and a set of activities or practices congruent with them. The freshmen defined their situation as one in which there was more work than they could possibly do. They developed the idea that they must necessarily learn what the faculty wanted them to learn, although it sometimes seemed to them that these were not the things they themselves would have thought necessary for a medical practitioner. They developed ways of acting, studying, and working which made it possible for them to achieve this goal in the situation they had defined. Similarly the students in the clinical years saw their situation as one in which the goal of learning what was necessary for the practice of medicine might be interfered with by the structure of the hospital and by the necessity of making a good impression on the faculty. As they came in contact with clinical medicine, they developed new goals that were more specific than those they had before. They learned to want clinical experience and to want the opportunity of exercising medical responsibility but were often frustrated in their attempts to realize these desires by the necessary constraints imposed by the organization of the hospital. They developed ideas about how they must deal with the faculty, with patients, and with each other, and modes of activity in which these ideas are put into practice. They developed ways of co-operating among themselves to handle the work they must do, to deal with the problem of making a good impression on the faculty and of getting as much clinical experience and medical responsibility as possible. These perspectives, taken together, constitute student culture in the medical school.

Note

1. The Johns Hopkins University has already adopted a plan to allow students to enter medical school a year earlier. Other schools are said to be considering similar steps. While such a change will, in the absence of further lengthening of specialty residencies, get young men into practice earlier, it also requires of them a still earlier decision to enter the profession.

Reprinted by permission of The University of Chicago Press, Chicago. Howard S. Becker *et al.* (1961) *Boys in White: Student Culture in Medical School*, University of Chicago Press, Chicago, pp. 7–8, 421–424, 435–436.

Chapter 25

The silent dialogue: a study in the social psychology of professional socialization

Virginia L. Olesen and Elvi W. Whittaker

Our sketch of professional socialization begins with the student arriving at the door of the institution as pristine and virginal as though untouched by Original Sin: no hint of being male or female, no taint of social class membership, no attributes of brilliance, stupidity, or simple ability. The formal start of school is the beginning of the aspirant's professional life. He has never, until now, thought of himself as doctor, social worker, pharmacist, schoolteacher, or lawyer, because he has presumably never thought about himself in any connection.

One student is like another with respect to ability, experience, interest in and expectations of the chosen profession. Identical, too, are the schools: the small, Midwestern divinity school is comparable to the large one in New York City; the normal school of twenty years ago is akin to the university education department of today; the social work department with strong Freudian emphasis differs not from the school which espouses Rogerian theories.

The faceless, ahistorical student, having forsaken or never having considered private interests, the possibilities of marriage, or activities as a citizen, looks to life only as a professional person in the institutional years. Immersed in the profession, he converses only with faculty, who presumably speak only to the leaders of the profession. Neither students nor faculty, of course, have any commerce with such lesser beings as spouses, children, fellow citizens, parents, or clients. The only significant statements heard by the student are gleaned from the faculty, who have only significant statements to make.

Once the educational system has formally started work on the student, his empty head is filled with values, behaviors, and viewpoints of the profession, the knowledge being perfect and complete by the time of graduation. To achieve this state of grace, the student has smoothly moved ever away from the unholy posture of layman, upward to the sanctified status of the professional, being divested of worldly care and attributes along the way.

The result: 'the true professional', 'the finished product', 'the outcome of the system', 'the end product'. These phases and concepts are actually to be found in literature on professional socialization (Olesen and Whittaker, 1966).

Our sketch terminates with the day of graduation when, like the dolls in nurse–doctor play kits, young professionals move as equally substitutable units from the school assembly line into a world where no further change can be wrought upon or with them, they being now fully garbed with the indisputable trappings of the professional.

Being well embedded in sociological thinking about professional socialization, these images guide the researcher's use of theory and method, influence his expectations for results, and generally shape the literature in the field. Their influence leads to research questions like '*What* is the effect of professional education on the student?' '*How much* role learning do students do?' '*What* kind of professional role do students learn?' '*How much* of the profession's values do students acquire?' Attached to the images and the questions are research methods that call for before–after designs, instruments to measure amount of role or value acquisition and tests to assess the contours of a 'true professional'. Not infrequently, these research enterprises come to nothing, partly because these assumptions and questions are unrelated to the actual experiences of both faculty and students in professional socialization.

Young students in any professional school participate in their own education by making choices to meet faculty demands, to handle non-institutional pressures, and to work out situations of their own creating. Students may choose foolishly or wisely, depending on the perspective they or the faculty take. They may later regret or be satisfied with their choices, but they are constantly choosing among the degrees and ranges of alternatives open to them and those which they open for themselves in the institutional setting.[1] The students do more than simply talk back: they are, in fact, actively involved in the shaping of existential situations in which acquisition of professional and adult role behaviors occur.

To describe student professionals thus is to speak only of one sector of the socialization process during the student years. The student encounters others who have many roles both within and outside of the formal institutional structure. Medical students, for example, may learn from their patients a great deal that the instructors do not wish them to assimilate; furthermore, such knowledge may be more easily learned from the faculty (Hughes, 1958). Thus there is in every profession a kind of bootlegging, in which the student, unwittingly or not, acquires from non-official vendors the ideas, values, and ways of behaving and thinking that are attributed, sometimes legitimately and sometimes not, to the profession.[2]

... Embedded in the frequently banal, sometimes dreary, often uninteresting world of everyday living, professional socialization was of the commonplace.[3] In the mundane, not in the abstract or exalted, occurred the minute starts and stops, the bits of progress and backsliding, the moments of reluctant acquisition of a new self and the tenacious relinquishing of the old: the flush of pride and elation when telling a fellow student about a good evaluation or listening silently and painfully when being told of someone else's good marks; the feeling of relief that one had not been the object of group laughter in conference; the sense of anxiety when learning from a classmate that yet another student had married or become engaged; the right look at the right time when discussing the patient with the instructor.

These matters constitute the silent dialogue wherein are fused person, situation, and institution. Therein lies the heart of professional socialization.

Notes

1. This image of the student professional assumes an underlying philosophy of 'soft determinism,' 'foresight,' or 'prehension.' Among the many sources which analyze this position are Matza, D. (1964) *Delinquency and Drift*, Wiley, New York, especially p.11; Sullivan, H. S. (1964) Tensions interpersonal and international: a psychiatrist's view. In *The Fusion of Psychiatry and Social Sciences* (Perry, H. S., ed.), Norton, New York, especially p.303; Whitehead, A. N. (1933) *Adventures of Ideas*, Macmillan, New York; Sperry, R. W. (1964) Mind, brain and humanist values. In *New Views of The Nature of Man* (Platt, J. R., ed.), University of Chicago Press, Chicago, pp. 71–92, especially p.87.
2. On parents as sources of information and support, see Dornbusch, S. M. (1955) The military academy as an assimilating institution, *Social Forces*, 32 (March), 321.
3. Consider Sartre on the commonplace: 'For this excellent word (commonplace) has several meanings. It designates, of course, our most hackneyed thoughts, inasmuch as these thoughts have become the meeting place of the community. It is here that each of us finds himself as well as the others. The commonplace belongs to everybody, it is the presence of everybody in me.' (Sartre, 1956, *Situations*, trans. by Benita Eisler, Fawcett, New York, p.137.)

References

Hughes, E. (1958) *Men and Their Work*, Free Press, Glencoe, Ill
Olesen, V. and Whittaker, E. (1966) Some images of man implicit in studies of professional socialization. Presented at the Sixth World Congress of Sociology, Evian, France, September

Chapter 26

The reproduction of the professional community

Paul Atkinson

Students do not learn what the school proposes to teach them. Colleges do not make students more liberal and humane...nor do they have any great effect on students' intellectual development and learning.... Medical school training has little effect on the quality of medicine a doctor practices.... Actors considered expert by their peers have seldom gone to drama school.... The spectacle of elementary and secondary education gives credence to Herndon's...wry hypothesis that nobody learns anything in school, but middle-class children learn enough elsewhere to make it appear that schooling is effective....

The title of Becker's piece sums up his argument: 'School is a Lousy Place to Learn Anything.'

Now I am sure that Becker is deliberately and self-consciously engaging in hyperbole – trailing his coat. But he is clearly in danger of adopting a nonsensical position – one which is only a slight exaggeration of the interactionist stance. There have from time to time been stories of individuals operating as successful and apparently competent doctors, dentists and so on who turn out to have no formal qualifications. Commentators never overlook the irony of such revelations. But it would nevertheless be quite absurd to extend the argument – as Becker appears to – and suggest that medical students do not learn medicine in medical school.

It is undoubtedly true that students do not 'learn medicine' in any absolute sense. They certainly do not assimilate a package of knowledge and skills which they then proceed to apply throughout their subsequent working lives as medical practitioners. There is no ideal 'medicine' which exists absolutely and independently from the practicalities of day-to-day practice in actual medical settings. On the other hand there can surely be no doubt that medical students do learn medicine – or at least some version or versions of medicine – and it may seem banal and even bizarre that one should need to emphasize the point in this context.

If Becker can be taken to mean that 'medical school is a lousy place to learn medicine', then one assumes that he has some idealized view of how it should be taught, and that present educational practice falls some way short of that. A corollary of that might be to argue that 'medical school is a place to learn lousy medicine'. That is certainly a view worth canvassing. But here again Becker's overall position would preclude such a view, since he and his interactionist colleagues foreclose any principled exploration of the relationship between training and work.

In effect this issue boils down to the interactionists' failure adequately to cope with problems of knowledge and to produce a sociology of the curriculum. This is in fact is a point of departure where later developments in the sociology of education diverge from earlier interactionist influences. For a direct consideration of school knowledge has become a major strand in the so-called 'new sociology of education'.[1] It was a legacy of both the functionalist and interactionist approaches that there should be a concern with the latent functions of education and aspects of the hidden curriculum. These were both, in their way, 'demystifying' – stripping away the rhetoric of educational provision in order to disclose its actual practice. But in the process the manifest function of education – the transmission and management of knowledge, the manifest curriculum – became overlooked. I want to argue that such a reappraisal is necessary in the context of 'professional' education, without necessarily abandoning the insights derived from the interactionist ethnographies of educational settings.

What is implied by the remarks so far is this: despite the apparent cleavage between thee two major schools in this field, there have in fact been convergences – both in terms of what has been done, and what has not been done. Fundamentally, both positions treat 'the profession' as unproblematic. The functionalists do so by taking on trust the characteristics the professions claim, and assimilating their view of education to that perspective. The interactionists effectively treat it as unproblematic by default, since they fail systematically to question the relationship between education, practice and the organization of occupational groups.

In effect, then, what has been lacking is an adequate treatment of cultural transmission and knowledge management in the reproduction of the professions. Yet this is odd, as all observers are moved to remark on the extent to which professions are potent self-replicating collectivities. We have been in danger of abandoning 'socialisation' only to leave ourselves with no room adequately to cope with issues of cultural reproduction.

———

Hence the production and reproduction of knowledge – legal, medical, religious, educational and so on – will become the *leitmotiv* for a sociology of professional education.

We must recognize that all educational knowledge – be it that of primary schools or universities – is in a sense *arbitrary*. There is no absolute, pre-given corpus of knowledge which self-evidently presents itself as a 'curriculum', and which is inherently endowed with order, sequential organization and so on. The curriculum is a device whereby knowledge is classified and combined: it is a cultural imposition. There is no ideal 'law', 'medicine', 'theology' or whatever 'out there' to which the curriculum corresponds as a mere reflection or copy.

Educational knowledge separates what is thinkable from what is unthinkable; it identifies what is deemed important and attempts to distinguish it from what is trivial; it marks out what is introductory from what is specialized and advanced; it may construct an essential 'core' as opposed to the peripheral or optional. In the course of setting up and legitimating such definitions of knowledge curricula portray the essentially arbitrary as *natural*: natural, that is, in that they appear to reflect a given order in the domain of knowledge and in the world of work. Hence its status as a cultural artefact remains hidden. (Though this is not to deny that there may be occasions on which some conscious questioning may take place.)

Note

1. The title 'new sociology of education' has been applied to a somewhat diverse collection of theoretical approaches and empirical studies, variously inspired by phenomenology and Marxism. The main programmatic statements can be found in Young, M. F. D. (ed.) (1971) *Knowledge and Control: New Directions for the Sociology of Education*, Collier-Macmillan, London. A useful review is Demaine, J. (1977) On the new sociology of education. *Economy and Society*, 6.

Reprinted by permission of Macmillan Ltd, Basingstoke. Paul Atkinson (1983) The reproduction of the professional community. In *The Sociology of the Professions: Lawyers, Doctors and Others* (Dingwall, R. and Lewis, P., eds), Macmillan Press, Basingstoke, pp. 233–235.

Chapter 27

Learning and working: the occupational socialization of nurses

Kath M. Melia

One of the abiding problems of occupational socialization has to do with the differences between the idealized version of work as it is presented to new recruits and the work as it is practised daily by members of the occupation. This book is about occupational socialization in nursing. Its chief concern has to do with how newcomers to nursing are made aware not only of the activities involved in nursing, but also of how nursing is practised on a daily basis by qualified nurses. It takes as its starting point the accounts of nursing which students in training gave of their experiences of becoming nurses.

A central feature of the students' accounts of nursing is the division which they saw between nursing, as it was presented to them in the college, and nursing as they observed and practised it on the hospital wards. It is clear enough what kind of a difficulty this situation presents for students of nursing. However, if we take a closer look at this division it can be seen to be of interest to nursing in general. By pointing to the division within the occupation, the students have directed attention to a long-standing problem which is inherent in the apprenticeship approach to the training of nurses and staffing of hospital wards.

The structure of nurse training is an historical compromise between the provision of a nursing service and the education of nurses. This compromise makes student nurses both learners and workers. The compromise is rooted in the way in which the nursing service operates in Britain, that is by employing large numbers of students who work under the direction of a much smaller number of qualified staff.

Hughes (1971, p.357) ... says that occupations contain such a variety of members with varying perceptions of the work that 'to call them by one name is close to misleading'. We have not got, according to Hughes, 'a fully worked out anatomy of occupational prestige, including all contacts and interactions out of which the images of the various occupations develop'.

Following Bucher and her colleagues, I have used the notion of segmentation as an analytic and organizing device. I shall argue that nursing is an occupation which contains segments similar to those Bucher *et al.* describe in the professions; each with its own particular reason for canvassing the version of nursing which it has made its own. The two main segments are *service* and *education*.

'Fitting in' emerges as a theme which runs through the analysis as the students described how throughout their training they tried to behave in the way that any given situation demanded. Their concern was to meet the expectations of those in authority and so 'fitting in' constitutes a major part of the students' efforts in negotiating their way through training.

Throughout this book I have argued that nursing is too diverse an enterprise to be embraced by one name, and that the occupational group of nurses is too large and heterogeneous a group for its members to share the same view of what their work should be and how it should be organized. It is this segmentation which is responsible for the existence of two different versions of nursing encountered by the students.

In some sense the students' accounts can be viewed as an elaborate and protracted way of addressing the much vaunted question 'what is nursing?' The answer for the students, in so far as there is one, seems to be that nursing resembles neither the 'professional' nor the 'workload' approach to nursing as canvassed respectively by the education and service segments. This puts into question the whole business of occupational socialization, because students are being socialized into neither version of nursing. Instead they learn to recognize when one form of nursing rather than the other is appropriate, and 'fit in' accordingly. In other words, they learn how to be *student* nurses and not how to be *nurses*.

Carpenter [1977] describes three main groups within nursing: 'new managers', 'new professionals', and the 'rank and file'. To these I have added the 'academic professionalizers'. The new managers emerged, according to Carpenter, after the Salmon Report recommendations (DHSS, 1966). They operate according to an industrial model of professionalized management and their organizational structure takes the form of bureaucratic line management rather than a collegial model of professional behaviour. The *new professionals* are, as yet, a relatively small group of clinical nurse specialists who emerged, according to Carpenter, as a response to the 'new managerialism'. These clinical specialists, who are independent of line management, stand outside the hierarchical structure of nursing. This clinical development, Carpenter suggests, is modelled on the American notion of the clinical nurse consultant, who 'creams off' the more complex parts of nursing. Carpenter also says that this group of 'new professionals' may well push for the delegation of the more routine work of medicine. The position of clinical specialisms in nursing might be said to have been formalized with the proliferation of post-basic courses and their national recognition in the early 1970s. The *rank and file* can be regarded as the mainstream of nursing. These are nurses who enjoy both doctor-devolved work and the reflected status which comes with working alongside the medical profession. The *academic professionalizers* are to be found in the main in academic circles, and tend to be rather removed from the patients. The work of this group centres mainly on research and the teaching of undergraduate nurses. They seek to achieve autonomy for nursing by elevating the status of 'basic' or 'primary' care, and placing less emphasis upon medically prescribed work. In short, their aim is to promote a style of nursing founded on 'nursing theory', which can take its place among other academic writings, rather than nursing which is founded merely upon tradition and medical dominance.

These four descriptive groups can be considered rather more easily if we adopt as an analytic device the concept of segmentation (Bucher and Strauss, 1961; Bucher and Stelling, 1977) This allows us to focus upon the interests of each segment, instead of being overly concerned with description. What we have is a straight divide between the *education* segment, which embraces the academic professionalizers and the college tutors, with whom the students come into contact, and the *service* segment, which includes the 'new managers', the 'rank and file', and the 'new professionals'. These two segments canvass distinctly different approaches to the work. Each segment has its more vocal and prominent sections among the membership – the 'academic professionalizers' for the education segment and the 'new managers' for the service. Indeed, it might be more accurate to view the segments in this more narrowly defined way rather than to divide the whole occupational group neatly into just two segments. For the purpose of this analysis, though, I have chosen to view nursing in terms of two segments, each containing more and less committed members. I recognize the limitations of this approach, but proffer it as a start.

The apparent compartmentalization of nursing clearly presents problems for student nurses, who by the very organization of their training have to cross from one segment to another. As the students move between the worlds of education and service, they have to come to terms with two versions of nursing, each with its own rationality and its own structural constraints.

———

Having mastered the professional nursing rhetoric of the education segment and the practicalities of the service way of nursing, the students discover that, by and large, the best way to get through the training programme is to fit in with the trained staff on the wards. So, while the educators might have the edge on the service segment in so far as they, the educators, are seen to be largely responsible for the control of the training, it seems that, in the students' view, there is more to be gained from accommodating the needs of the service segment. This allegiance is perhaps not surprising since the students, when they qualify, will no longer move between segments, rather they will be located in the service segment.

A segmented occupational group has to find ways of containing its differences when it operates publicly. In other words whilst differences of ideology and work organization may be possible to sustain within the group, when it comes to its dealings with other health care disciplines the group must be able to produce and rely upon a united front.

... the notion of various internal differences existing within an occupation is useful. The united front is clearly required when nursing deals with other groups. The students learn not to expose the differences as they pass between segments during their training – instead, they 'fit in' and move on.

It is difficult, and ultimately unhelpful, to draw any succinct conclusions from this analysis of the students' wide-ranging accounts of nursing. I am conscious of the fact that one response to this detailed exposition of the student nurses' world might well be to say 'now what?', or even 'so what?' I will conclude, then, by posing the question which, as I see it, nursing urgently needs to address. Stated briefly, this would be: How best can such a heterogeneous group as nurses be organized in order to provide its service? From this stems a further question – Should nurses continue as this heterogeneous group, making various claims to profession?

It seems that there are at least two possible alternative structures which nurses might consider. The first scenario involves a reduction in number, and a rise in educational standards. The aim would be to produce 'professional' nurses charged with effecting patient care through a mixed workforce, which would include some grade of trained nursing auxiliary. The effort would, then, be directed towards the production of 'scientific manager' sisters, rather than, as is currently the case, producing large numbers of nurses, many of whom function at a lower level than the one proposed here. With a smaller and more homogeneous group, educated to a higher level, claims to 'profession' might be more successful. At the moment the sheer numbers involved make claims to professional status little more than pipe dreams. The second option would involve a drawing away from attempts to gain professional status for nursing. Instead nursing would be characterized as a craft. Emphasis would be placed on the perfection of the skilled work of nursing and less stress placed on achieving a place for the occupation among 'the professions'.

Nurse theorists derive their satisfaction from the intellectual exercise of promoting nursing as an autonomous activity, which is free of medical dominance. Whether or not this group would sustain their interest if they were to find themselves practising according to their reconstruction of 'basic nursing care' is probably another matter. But the question still remains. Is this intellectual activity undertaken for altruistic reasons concerning patient welfare, or is it a means of achieving academic and professional status of nursing (which would perhaps be no bad thing). Professional status brings with it power, and this could be an important factor in getting the provision of nursing care right for the changing needs of the population.

A concentration on skills, with appropriate reference to theoretical ideas, would fit nicely into the craftsman approach to nursing. Craftsmen, having served an apprenticeship, are the masters of their trade or craft. Braverman (1974, p.443) in his discussion of degraded work, catalogues the demise of the craftsman who he says was 'tied to the technical and scientific knowledge of his time in the daily practice of his craft'.

Characterization of nursing as a craft would entail less emphasis upon drawing away from medicine. There would, nevertheless, be organizational implications. Braverman's (1974, p.443) comment is pertinent here:

> For the worker the concept of skill is traditionally bound up with craft mastery – that is to say, the combination of knowledge of materials and processes with the practised manual dexterities required to carry out a specific branch of production. The breakup of craft skills and the reconstruction of production as a collective or social process have destroyed the traditional concept of skill and opened up only one way for mastery over labor processes: in and through scientific, technical and engineering knowledge.... What is left to workers is a reinterpreted and woefully inadequate concept of skill: a specific dexterity, a limited and repetitious operation 'speed as skill', etc.

A concentration on craft and skills would produce a nursing workforce which could operate along the lines Stinchcombe (1959) describes in the construction industry. These were skilled craftsmen who needed little in the way of supervision in their tasks as their work is guided by standards of craftsmanship, which Stinchcombe argues are similar to professional standards.

As things stand, though, the occupational group which operates under the name 'nursing' must accept, if it is to continue as one group, that there exists within it a wide range of interests, skills, and academic ability. Much of the difficulty in defining what nursing is, both in terms of activity and professional status, lies in the heterogeneity of the group. Recognition of the abilities and limitations, and of the ambitions and motivations of the different segments within the totality of nursing provides at least a starting point from which to consider the future of nursing as a united group. Nursing's future will, to a large extent, also be dependent upon the changes both within the medical profession and society as a whole. Changes in age structure, disease patterns, population trends, economic and social constraints which result in less emphasis on the technological and more on the social and community-based aspects of care will, in all probability, lead to nursing coming into the forefront of health care. In this event there must exist a united nursing service, which will not only be able to represent its needs at government level, but will also be able to provide care of all kinds, requiring different levels of skill, safety and efficiency.

———————

Ultimately, it is an occupation's ambitions and self-image that will, more than anything else, shape the nature of the work it undertakes or the service it provides. In the case of nursing, the occupation's views on the status of the auxiliary workers who undertake patient care will be crucial in the restructuring of the group. Debates about nursing's self-image, about professionalism and professional status, extend well beyond semantics. The organizational structure and, indeed, the survival of nursing as an occupational group depend upon the outcome of such deliberations.

References

Braverman, H. (1974) *Labor and Monopoly Capital. The Degradation of Work in the Twentieth Century*, Monthly Review Press, New York
Bucher, R. and Stelling, J.G. (1977) *Becoming Professional*, Sage, Beverly Hills
Bucher, R. and Strauss, A.L. (1961) Professions in process. *American Journal of Sociology*, 66, 325–334
Carpenter, M. (1977) The new managerialism and professionalism in nursing. In *Health and the Division of Labour* (Stacey, M., Reid, M., Heath, C. and Dingwall, R., eds), Croom Helm, London
Hughes, E.C. (1971) *The Sociological Eye*, Aldine, Chicago
Stinchcombe, A.L. (1959) Bureaucratic and craft administration of production: a comparative study. *Administrative Science Quarterly*, 4

Reprinted by permission of Routledge (Tavistock Publications), Andover. Kath M. Melia (1987) *Learning and Working: The Occupational Socialization of Nurses*, Tavistock, London, pp.1, 2, 4, 5, 162–164, 165, 182, 183–185, 187, 197–201.

Chapter 28

Professions in process

Rue Bucher and Anselm Strauss

Functionalism sees a profession largely as a relatively homogeneous community whose members share identity, values, definitions of role, and interests.[1] There is room in this conception for some variation, some differentiation, some out-of-line members, even some conflict; but, by and large, there is a steadfast core which defines the profession, deviations from which are but temporary dislocations. Socialization of recruits consists of induction into the common core. There are norms, codes, which govern the behaviour of the professional to insiders and outsiders. In short, the sociology of professions has largely been focused upon the mechanics of cohesiveness and upon detailing the social structure (and/or social organization) of given professions. Those tasks a structural-functional sociology is prepared to do, and do relatively well.

But this kind of focus and theory tend to lead one to overlook many significant aspects of professions and professional life. Particularly does it bias the observer against appreciating the conflict – or at least difference – of interests within the profession; this leads him to overlook certain of the more subtle features of the profession's 'organization' as well as to fail to appreciate how consequential for changes in the profession and its practitioners differential interests may be.

In actuality, the assumption of relative homogeneity within the profession is not entirely useful: there are many identities, many values, and many interests. These amount not merely to differentiation or simple variation. They tend to become patterned and shared; coalitions develop and flourish – and in opposition to some others. We shall call these groupings which emerge within a profession 'segments'. (Specialties might be thought of as major segments, except that a close look at a specialty betrays its claim to unity, revealing that specialties, too, usually contain segments, and, if they ever did have common definitions along all lines of professional identity, it was probably at a very special, and early, period in their development.) We shall develop the idea of professions as loose amalgamations of segments pursuing different objectives in different manners and more or less delicately held together under a common name at a particular period in history.

'Organized medicine'

Medicine is usually considered the prototype of the professions, the one upon which current sociological conceptions of professions tend to be based; hence, our illustrative points in this paper will be taken from medicine, but they could just as pertinently have come from some other profession. Of the medical profession as a whole a great deal could be, and has been, said: its institutions (hospitals, schools, clinics); its personnel (physicians and paramedical personnel); its organizations (the American Medical Association, the state and county societies); its recruitment policies; its standards and codes; its political activities; its relations with the public; not to mention the professions' informal mechanisms of sociability and control. All this minimal 'structure' certainly exists.

But we should also recognize the great divergency of enterprise and endeavour that mark the profession; the cleavages that exist along with the division of labor; and the intellectual and specialist movements that occur within the broad rubric called 'organized medicine'. It might seem as if the physicians certainly share common ends, if ever any profession did. When backed to the wall, any physician would probably agree that his long-run objective is better care of the patient. But this is a misrepresentation of the actual values and organization of activity as undertaken by various segments of the profession. Not all the ends shared by all physicians are distinctive to the medical profession or intimately related to what many physicians do, as their work. What is distinctive of medicine belongs to certain segments of it – groupings not necessarily even specialties – and may not actually be shared with other physicians. We turn now to a consideration of some of those values which these segments do *not* share and about which they may actually be in conflict.

The sense of mission

It is characteristic of the growth of specialties that early in their development they carve out for themselves and proclaim unique missions. They issue a statement of the contribution that the specialty, and it alone, can make in the total scheme of values and, frequently, with it an argument to show why it is peculiarly fitted for this task. The statement of mission tends to take a rhetorical form, probably because it arises in the context of a battle for recognition and institutional status. Thus, when surgical specialties, such as urology and proctology, were struggling to attain identities independent of general surgery they developed the argument that the particular anatomical areas in which they were interested required special attention and that only physicians with their particular background were competent to give it. Anesthesiologists developed a similar argument. This kind of claim separates a given area out of the general stream of medicine, gives it special emphasis and a new dignity and, more important for our purposes, separates the specialty group from other physicians. Insofar as they claim an area for themselves, they aim to exclude others from it. It is theirs alone.

Colleagueship

Colleagueship may be one of the most sensitive indicators of segmentation within a profession. Whom a man considers to be his colleagues is ultimately linked with his own place within his profession. There is considerable ambiguity among sociologists over the meaning of the term 'colleague'. Occasionally the word is used to refer to co-workers, and other times simply to indicate formal membership in an occupation – possession of the social signs. Thus, all members of the occupation are colleagues. But sociological theory is also likely to stress colleagueship as a brotherhood. Gross, for example, writes about the colleague group characterized by *esprit de corps* and a sense of 'being in the same boat'. This deeper colleague relationship, he says, is fostered by such things as control of entry to the occupation, development of a unique mission, shared attitudes toward clients and society, and the formation of informal and formal associations (Gross, 1958).

This conception of colleagueship stresses occupational unity. Once entry to the occupation is controlled, it is assumed that all members of the occupation can be colleagues; they can rally around common symbols. However, the difficulty is that the very aspects of occupational life which Gross writes about as unifying the profession also break it into segments. What ties a man more closely to one member of his profession may alienate him from another: when his group develops a unique mission, he may no longer share a mission with others in the same profession.

Insofar as colleagueship refers to a relationship characterized by a high degree of shared interests and common symbols, it is probably rare that all members of a profession are even potentially colleagues. It is more feasible, instead, to work with a notion of circles of colleagueship. In the past, sociologists have recognized such circles of colleagueship, but from the viewpoint of the selective influence of such social circumstances as class and ethnicity. The professional identity shared by colleagues, though, contains far more than the kinds of people they desire as fellows. More fundamentally, they hold in common notions concerning the ends served by their work and attitudes and problems centering on it. The existence of what we have called segments thus limits and directs colleagueship.

Segments are not fixed, perpetually defined parts of the body professional. They tend to be more or less continually undergoing change. They take form and develop, they are modified, and they disappear. Movement is forced upon them by changes in their conceptual and technical apparatus, in the institutional conditions of work, and in their relationship to other segments and occupations. Each generation engages in spelling out, again, what it is about and where it is going. In this process, boundaries become diffuse as generations overlap, and different loci of professional activity articulate somewhat different definitions of the work situation. Out of this fluidity new groupings may emerge.

Note

1. Cf. Goode, W.J. (1957) Community within a community: the professions. *American Socio-logical Review*, **XX**, 194–200.

Reference

Gross, E. (1958) *Work and Society*, Thomas Y. Crowell Co., New York, pp.223–235

Reprinted by permission of The University of Chicago Press, Chicago. Rue Bucher and Anselm Strauss (1960–61) Professions in process. *The American Journal of Sociology*, **LXVI**, 325–327, 330, 332.

Chapter 29

The reflective practitioner: how professionals think in action

Donald A. Schön

When people use terms such 'art' and 'intuition', they usually intend to terminate discussion rather than to open up inquiry. It is as though the practitioner says to his academic colleague, 'While I do not accept *your* view of knowledge, I cannot describe my own'. Sometimes, indeed, the practitioner appears to say, 'My kind of knowledge is indescribable,' or even, 'I will not attempt to describe it lest I paralyze myself'. These attitudes have contributed to a widening rift between the universities and the professions, research and practice, thought and action. They feed into the university's familiar dichotomy between the 'hard' knowledge of science and scholarship and the 'soft' knowledge of artistry and unvarnished opinion. There is nothing here to guide practitioners who wish to gain a better understanding of the practical uses and limits of research–based knowledge, or to help scholars who wish to take a new view of professional action.

We are in need of inquiry into the epistemology of practice. What is the kind of knowing in which competent practitioners engage? How is professional knowing like and unlike the kinds of knowledge presented in academic textbooks, scientific papers, and learned journals? In what sense, if any, is there intellectual rigor in professional practice?

In this book I offer an approach to epistemology of practice based on a close examination of what some practitioner – architects, psychotherapists, engineers, planners, and managers – actually do. I have collected a sample of vignettes of practice, concentrating on episodes in which a senior practitioner tries to help a junior one learn to do something. In my analysis of these cases, I begin with the assumption that competent practitioners usually know more than they can say. They exhibit a kind of knowing-in-practice, most of which is tacit. Nevertheless, starting with protocols of actual performance, it is possible to construct and test models of knowing. Indeed, practitioners themselves often reveal a capacity for reflection on their intuitive knowing in the midst of action and sometimes use this capacity to cope with the unique, uncertain, and conflicted situations of practice.

=========

The professions have become essential to the very functioning of our society. We conduct society's principal business through professionals specially trained to carry out that business, whether it be making war and defending the nation, educating our children, diagnosing and curing disease, judging and punishing those who violate the law, settling disputes, managing industry and business, designing and constructing buildings, helping those who for one reason or another are unable to fend for themselves. Our principal formal institutions – schools, hospitals, government agencies, courts of law, armies – are arenas for the exercise of professional activity. We look to professionals for the definition and solution of our problems, and it is through them that we strive for social progress. In all of these functions we honor what Everett Hughes (1959) has called 'the professions' claim to extraordinary knowledge in matters of great social importance'; and in return, we grant professionals extraordinary rights and privileges. Hence, professional careers are among the most coveted and remunerative, and there are few occupations that have failed to seek out professional status. As one author asked, are we seeing the professionalization of nearly everyone? (Wilensky, 1964).

But although we are wholly dependent on them, there are increasing signs of a crisis of confidence in the professions. Not only have we witnessed well-publicised scandals in which highly esteemed professionals have misused their autonomy – where doctors and lawyers, for example, have used their positions illegitimately for private gain – but we are also encountering visible failures of professional action. Professionally designed solutions to public problems have had unanticipated consequences, sometimes worse than the problems they were designed to solve. Newly invented technologies, professionally conceived and evaluated, have turned out to produce unintended side effects unacceptable to large segments of our society. A professionally conceived and managed war has been widely perceived as a national disaster. Professionals themselves have delivered widely disparate and conflicting recommendations concerning problems of national importance, including those to which professional activities have contributed.

As a result, there has been a disposition to blame the professions for their failures and a loss of faith in professional judgment. There have been strident public calls for external regulation of professional activity, efforts to create public organizations to protest and protect against professionally recommended policies, and appeals to the courts for recourse against professional incompetence. Even in the most hallowed professional school of medicine and law, rebellious students have written popular exposés of the amoral, irrelevant, or coercive aspects of professional education.[1]

But the questioning of professionals' rights and freedoms – their license to determine who shall be allowed to practice, their mandate for social control, their autonomy – has been rooted in a deeper questioning of the professionals' claim to extraordinary knowledge in matters of human importance. This skepticism has taken several forms. In addition to the public loss of confidence noted above, there has been a virulent ideological attack on the professions, mostly from the Left. Some critics, like Ivan Illich (1970), have engaged in a wholesale debunking of professional claims to special expertise. Others have tried to show that professionals misappropriate specialized knowledge in their own interests and the interest of a power elite intent on preserving its dominance over the rest of the society.[2] Finally, and most significantly, professionals themselves have shown signs recently of a loss of confidence in their claims to extraordinary knowledge.

Knowing-in-action which the child may represent to himself in terms of a 'feel for the blocks', the observers redescribe in terms of 'theories'. I shall say that they convert the child's know*ing*-in-action to know*ledge*-in-action.

A conversion of this kind seems to be inevitable in any attempt to talk about reflection-in-action. One must use words to describe a kind of knowing, and a change of knowing, which are probably not originally represented in words at all. Thus, from their observations of the children's behavior, the authors make verbal descriptions of the children's intuitive understandings. These are the authors' theories about the children's knowing-in-action. Like all such theories, they are deliberate, idiosyncratic constructions, and they can be put to experimental test:

> just as the child was constructing a theory-in-action in his endeavor to balance the blocks, so we, too, were making on-the-spot hypotheses about the child's theories and providing opportunities for negative and positive responses in order to verify our own theories![3]

Reflecting-in-practice

The block-balancing experiment is a beautiful example of reflection-in-action, but it is very far removed from our usual images of professional practice. If we are to relate the idea of reflection-in-action to professional practice, we must consider what a practice is and how it is like and unlike the kinds of action we have been discussing.

The word 'practice' is ambiguous. When we speak of a lawyer's practice, we mean the kinds of things he does, the kinds of clients he has, the range of cases he is called upon to handle. When we speak of someone practicing the piano, however, we mean the repetitive or experimental activity by which he tries to increase his proficiency on the instrument. In the first sense, 'practice' refers to performance in a range of professional situations. In the second, it refers to preparation for performance. But professional practice also includes an element of repetition. A professional practitioner is a specialist who encounters certain types of situations again and again. This is suggested by the way in which professionals use the word 'case' – or project, account, commission, or deal, depending on the profession. All such terms denote the units which make up a practice, and they denote types of family-resembling examples. Thus a physician may encounter many different 'cases of measles'; a lawyer, many different 'cases of libel.' As a practitioner experiences many variations of a small number of types of cases, he is able to 'practice' his practice. He develops a repertoire of expectations, images, and techniques. He learns what to look for and how to respond to what he finds. As long as his practice is stable, in the sense that it brings him the same types of cases, he becomes less and less subject to surprise. His knowing-in-practice tends to become increasingly tacit, spontaneous, and automatic, thereby conferring upon him and his clients the benefits of specialization.

On the other hand, professional specialization can have negative effects. In the individual, a high degree of specialization can lead to a parochial narrowness of vision. When a profession divides into subspecialties, it can break apart an earlier wholeness of experience and understanding. Thus people sometimes yearn for the general practitioner of earlier days, who is thought to have concerned himself with the 'whole patient' and they sometimes accuse contemporary specialists of treating particular illnesses in isolation from the rest of the patient's life experience. Further, as a practice becomes more repetitive and routine, and as knowing-in-practice becomes increasingly tacit and spontaneous, the practitioner may miss important opportunities to think about what he is doing. He may find that, like the younger children in the block-balancing experiment, he is drawn into patterns of error which he cannot correct. And if he learns, as often happens, to be selectively inattentive to phenomena that do not fit the categories of his knowing-in-action, then he may suffer from boredom or 'burn-out' and afflict his clients with the consequences of his narrowness and rigidity. When this happens, the practitioner has 'over-learned' what he knows.

A practitioner's reflection can serve as a corrective to over-learning. Through reflection, he can surface and criticize the tacit understandings that have grown up around the repetitive experiences of a specialized practice, and can make new sense of the situations of uncertainty or uniqueness which he may allow himself to experience.

Practitioners do reflect on their knowing-in-practice. Sometimes, in the relative tranquility of a postmortem, they think back on a project they have undertaken, a situation they have lived through, and they explore the understandings they have brought to their handling of the case. They may do this in a mood of idle speculation, or in a deliberate effort to prepare themselves for future cases.

But they may also reflect on practice while they are in the midst of it. Here they reflect-in-action, but the meaning of this term needs now to be considered in terms of the complexity of knowing-in-practice.

A practitioner's reflection-in-action may not be very rapid. It is bounded by the 'action-present', the zone of time in which action can still make a difference to the situation. The action-present may stretch over minutes, hours, days, or even weeks or months, depending on the pace of activity and the situational boundaries that are characteristic of the practice. Within the give-and-take of courtroom behavior, for example, a lawyer's reflection-in-action may take place in seconds; but when the context is that of an antitrust case that drags on over years, reflection-in-action may proceed in leisurely fashion over the course of several months. An orchestra conductor may think of a single performance as a unit of practice, but in other sense a whole season is his unit. The pace and duration of episodes of reflection-in-action vary with the pace and duration of the situations of practice.

When a practitioner reflects in and on his practice, the possible objects of his reflection are as varied as the kinds of phenomena before him and the systems of knowing-in-practice which he brings to them. He may reflect on the tacit norms and appreciations which underlie a judgment, or on the strategies and theories implicit in a pattern of behavior. He may reflect on the feeling for a situation which has led him adopt a particular course of action, on the way in which he has framed the problem he is trying to solve, or on the role he has constructed for himself within a larger institutional context.

Reflection-in-action, in these several modes, is central to the art through which practitioners sometimes cope with the troublesome 'divergent' situations of practice.

When the phenomenon at hand eludes the ordinary categories of knowledge-in-practice, presenting itself as unique or unstable, the practitioner may surface and criticize his initial understanding of the phenomenon, construct a new description of it, and test the new description by an on-the-spot experiment. Sometimes he arrives at a new theory of the phenomenon by articulating a feeling he has about it.

Notes

1. For example, Throw, S. (1977) *One L: Inside Account of Life in the First Year at Harvard Law School*, G. P. Putnam's Sons, New York.
2. See, for example, *The New Professionals* (Gross and Osterman, eds), Simon and Schuster, 1972, New York.
3. Barbel Inhelder and Annette Karmiloff-Smith, 'If you want to get ahead, get a theory. *Cognition*, 3(3), 195–212.

References

Hughes, E. (1959) The study of occupations. In *Sociology Today* (Merton, R. K. Broom, L. and Cottrell. L. S., eds), Basic Books, New York

Illich, I. (1970) *A Celebration of Awareness: A Call for Institutional Revolution* Doubleday, Garden City, N.Y.

Wilensky, H. L. (1964) The professionalization of everyone? *American Journal of Sociology*, **70**, 137–158.

Chapter 30

Profession of medicine: a study of the sociology of applied knowledge

Eliot Freidson

Introduction

This book presents an extended analysis of a profession. As its title implies, emphasis is on both sides of the meaning of the word – 'profession' as a special kind of occupation, and 'profession' as an avowal or promise. As I shall try to show in the chapters that follow, it is useful to think of a profession as an occupation which has assumed a dominant position in a division of labor, so that it gains control over the determination of the substance of its own work. Unlike most occupations, it is autonomous or self-directing. The occupation sustains this special status by its persuasive profession of the extraordinary trustworthiness of its members. The trustworthiness it professes naturally includes ethicality and also knowledgeable skill. In fact, the profession claims to be the most reliable authority on the nature of the reality it deals with. When its characteristic work lies in the attempt to deal with the problems people bring to it, the profession develops its own independent conception of those problems and tries to manage both clients and problems in its own way. In developing its own 'professional' approach, the profession changes the definition and shape of problems as experienced and interpreted by the layman. The layman's problem is re-created as it is managed – a new social reality is created by the profession. It is the autonomous position of the profession in society which permits it to re-create the layman's world.

From these observations it is possible to identify two major problems for analysis presented to the sociologist by the profession. First, one must understand how the profession's self-direction or autonomy is developed, organized, and maintained. Second, one must understand the relation of the profession's knowledge and procedures to professional organization as such and to the lay world. The first is a problem of social organization; the second a problem of the sociology of knowledge.[1] These are the problems I shall attempt to deal with in my analysis of one of the major professions of modern society – medicine.

Medicine, however, is not merely one of the major professions of our time. Among the traditional professions established in the European universities of the Middle Ages, it alone has developed a systematic connection with science and technology. Unlike law and the ministry, which have no important connection with modern science and technology, medicine has developed into a very complex division of labor, organizing an increasingly large number of technical and service workers around its central task of diagnosing and managing the ills of mankind. Too, it has surpassed the others in prominence. Since the production of goods and other forms of real property are far less of a problem to postindustrial societies than is the welfare of their citizens, since welfare has come to be defined in wholly secular terms, and since the notion of illness has itself been expanded to include many more facets of human welfare than it did in earlier times, medicine has displaced the law and the ministry from their once dominant positions. Indeed, in one way or another, the profession of medicine, not that of law or the ministry or any other, has come to be the prototype upon which occupations seeking a privileged status today are modeling their aspirations. The better we understand medicine, then, the better we will be able to understand the problems that may be posed by the professionalization of the key service workers of the welfare state.

The flaw of professional autonomy

Autonomy is the prize sought by virtually all occupational groups, for it represents freedom from direction from others, freedom to perform one's work the way one desires. In industrial work, the restriction of output represents crudely the efforts of workers to exercise control over their work and thereby gain a degree of autonomy. Similar efforts are found among all who work for others – among waitresses, physicians, students, soldiers, professors, or whatever.[2] However, only those who advance the claim to be professionals assert that their efforts to control the terms and content of work are justified because of the benefit accruing to those clients they work with or on. The freedom they ask for is the same as others: they ask to determine their own working hours, work load, compensation, the kind of work they do, and the way they do it. Unlike lesser workers, however, professionals claim that self-interest is not at issue; they claim to serve humanity before self. But unlike mere amateur humanitarians, they claim that their esoteric expertise is such that only they are able to determine what is wrong with humanity, how it may best be served, and at what price. This claim is what makes professions special, and it is what justifies the autonomy distinguishing them from other occupations. At the heart of most questions of social policy bearing on the professions lies this central question of autonomy, for it bears on who may determine what the problem is, how the problem is to be dealt with, and what price is to be paid for dealing with it.

It is important to understand what professional autonomy is. It is always limited to some degree by the political power which it needs to create and protect it, and those limits vary from time to and from place to place.[3] Structurally, the autonomy of the consulting profession, when it is great, is an officially created *organized autonomy*, not the autonomy one might gain by evading attention, by being inconspicuous and unimportant. Second, that organized autonomy is not merely freedom from the competition or regulation of other workers, but in the case of such a profession as medicine if not that of less well-established claimants, it is also freedom to regulate other occupations. Where we find one occupation with organized autonomy in a division of labor, it dominates the others. Immune from legitimate regulation or evaluation by other occupations, it can itself legitimately evaluate and order the work of others. By its position in the division of labor we can designate it as a *dominant profession*. Third, insofar as it regulates itself and is not subject to the evaluation and regulation of others, it also *educates itself*. This is to say, its educational or training institutions tend to be self-sufficient and segregated from others – professional schools with their own independent resources and faculties. Those educated for the profession get their training in such schools largely protected from contact with faculties and students from other schools. And finally, when it is a consulting rather than scholarly profession, having the right to regulate its own work also implies that it has been granted the legitimate right to in some way *regulate the clientele* with which it works, rather than having to be finely responsive to the clientele's notions of its needs, like a mere salesman. Thus, the characteristics of professional autonomy are such as to give professions a splendid isolation, indeed, the opportunity to develop a protected insularity without peer among occupations lacking the same privileges.

This is the critical flaw in professional autonomy: by allowing and encouraging the development of self-sufficient institutions, it develops and maintains in the profession a self-deceiving view of the objectivity and reliability of its knowledge and of the virtues of its members. Furthermore, it encourages the profession to see itself as the sole possessor of knowledge and virtue, to be somewhat suspicious of the technical and moral capacity of other occupations, and to be at best patronizing and at worst contemptuous of its clientele. Protecting the profession from the demands of interaction on a free and equal basis with those in the world outside, its autonomy leads the profession to so distinguish its own virtues from those outside as to be unable to even perceive the need for, let alone undertake, the self-regulation it promises.

I do not mean to deprecate either the real knowledge or the intent of the profession at large. Both its knowledge and its intent are admirable. The problem is that once given its special status, the profession quite naturally forms a perspective of its own, a perspective all the more distorted and narrow by its source in a status answerable to no one but itself. Once the profession forms such a self-sustaining perspective, protected from others' perspectives, insulated from the necessity of justifying itself to outsiders, it cannot reasonably be expected to see itself and its mission with clear eyes, nor can it be reasonably expected to assume the perspective of its clientele. If it cannot assume the perspective of its clientele, how can it pretend to serve it well? Its very autonomy has led to insularity and a mistaken arrogance about its mission in the world. Consulting professions are not baldly self-interested unions struggling for their resources at the expense of others and of the public interest. Rather, they are well-meaning groups which are protected from the public by their organized autonomy and at the same time protected from their own honest self-scrutiny by their sanctimonious myths of the inherently superior qualities of themselves as professionals – of their knowledge and of their work. Their autonomy has created their narrow perspective and their self-deceiving views of themselves and their work, their conviction that they know best what humanity needs. It is time that their autonomy be tempered.

Historically, the profession's development of a valuable body of knowledge, pure and applied, seems to have required protection from the urgent ignorance of its clientele, the mischief of low-class competitors, and other forces destructive to an infant discipline. The profession had to be protected against the very consequences of its prime reason for being – its dependence upon a clientele which is prejudiced about what it wants and needs at a time when knowledge of how to treat wants and needs had no firm foundation. Freed from trade and competition, supported by the state, institutionalized, it was able to develop its own foundation for knowledge – its own concepts and science – independently of its clientele. So protected, it was also able to develop the capacity to nourish itself, like science and scholarship, pretty much on its own: it developed a body of colleague opinion and colleague-dependent practices. So sustained, it made enormous strides in knowledge and technique. Without its autonomy, medicine may never have made the great discoveries of the past century. But advances in knowledge are one thing, and those in practice are quite another.

No one is nostalgic for the bleeding and purging of nineteenth-century medical treatment: what we have now is patently better. But as the nostalgia for the no doubt mythical GP of the past indicates, the *practice* of medicine has not half so obviously advanced. It is precisely in practice – in the designation of disease, in the management of treatment, in the economic organization of medical care, and in the social organization of medical care – where medicine has not advanced. *While the profession's autonomy seems to have facilitated the improvement of scientific knowledge about disease and its treatment, it seems to have impeded the improvement of the social modes of applying that knowledge.* It is precisely in applying knowledge to human affairs, I submit, where extensive professional autonomy is justified neither morally nor functionally. It is not justified morally because I believe that human beings, even if laymen, have a right to determine what their own problems are and to have a voice in how they are to be managed. It is not justified functionally, I have argued, because it leads the profession to be blind to its own shortcomings and unable to regulate its practices adequately. From these conclusions follows the question of how the application of knowledge to human affairs by professional experts should be organized in the public interest.

Notes

1. Berger, P. L. and Luckmann, T. (1966) *The Social Construction of Reality*, Doubleday and Co., Garden City, New York, and particularly Holzner, B. (1968) *Reality Construction in Society*, Schenkman Publishing Co., Cambridge, Mass.
2. Perhaps the most pertinent general comments on this phenomenon have been made by Hughes, E. C. (1958) *Men and Their Work*, The Free Press, New York.
3. Gilb, C. L. (1966) *Hidden Hierarchies: The Professions and Government*, Harper and Row, New York, has made a major contribution to the political analysis of professions.

Reprinted by permission of The University of Chicago Press, Chicago. Eliot Freidson (1988) *Profession of Medicine: A Study of the Sociology of Applied Knowledge*, University of Chicago Press, Chicago, pp.xvii–xviii, 368–371.

Chapter 31

Teachers, nurses, social workers

Amitai Etzioni

This book attempts to increase sociological knowledge about the *professions* by focusing on a group of new professions whose claim to the status of doctors and lawyers is neither fully established nor fully desired. Lacking a better term, we shall refer to those professions as *semi*-professions. Their training is shorter, their status is less legitimated, their right to privileged communication less established, there is less of a specialized body of knowledge, and they have less autonomy from supervision or societal control than 'the' professions.[1] We use the term semi-professions without any derogatory implications. Other terms which have been suggested are either more derogatory in their connotations (e.g. sub-professions or pseudo-professions) or much less established and communicative (e.g. 'heteronomous' professions, a concept used by Max Weber).[2]

By focusing on semi-professions, we also enter willy-nilly three other areas of sociological study: that of *organizations*, in which practically all semi-professionals are employed; that of *demography*, because the large majority of the labor force we deal with is female and its demographic attributes significantly affect our subject; and that of *conflict analysis*, because – as we shall see – the normative principles and cultural values of professions, organizations, and female employment are not compatible. Hence this may also be seen as a study of societal sources of tension, adaptations, and their limitations.

An intriguing policy recommendation arises from the following analysis: as we see it, a significant segment of the semi-professions aspire to a full-fledged professional status and sustain a professional self-image, despite the fact that they themselves are often aware that they do not deserve such a status, and despite the fact that they objectively do not qualify for reasons that will be discussed. One reason, it seems, they aspire to professional status is because the only alternative status is that of the non-professional employee, specifically the white collar and blue collar worker. As semi-professionals see it, they obviously are 'more' than secretaries, salesgirls, or office clerks. Unable to find a niche between these white collar statuses and the professions, and not wishing to be identified with the lower-status group, they cling to the higher aspiration of being a full professional.[3]

This unrealistic aspiration is not without cost. The costs are those typically associated with persons seeking to pass for what they are not: a guilty feeling for floating a status claim without sufficient base and a rejection by those who hold the status legitimately. The semi-professionals' efforts to change themselves, more fully to live up to the claim floated, generate a major source of tensions because there are several powerful, societal limitations on the extent to which these occupations can be fully professionalized. Various rationalizations are provided to justify continued attempts to reach the unreachable; for example, semi-professional ideologues argue that, since the line marking professional from the semi-professional is a murky one, how is one to tell who is 'in' and who is not? (The correct observation is that although the borderlines are not sharply delineated, the parties involved are not prevented from recognizing those who are manifestly, on several accounts, on one side or the other.) Finally, as in other such status groups, the desire to pass for a higher-status group produces pressures which split the group into those closer to the 'passing' limit and those more remote, thus weakening both subgroupings in the societal give-and-take.

Memo to participants[4]

ADMINISTRATIVE VS. PROFESSIONAL AUTHORITY

Administration assumes a power hierarchy. Without a clear ordering of higher and lower in rank, in which the higher in rank have more power than the lower ones and hence can control and coordinate the latter's activities, the basic principle of administration is violated; the organization ceases to be a coordinated tool. However knowledge is largely an individual property; unlike other organizational means, it cannot be transferred from one person to another by decree. Creativity is basically individual and can only to a very limited degree be ordered and coordinated by the superior in rank. Even the application of knowledge is basically an individual act, at least in the sense that the individual professional has the ultimate responsibility for his professional decision. The surgeon has to decide whether or not to operate. Students of the professions have pointed out that the autonomy granted to professionals who are basically responsible to their consciences (though they may be censured by their peers and in extreme cases by the courts) is necessary for effective professional work. Only if immune from ordinary social pressures and free to innovate, to experiment, to take risks without the usual social repercussions of failure, can a professional carry out his work effectively. It is this highly individualized principle which is diametrically opposed to the very essence of the organizational principle of control and coordination by superiors – i.e. the principle of administrative authority. In other words the ultimate justification for a professional act is that it is, to the best of the professional's knowledge, the right act. He might consult his colleagues before he acts but the decision is his. If he errs, he still will be defended by his peers. The ultimate justification of an administrative act, however, is that it is in line with the organization's rules and regulations, and that it has been approved – directly or by implication – by a superior rank.

THE SEMI-PROFESSIONAL ORGANIZATIONS

The basis of professional authority is knowledge, and the relationship between administrative and professional authority is largely affected by the amount and kind of knowledge the professional has. The relationship described above holds largely for organizations in which professional authority is based on long training (five years or more), when questions of life and death and/or privileged communication are involved, and when knowledge is created or applied rather than communicated. When professional authority is based on shorter training, involves values other than life or privacy, and covers the communication of knowledge, we find that it is related to administrative authority in a different way. First, professional work here has less autonomy; that is, it is more controlled by those higher in ranks and less subject to the discretion of the professional than in full-fledged professional organizations, though it is still characterized by greater autonomy than blue- or white-collar work. Second, the semi-professionals often have skills and personality traits more compatible with administration, especially since the qualities required for communication of knowledge are more like those needed for administration than those required for the creation, and to a degree, application of knowledge. Hence these organizations are run much more frequently by the semi-professionals themselves than by others.

The most typical semi-professional organization is the primary school. The social-work agency is the other major semi-professional organization. A semi-professional sector, rather than full-fledged organization, is found in the nursing service of hospitals.

The goal of the primary school is largely to communicate rather than to create or apply knowledge. The training of its professionals on the average falls well below five years of professional education. The social-work agency is less typical since it applies knowledge but is semi-professional in the fairly short training involved, in the fact that no questions of life and death are involved, and that privileged communication is not strictly maintained (e.g., vis-á-vis the courts). Among social workers, the longer the training and the more professional the orientation, the greater the tendency to orient to the social-work 'profession' and not to the agency (the organization).

Nurses apply knowledge, but their training is much shorter than doctors, and the question of what therapy to administer is concentrated in the hands of the doctors; in this sense the nursing service is not directly related to professional decisions of life or death, although nurses have much more effect on it than teacher or social worker, and in this sense are less typical semi-professionals.

The work of these three groups has less autonomy than that of the professions discussed earlier. Their work day is tightly regulated by the cases where performance is not visible – e.g., in the case of social work because it is done in the field, or teaching because it is conducted in the classroom – detailed reporting on performance is required, and supervisors are allowed to make surprise visits to check on work being done. Nurses are directly observed and corrected by doctors and by superior nurses. Such supervision is not characteristic of the mechanisms of control found in the full-fledged professions. Inspectors are not widely used to drop in on a professor's classroom to check his teaching, especially not in the better universities. No doctor will be asked to report to an administrative superior on why he carried out his medical duties in the way he did or stand corrected by him. External examinations used in schools to check on teachers as well as students are very rare in universities.

Furthermore, much of the supervision is done by people who are themselves semi-professionals or professionals. Almost all school principals have been teachers; few have been recruited directly from training courses for school administration, and almost none are lay administrators. Virtually all social-work supervisors have been social workers. Few have assumed supervisory positions early in their careers and again almost none are lay administrators. The same is true of nursing. Thus while the semi-professionals are more supervised than the professionals, supervision is more often conducted by their own kind.

Some de-professionalization occurs in these organizations, as it does in full professional ones. Those teachers who are less committed to children, that is, the least 'client-oriented', are more administration conscious, and more likely to become principals. Few principals, unless the school is particularly small, keep teaching other than in a very limited, ritualistic way. Similarly, the social-work supervisors tend to be more organization-oriented, less client-oriented even in their field-work days, and they see few cases, if any, once they move up in the hierarchy.

Not all the differences between professional and semi-professional organizations can be traced to the difference in the nature of the professional authority. Part of the problem is due to the fact that the typical professional is a male where the typical semi-professional is a female. Despite the effects of emancipation, women on the average are more amenable to administrative control than men. It seems that on the average, women are also less conscious of organizational status and more submissive in this context than men. They also, on the average, have fewer years of higher education than men, and their acceptance into the medical profession or university teaching is sharply limited. It is difficult to determine if the semi-professional organizations have taken the form they have because of the high percentage of female employees, or if they recruit females because of organizational reasons; in all likelihood these factors support each other.

Whatever the deeper reasons, the fact is that the professional and administrative authority are here related in a different way from professional organizations. Control through organization regulations and superiors is much more extensive, though not as extensive as that of blue- or white-collar workers, and it is done mainly by semi-professionals themselves. As in professional organizations, the articulation of the two modes of authority is not without strain. Here, the semi-professional subordinates tend to adopt the full-fledged professions as their reference group in the sense that they view themselves as full-fledged professionals and feel that they should be given more discretion and be less controlled. Teachers resent the 'interference' of principals and many principals try to minimize it. Social workers rebel against their supervisors. Nurses often feel that they are more experienced than the young intern or more knowledgeable than the older supervisor, and hence should not be expected to submit themselves to the command of either. [*End of reprinted material.*]

Notes

1. On the relevant dimensions, see Greenwood, E. (1962) Attributes of a profession. *In Man,*

Work, and Society (Nosow, S. and Form, W. H., eds), Basic Books, New York, pp.207–218, and Goode, W. J. (1957) Community within a community: the professions. *American Sociological Review*, 22, 194–200. On the dynamics involved, see Goode's (1960) Encroachment, charlatanism, and the emerging professions: psychology, sociology, and medicine. *American Sociological Review*, 25, 902–914; Wilensky, H. L. The professionalization of everyone? *American Journal of Sociology*, 70(2), 137–158.

2. Weber, M. (1947) *The Theory of Social and Economic Organization* (trans. A. M. Henderson and Talcott Parsons), Free Press, New York, p.148. See also Scott, W. R. (1965) Reactions to supervision in a heteronomous professional organization. *Administrative Science Quarterly*, June, 65–81.

3. On this points, see Leonard, P. (1966) Social workers and bureaucracy. *New Society*, 2 June, 12–13, and Cohen, W. J. (1966) What every social workers should know about political action. *Social Work*, 11(3) 3–11.

4. The bulk of this memorandum is taken from Etzioni, A. (1964) *Modern Organizations*, pp. 76 ff., © 1964. Reprinted by permission of Prentice-Hall, Inc., Englewood Cliffs, N.J.

Chapter 32

The new managerialism and professionalism in nursing
Michael Carpenter

...The further one travels from the ward the less one can talk of 'nursing' or even 'nursing management', but rather management which applies the techniques derived from aspects of capitalist rationality to an area which just happens to be nursing. In the future the new managerial élite may increasingly feel themselves to be managers first and nurses second, or simply managers who are ex-nurses. By contrast, under traditional definitions, the matrons of the traditional élite were always nurses first. Reorganization carries these tendencies much further. The teaching hospitals are brought firmly within the same management structure which can only narrow the social distance between them and other types of hospitals so characteristic of the traditional system.

The inclusion of nurses as full members of the consensus teams at district level and above will create strong pressures towards the adoption of managerial rather than nursing reference groups. For example, the District Nursing Officer is able to include himself or herself in the same group as the District Administrator in order to obtain personal advancement in ways simply not open to a Matron in relation to a Group Secretary. In this the new structure continues and amplifies a feature of all previous structures. To achieve any kind of meaningful equality with other élite groups on the health service, nurses have had to remove themselves from the sphere of clinical decision-making and enter the political sphere. This is a contradiction the medical profession had not yet had to face. It has used its dominance in the clinical sphere as a lever to maintain much of its political power within the reorganized NHS, even though it was only retained by granting, for the first time' formal equality to other groups on the management teams.[1]

The traditional élite always maintained the pretence that in pursuing such a strategy of control outside the clinical sphere they were attempting not merely to further their own sectional interests but to uplift the profession as a whole. To date the newer élite based on the new managerialism has been no different from its predecessors in this respect, though it has been prepared to use more activist methods. Whilst the traditional élite typically suppressed most forms of activity by subordinates, the new élite has on occasions promoted its expression within clearly defined limits. During the Rcns 'Raise the Roof' campaign at the tail end of the 1960s the emergent élite sponsored considerable militancy by student nurses on a pay claim largely designed to widen differentials. This was said to be necessary to attract good recruits and in order to create a new opportunity structure. However the new equality with other élite groups does not entail an uplifting of nursing as a whole. It is an equality won by virtue of the élite's domination over the nursing labour force, an equality which poses no real threat to medical dominance in the clinical sphere.

The new professionalism?

Such factors have helped to generate considerable disillusion with Salmon at the lower levels of the nursing hierarchy. Amongst trained nurses at ward sister and nursing officer level there has been increasing disquiet at the effects of the full-blooded managerialist solution. 'Inbred attitudes' may play a part, but equally important is the desire of many of these disaffected elements for a clinical solution to their status problem. The Salmon reforms overemphasized the importance of managerial changes in job content to the detriment of clinical changes. It created a formal structure in which power, prestige and remuneration increase with distance from the point of patient contact. Yet with increasing specialization and advances in medical knowledge nursing administrators are sometimes embarrassingly ignorant of the complexities of the ward situation and this tends to lead ward level staff to resent what appears to them to be a power structure which does not accord with this situation. As Manson (1977) argues, there appears to be increasing resentment against interference from senior nursing managers. It is not so much that this interference is new, for the power of the matron at crucial times depended on just that. Nevertheless, a 'custom and practice' of considerable ward-sister autonomy had grown up over the years, which Salmon breached in very important respects.

It is undoubtedly the case that, at these levels, the professional model is being revived. The *ad hoc* growth of postgraduate nurse training, to some extent formalized by the formation of a coordinating Joint Board of Clinical Nursing Studies in 1970, is an important factor behind this revival. Historical figures in nursing history such as Mrs Bedford Fenwick, who was one of the militantly professional nursing reformers, are being 'rehabilitated' (Hector, 1973). The proposals of the Briggs Report on nurse education pose these questions most directly, not by overturning 'managerialism', but by adding other clinical avenues of advancement (Report of the Committee on Nursing, 1972). Briggs argues for the ending of the SEN/SRN division in nurse training in favour of a series of modules built around a basic nursing course, followed in Colleges of Nursing independent of service organizations. The major insight of the report is its recognition of nursing diversity, and it represents in many ways a bold attempt to devise a training scheme to cope with this fact. It tries to erase the status distinction between nursing fields that dates from the 1919 Act by making all fields into 'options' and displacing general training from its former pre-eminent position. Ironically, some of the most vocal opposition to the report has come from nurses in fields previously defined as low status. They seem to be worried that old distinctions will continue in practice, because students will not choose to specialize in 'inferior' options. Under the old system, lack of easy mobility from one sector to another created an almost 'captive' labour force.

The most important proposal of the Briggs Report for the new professionalism is by no means novel: the greater separation of education from service needs. Although not novel, the forces favouring some kind of separation are much greater than in the past. However, implementation would, in the short run at least, be quite costly, in that far greater numbers of auxiliary nurses would have to be recruited to replace student labour. Such a separation between 'clinical' and 'basic' nursing would represent a final break with traditional nursing values. No longer would the performance of basic nursing tasks be seen as noble or worthy in its own right, but as something to be performed only so long as is necessary to learn how to do it. Because more complex tasks take longer to learn than others, more prestige attaches to them. Furthermore, the creation of separate schools would aid the development of an ideology of professionalism. There has, for many years, been a tendency for the 'cosmopolitanism' of the school to come into conflict with the 'localism'[2] of the hospital or service agency. The creation of a group of largely autonomous nurse educators would widen this rift. Under the traditional system, it will be recalled, the authority of the matron seemed to embody both the qualities of the local and the cosmopolitan. The roles of administrator and educator were originally combined, and have subsequently become differentiated.[3]

Because of the economic crisis, Briggs is unlikely to be implemented, except in a diluted form. Nevertheless a general trend of new rifts between managers and clinicians are emerging, as well as the now established rifts between managers and wage workers. These are not hard and fast categories, except at the extreme. The wage worker model fits the nursing auxiliary most, but also fits the large numbers of staff nurses and ward sisters who would not call themselves 'career minded'.[4] As yet, there are few 'pure' clinicians among trained nurses. There are, however, those ward sisters who combine in varying degrees clinical and managerial responsibilities, and those above them in the hierarchy whose responsibilities are almost entirely managerial.

In the mid-1960s managerialism was very much in the ascendent. The new administrative posts suddenly provided an outlet for frustrated elements at ward level. Social mobility on such a scale could only be a once-and-for-all phenomenon. For those passed over, and for new generations of trained staff, career advancement up a non-clinical hierarchy will not be such an open possibility. During the late 1960s there was almost an excess of posts over applicants. In future the situation might be reversed, especially if larger numbers of graduates are recruited. In any case, higher unemployment and the fact that traditional outlets for middle class girls, such as teaching, are becoming much more insecure may mean that nursing will be able to gain the kinds of recruits that élite members have always wanted. If there are not enough non-clinical posts to meet their aspirations it will hardly escape their notice that many present incumbents are people who got there primarily because there was so little competition.

The complex restructuring of the labour force and the decline in traditional forms of leadership are therefore dialectically linked, making the claim by the new managerialists to occupational leadership much weaker. It will not, however, necessarily lead to nurse managers making a complete break from nursing. The resulting vacuum has in part been filled by renewed clinical aspirations by some elements. It has also led to the rapid growth of trade unionism among nurses. Emergent trade union consciousness was closely linked to the restructuring of the labour force. Trade unions were swelled by the growing army of auxiliary and assistant nurses who, whatever their predispositions, were excluded from the professional organizations. They were joined by increasing numbers of rank-and-file trained nurses, who became disenchanted by the careerist ethos of professional associations and their apparent lack of concern with the problems nurses faced as workers. Sometimes this combined with external factors, such as in 1974 when frustration mounted over the effect of successive incomes policies. As a result, it seems almost certain that trade unions have more nurses in membership than the professional associations, even allowing for some degree of joint membership.[5]

Notes

1. As Celia Davies (1972) notes (in Professionals in organisations: some preliminary observations in hospital consultants. *Sociological Review*, pp.553–67), the growth in the complexity of the health services, although in theory making doctors more dependent on other occupations and lay management, in fact strengthens their power and position because it is they who are legally responsible for patient care.
2. As introduced into occupational sociology by Gouldner, A. (1957–58) in Cosmopolitans and locals: toward an analysis of latent social roles – I, *Administrative Science Quarterly*, 2, 281–306.
3. This is in marked contrast to the historical development of nursing in the USA. For a discussion of the implications, see Glaser, W. A. (1966) Nursing leadership and policy: some cross-national comparisons. In *The Nursing Profession* (Davis, F., ed), John Wiley, New York.
4. The postal survey of the Briggs Report, op. cit., showed that many respondents, trained and untrained, were not actively seeking promotion (Table 45, paras 526–529).
5. The response of the Rcn to this fact is to point out that many union members are auxiliary nurses. Given a unified bargaining structure this is hardly relevant. However, it is by no

means certain that the professional associations now have a majority of trained nurses. Significant sections of their membership include students and retired nurses. At the time of writing, the Rcn is in the process of seeking registration as a trade union. Whether in the long run this will mean more than just a formal change in status for instrumental purposes, remains to be seen.

References

Hector, W. (1973) *The Work of Mrs. Bedford Fenwick and the Rise of Professional Nursing*, RCN, London

Manson, T. (1977) Management, the professions and the unions: a social analysis of change in the NHS. In *Health and the Division of Labour* (Stacey, M., Reid, M., Heath, C. and Dingwall, R., eds), Croom Helm, London

Report of the Committee on Nursing (Briggs Report) (1972) HMSO, London

Reprinted from Michael Carpenter (1977) The new managerialism and professionalism in nursing. In *Health and the Division of Labour* (Stacey, M., Reid, M, Heath, C. and Dingwall, R.), Croom Helm, London/Prodist, New York, pp.184–188, 192, 193 (out of print).

Chapter 33

Sexual division of labour: the case of nursing

Eva Gamarnikow

This paper is concerned with the structural determinants of the sexual division of labour, with particular reference to the occupational structure of nineteenth- and early twentieth-century nursing. The period I shall be looking at stretches from 1860, the year in which Florence Nightingale opened the Nightingale Fund School of Nursing at St Thomas's Hospital (a traditional landmark in the history of modern nursing), to 1923 when the profession elected its first General Nursing Council. I shall argue that the patriarchal character of the sexual division of labour manifests itself in the nursing profession in a number of interrelated ways. First, in the total operation of health care, nursing occupies a role in subordination to medicine, in that it is the medical profession which possesses the sole right of decision as to who is to be defined as a patient. This subordination structures the nurse–doctor–patient relationship, which comes to take on the ideological resonances of power relations between men, women and children within the patriarchal family – the doctor being the incumbent of the 'rule of the father'. The female dominance of the nursing profession and the male dominance of medicine are of obvious relevance to the situation, the implications of which none the less obtain in the 'anomalous' instances of women doctors and, particularly, male nurses – although in such cases the tensions and contradictions in the situation are perhaps more likely to surface in the doctor–nurse relationship. Moreover, in the period under consideration, the moral traits of the 'good nurse' were evidently seen within the profession itself as identical with the characteristics desirable in a 'good woman'. Finally, I shall argue that the character of nursing as a profession for 'good women', together with the patriarchal and familial character of authority relations within the health care professions, meant that many aspects of the nurse's work became identifiable with domestic labour; but that because of the claim of nursing to some professional status, certain tasks commonly defined as within the province of domestic labour –

cleaning and 'hygiene' in particular – come to occupy a central, but at the same time a problematic, position.

... biologistic explanations treat the sexual division of labour as a natural division, springing from or ultimately rooted in reproductive functions. This 'naturalism' is seen to underpin women's labour in both the family and the wage sector, because both are characterized by sex specific task and job allocation. The ideology of naturalism, therefore, represents labour processes, or parts of labour processes, as specifically 'feminine' or 'masculine'. This is achieved either by direct reference to biology (motherhood, for example), or by drawing analogies between such apparently biologically determined activities as motherhood and particular types of work – such as, say, nursing which is frequently defined as 'maternal' caring for the sick. Biological determinism, or naturalism, underpins technological determinism, which locates divisions in the labour process in terms of technological imperatives rather than relations of production. In the particular case of health care as a labour process a distinction is made in this frame of reference between caring and curing tasks and functions which are allocated to nurses and doctors respectively because they seem to coincide with 'natural' biological functions (Thorner, 1955; Schulman, 1958; Maclean, 1974).

The sexual division of labour treats all women as potential wives-mothers – that is, as dependent on men – precisely because they are biological females. The ideologically implicated nature of this mode of work and task allocation lies in its emphasis on sex differences rather than on, say, human similarities (Pedinielli-Plaza, 1977); and the priority granted to biological differences rather than human similarities provides a focus and a legitimation for hierarchical differentiation between men and women. The sexual division of labour as ideology is articulated at the point of differentiation and hierarchization in the patriarchal labour process.

Thus the sexual division of labour identifies *all* women as a separate category of worker and integrates into patriarchy women who are not married and therefore not subject to direct patriarchal exploitation within the family. As a mode of work organization, the sexual division of labour divides all discrete work processes into male and female tasks and jobs. As a patriarchal structure, it subordinates – either directly (secretarial work) or indirectly (low-paid women's work in industry) – tasks defined as female to those defined as male. The 'maleness' or 'femaleness' of a task is thus not inherent in the operation itself but in the ideological identification and distribution of tasks. The sexual division of labour then situates individuals in jobs and designates jobs as sex specific. This is an ideological operation specific to patriarchy. It is not an *ex post facto* description of occupational sex ratios. Thus it is possible for some women to enter 'male' jobs and vice versa without these jobs losing their ideological designation as sex specific: rather, this becomes an individualized act, frequently resulting in contradictory and difficult work relations – female executives and male nurses being cases in point.

==========

The pivotal interprofessional relationship within health care is that between the nurse and doctor. However, the division of labour between these two occupations is not primarily a technical one. The dividing line between their tasks is flexible, both historically and across the range of institutions in any given period. Rather, the division of labour must be located in the division of health care into two spheres of competence, based on unequal interprofessional relations. That this division was resolved into a sexual division of labour can be understood in terms of the fact that it was women who entered nursing. Professional power relations were overdetermined by the patriarchal relations implied in the sexual division of labour: hence the subordination of nursing – whose tasks were defined and practices limited – to medicine. The justification for this division of labour in health care drew upon existing representations around 'naturalism' within patriarchal ideology.

Nineteenth-century nursing reforms had two aims. The first was to establish a single stratified occupation with responsibility for patient care and the organization and management of nursing; and the other was to introduce this occupation into existing health care institutions or to reform nursing arrangements to accord with the Nightingale blueprint. The growth of reformed nursing, therefore, also brought with it the organisationally autonomous nursing hierarchy, located in a separate department:

> Vest the whole responsibility for nursing internal management, for discipline and training (if there is to be a Training School) of nurses in one female head of the nursing staff. ... The Matron (Superintendent) should be responsible to the governor of the infirmary alone for the efficient discharge of her duties; and the Nurses should be responsible to the Matron alone for the discharge of their duties (Nightingale, 1874, pp.5 and 9).

Moreover, this autonomous nursing hierarchy was responsible for the training and professional socialization of future nurses. The occupational hierarchy was constituted as a training hierarchy:

==========

Whatever the medical fears, the organizational autonomy of nursing hid its actual position of occupational dependence and subordination: nursing organization in effect supervised and taught a form of nursing care which established and maintained the hierarchical divisions between nursing and medicine, being based on the structure of the nurse–doctor relation which subordinated nursing to medicine in all matters defined as 'medical' by medicine itself. The divisions mapped out spheres of competence which made nursing practice dependent on medical intervention.

Nightingale entrusted nursing with two functions, 'nursing the room', or hygiene, and assisting the doctor:

> Nursing is performed usually by women, under scientific heads – physicians and surgeons. Nursing is putting us in the best possible conditions for Nature to restore or to preserve health. The physician or surgeon prescribes these conditions – the nurse carries them out. .... Sickness or disease is Nature's way of getting rid of the effects of conditions which have interfered with health. It is Nature's attempt to cure – we have to help her. Partly, perhaps mainly, upon nursing must depend whether Nature succeeds or fails in her attempt to cure by sickness. Nursing is therefore to help the patient to live. ... Nursing is an art, and an art requiring an organized practical and scientific training. For nursing is the skilled servant of medicine, surgery and hygiene. ... Nursing proper means, besides giving the medicines and stimulants prescribed, or applying the surgical dressing and other remedies ordered: – 1. The providing, the proper use of, fresh air, especially at night, that is ventilation, of warmth and coolness. 2. The securing of the health of the sickroom or ward, which includes light, cleanliness of floors and walls, of bed, bedding and utensils. 3. Personal cleanliness of patient and nurse, quiet, variety and cheerfulness. 4. The administering and sometimes preparation of diet (food and drink). 5. The application of remedies. In other words, all that is wanted to enable Nature to set up her restoration processes, to expel the intruder disturbing her rules of health and life. For it is Nature that cures: not the physician or nurse (Nightingale, 1882).

This dual role corresponds to tasks related to a specific nursing practice – providing a clean and comfortable environment – and those arising out of the relationship between nursing and medicine.

However, this double role is united in, and structured by, the fact that medical dominance in health care manifests itself by limiting the access to patients of practioners in other health occupations by means of monopolizing the initial intervention which designates the patient *qua* patient. Therefore both aspects of nursing care can be provided only after a medical diagnosis. Once the health care process is under way, nursing consists of a variety of tasks, some of which are ordered by the doctor, and others which reflect current ideas about providing a healthy environment. This conception of the function of nursing in health care prevailed throughout the period (and still exists today, though modified somewhat by the concept of the doctor as *primus inter pares* within a health care team). A 1904 *Hospital* editorial stated this succinctly:

> The nurse has no certificate which entitles her either to diagnose cases, or to judge whether a patient is so seriously ill as to need to be received into the wards; and the public have a right to demand that cases sent to a hospital should be treated by a registered practitioner and not by a nurse. ... The nurse cannot be too careful to keep a clear dividing line between her duties and those of the medical man, and she is culpable indeed if she rashly, and with her eyes open, grasps at responsibilities which are beyond her limit (26 November 1904, p.121).

Nurse training was preoccupied with professional socialization: teaching the limits of the role of the nurse in relation to medicine within the overall structure and provision of health care:

> Training is to teach a nurse to know her business, that is, to observe exactly, to understand, to know exactly, to tell exactly, in such stupendous issues as life and death, health and disease. ... Training has to make her, not servile, but loyal to medical orders and authorities. ... Training is to teach the nurse to handle the agencies within our control which restore health and life, in strict obedience to the physician's or surgeon's power and knowledge (Nightingale, 1882, p. 6).

> There is nothing to justify a nurse in going beyond her limit and diagnosing and treating patients. ... Her training ought to teach her above all things to keep within her own province (*Hospital*, 26 November 1904, p.121).

Thus the division of labour between nursing and medicine which mapped out nursing spheres of competence was not a neutral division, based on equal contribution to, and participation in, the healing process. Instead it created stratified health care and interprofessional inequality. The dominance of medicine in health care and its control over initiating and directing the healing process relegated nursing practice, in both its aspects, to a subordinate position. The nurse–doctor relation determined the division of labour between these two occupations.

Nursing is a unique non-industrial female occupation. It was established and designed for women, and located within a labour process – health care – already dominated by doctors, all of whom were men. Success depended on both creating paid jobs for women who needed them and situating and defining these jobs in a way which would pose no threat to medical authority. The particular form of the sexual division of labour which resulted from this conjuncture is specific to nursing: it is vivid and precise. It represents the patriarchal nature of the sexual division of labour in relatively pristine form, especially in that in many ways it cuts across capitalist class boundaries. The analysis of the sexual division of labour in health care demonstrates that technological determinism, the ideological representation of the capitalist division of labour, was less crucial than the ideology of naturalism in situating nursing within health care. Thus emphasis was placed on the interconnections between femininity, motherhood, housekeeping and nursing. Task division was circumscribed within the relationship between nursing and medicine. As such technological determinism was never the central issue.

The sexual division of labour is a patriarchal ideological structure in that it reproduces patriarchal relations in extra-familial labour processes. Thus women's labour in the family is based on the labour relations between husband and wife; in paid employment within capitalism her relationship to social production is on one level determined by the limits posed by the sexual division of labour. Any analysis seeking an explanation for the fact that women's work under capitalism is different from men's – both within marriage or the domestic mode of production and in wage labour in the capitalist mode of production – must unquestionably address itself to the pervasiveness of patriarchal relations. The form of these relations cannot be assumed to be self-evident, but must be analysed in their specificity.

References

Hospital (journal): 26 November 1904, Nursing Outlook: 'The nurse's limit'

Maclean, U. (1974) *Nursing in Contemporary Society*, Routledge and Kegan Paul, London

Florence Nightingale; some of her writings from the Nightingale Collection at the London School of Economics:
(1851) Institution of Kaiserswerth
(1867) Suggestions on the subject of providing, training, and organising nurses, for the sick poor in workhouse infirmaries. Letter to the President of the Poor Law Board
(1874) Suggestions for improving the nursing service of hospitals and on the method of training nurses for the sick poor
(1881) Letter to the probationer-nurses in the 'Nightingale Fund' Training School, at St Thomas's Hospital', 6 May
(1882) Training of nurses and nursing the sick poor. Reprinted from Dr Quain, *Dictionary of Medicine*.

Pedinielli-Plaza, M. (1977) Sex differences and women's reality – the patriarchal chain. Paper presented at the Anglo-French Seminar on Sexual Divisions, London

Rathbone, W. (1890) *History and Progress of District Nursing*, Macmillan, London

Schulman, S. (1958) Basic functional roles in nursing: mother surrogate and healer. In *Patients, Physicians and Illness* (Jaco, E. G., ed), Free Press, Chicago

Thorner, I. (1955) Nursing – the functional significance of an institutional pattern. *American Sociological Review*, **20**, 531–538

Reprinted by permission of HarperCollins Publishers Limited, London. Eva Gamarnikow (1978) Sexual division of labour: the case of nursing. In *Feminism and Materialism: Women and Modes of Production* (Kuhn, A. and Wolpe A. M., eds), Routledge, London, pp.97–100, 101–102, 105–107, 121.

Chapter 34

The importance of being a nurse

A. Oakley

What is especially important or distinctive about nursing? In what ways are nurses different kinds of people from doctors, patients, or other health care workers?

These questions are not merely academic. In many countries health services are now in a state of crisis. There is a growing failure to match the demand for medical services with available economic resources and at the same time there is a crisis of confidence in the ability of medicine to deliver the goods. Contributing to this new, more cynical view has been the rise of a so-called 'consumer' movement. Those at the receiving end of medical services have suddenly become much more articulate about what they want and need.

It has, at times, been enormously difficult for medical practitioners to ignore the potent relationships between bodies on the one hand, and minds and environments on the other. In order to do so, they have had to put on one side a great deal of evidence pointing to the social causation and prevention of disease – from studies showing the connections between life-events such as family arguments and the onset of infections such as streptococcal sore throats (Haggerty, 1980), to the presence of 'stress' chemicals in the blood and urine of unemployed men whose wives are not being especially kind to them (Cobb, 1974).

However, when we consider the history of nursing, we do not find the same relationship between what nurses do, or claim to do, on the one hand, and the curative model of medicine on the other. The origins of nursing lie in a different model of health and illness – based on environmental factors.

Nursing began to emerge as a separate occupation in the mid-19th century. At that time, it was no more, and no less, than a specialized form of domestic work.

Most hospital nurses were married women doing for patients what they did at home for their families. In addition, the dividing line between nurses and patients was blurred, and able-bodied convalescent patients were expected to help nurses with the domestic work of the ward.

Having been a domestic servant was the only qualification required at this time for ordinary nursing, except that, once taken on, these women were also taught how to make poultices, an absolute necessity in the pre-antibiotic era.

Conditions of work for the early nurses were poor; they were expected to sleep in the ward, and were not provided with meals when on duty. It was hardly surprising, therefore, that some were accused of stealing the patients' meals, and that Florence Nightingale remarked that nursing was done by those 'who were too old, too weak, too drunken, too dirty, too stolid, or too bad to do anything else'[1]. While food was not provided, alcohol was often given as part of the nurse's wages, or in return for particularly disagreeable work. A 19th century British nurse would get a glass of gin for laying out the dead, or two glasses of gin for one spell of night duty, though it is not clear whether these were to be drunk at the time or afterwards.

As with all histories, there is an official history of nursing which selects as important certain kinds of developments and not others (Davies, 1980). Hospital nursing training in Britain, for example, was begun before Florence Nightingale arrived on the scene, although in the orthodox history, the profession of nursing was created by Nightingale virtually single-handed. Florence Nightingale's achievements on behalf of nursing were, in reality, quite mixed. What she did was to wean nursing away from the cruder aspects of domestic work and attempt to establish it as a profession alongside the emerging profession of medicine.

Nightingale's efforts on behalf of nurses were aided by the growth of the demand for nurses in many countries at the end of the 19th century (in Britain the number of hospital beds tripled between 1861–1891 and 1891–1911) (Maggs, 1980), and by medicine's own insecurity about its professional credibility, and its consequent need to expand and control hospitals as places where captive patients could be used to teach future doctors. The new trained nurses were a particular problem for doctors, since they often came from a higher social class than the doctors themselves. This was one reason why the nurse's place in health care had to be very tightly controlled.

———

This historical division of labour between doctors and nurses presents today's nurse with a definite set of constraints as to what nurses are able to do for patients and for themselves. But almost an equal constraint – though it can be used as an advantage – is the gender division of labour in health care. The details of this vary between countries, but we may make two generalizations about it. First, the vast majority of the world's health care workers are women, not only in the Third World which relies heavily on untrained or partly-trained female health workers, but also in industrialized countries such as the United States and Britain, where 85% and 75% respectively of all workers in official health care are women.

The second generalization is that the medical profession is male-dominated. In most countries it is male-dominated in a statistical sense, but, even where it is not, the stereotype of a doctor conveyed in medical training and practice owes a great deal more to cultural notions of masculinity than femininity. Doctors are rational, scientific, unemotional and uninvolved.

Indeed, their very value is sometimes said to lie in their detachment from the personal needs of their patients. In talking about this gender division between medicine and nursing, we have to add that, although women may become doctors and men may become nurses, there is a tendency within both professions for men to monopolize the top jobs. While it is possible to understand why this happens in medicine – a science (or an art?) from which women were excluded so that they must now fight to be allowed back in – it is much harder to understand why nurses should allow their male colleagues to take an undue share of the top jobs. Do women know less about nursing than men? Of course this may seem a little provocative but there is no doubt that nurses, midwives, and women in general need assertiveness-training. If Florence Nightingale had trained her lady pupils in assertiveness rather than obedience, perhaps nurses would be in a different place now.

In surveys of people's attitudes to nurses, alertness to the needs of others is consistently picked out as the mark of a good nurse. This is also the mark of a good woman. When I observed earlier that the gender division of labour in health care – the masculinity of doctors and the femininity of nurses – is nurses' biggest problem and also their biggest opportunity today, I was referring to the altruistic aspect of womanhood and nursing. Altruism is a social strength (Titmuss, 1970). But, so far as the altruistic individual is concerned, it may well be weakness: altruism serves the community but often gets the individual nowhere.

The paradox of altruism is developed by Jean Baker Miller's (1977) argument about the personality characteristics that develop as a result of people belonging either to dominant or subordinate social groups. People who belong to subordinate groups, whether children, black people, women or nurses, tend to be socialized into a psychological pattern which emphasizes dependency, passivity, subservience, and thinking about other people's welfare.

On the other hand, people belonging to dominant social groups, whether adults, white people, men or doctors, develop qualities of independence, initiative, control, domination (not surprisingly), and putting their own welfare and development ahead of other people's.

Miller points out that 'serving others' is for losers, it is low-level stuff (Miller, 1977). But women's psychology and social roles are organized around the presumption that they will serve others, indeed, that from this serving of others will come the only self-enhancement that is culturally accepted as appropriate for women.

One of the most impressive mechanisms for denying the importance of caring work is to disenfranchise and disadvantage the people who do such work. The mechanism is effective, if not exactly subtle. The most outstanding example of it is childrearing, followed as a close second by housework. Both are unpaid occupations when located in the family and in conjunction with marriage, though, of course, in other circumstances both can be paid. But these occupations are not only normally financially unrewarded, they disenfranchise their holders in important ways: a woman who gives up employment to rear children will generally lose out on her pension rights for those years, and, if she is in professional work, the missing years will set her permanently behind on the career ladder.

The dilemmas of doing good and feeling bad apply to nurses just as they do to women in general. Insofar as caring is the signal quality and main work of nurses, nurses are likely to come up against two barriers. First, they will not achieve a social and financial status which underlines their inner feeling that nursing is good work – instead the external rewards of nursing are likely to undermine nurses' confidence in the performance of caring work. Second, it will be difficult to feel day-in and day-out, and in the face of so many counter challenges, that communication with patients is truly as valuable work as microsurgery, diagnoses with body scanners, and intricate immunological tests.

A simple message could be extracted from all this – that nursing needs to lose its association with femaleness in order to achieve full professional status. The logic is undeniable, and it certainly appears that male nurses are more likely to emphasize the professional status of nurses than are female nurses (Rosen, 1972).

If a profession is by definition male-dominated, then nurses might as well give up. Alternatively, nurses might ask the truly radical question as to what is so wonderful about being a professional anyway? This question is a bit like asking what is so wonderful about the family, motherhood, Father Christmas and the space programme. It is self-evident that being a professional is superior to not being one, just as living in a family or going to the moon are better than being a single parent (which would, in any case, disqualify one for training as an astronaut). The point is that the world takes the goodness of some people, activities and objects, and the badness of others for granted. Yet, the current crisis of confidence in medical care should tell us that professionalization is not only not the answer, but that it may, indeed, be positively damaging to health. It has been said that professions in the 20th century have, in general, created a 'dependent, cajoled and harassed, economically deprived and physically and mentally damaged' clientele. They are more entrenched and 'international than a world church, more stable than any labour union, endowed with wider competence than any shaman, and equipped with a tighter hold over those they claim as victims than any mafia' (Illich, 1977). This situation is disabling for everyone including the professionals themselves. Nurses owe it to themselves to lift off the veil that has made them invisible, and make everyone see and understand how important they really are.

Note

1. Cited in Abel-Smith, B. (1960) *A History of the Nursing Profession*, Heinemann, London.

References

Cobb, S. (1974) Physiologic changes in men whose jobs were abolished. *Journal of Psychosomatic Research*, 18, 245–258
Davies, C. (ed.) (1980) *Rewriting Nursing History*, Croom Helm, London
Haggerty, R.J. (1980) Life stress, illness and social supports. *Developmental Medicine and Child Neurology*, 22, 391–400
Illich, I. (1977) Disabling professions. In *Disabling Professions* (Illich, I. *et al.*, eds), Marion Boyars, London
Maggs, C. (1980) Nurse recruitment to four provincial hospitals 1881–1921. In *Rewriting Nursing History* (Davies, C., ed.), Croom Helm, London
Miller, J.B. (1977) *Towards a New Psychology of Women*, Beacon Press, Boston
Rosen, J.G. and Jones, K. (1972) The male nurse. *New Society*, 68, 493–494
Titmuss, R.M. (1970) *The Gift Relationship*, Allen and Unwin, London

Reproduced by kind permission of *Nursing Times*, where this article first appeared on 12 December 1984.

Chapter 35

The faces of Florence Nightingale: functions of the heroine legend in an occupational sub-culture

Elvi Whittaker and Virginia Olesen

... As might be expected with any occupational group, there are segments within the nursing profession which hold divergent philosophies about the meaning of nursing and the area of its responsibilities. How Florence Nightingale is perceived by these segments will be discussed from the point of view of the establishments which take upon themselves much of the responsibility for instigating ideology, namely the schools of nursing. The main focus will be on the faces of the legend presented by the university school as contrasted with the faces presented by the hospital school. These faces will be those that function to indoctrinate recruits, to justify change, and to suggest resolutions to some of the significant issues of the female work role.

Florence Nightingale as symbolic of cultural values

The popular conception of the Florence Nightingale story reveals a frail, delicate creature, dedicated and self-abnegating, moving alone, and at night, among rows of wounded and dying men. In her hand is the symbol of strength, a lamp, and as she passes by, soldiers in reverence and gratitude kiss the hem of her skirt. She is a saintly woman, who merely wants to serve. She is the heroine of the Crimea, but little else is known of her.

Generally speaking, the popular image of Florence Nightingale begins and ends with the incidents at Crimea. Many of the other deeds with which history credits Florence Nightingale are not included. The image does not encompass Florence Nightingale living an upper-class existence in England, Florence Nightingale receiving members of the Cabinet, or Florence Nightingale making authoritative demands and issuing voluminous reports from her sick-bed.

Florence Nightingale in history and biography

History, as the best available claim to objectivity, reveals a different Florence Nightingale. It shows an upper-class woman of substantial means and commendable intellectual abilities. It pictures not a personality gentle, saintly and feminine, but rather one which could be interpreted as power-loving, coolly manipulative and hypochondriacal. She is shown to be not self-abnegating as the woman of legend, but rather a woman of authority, a woman who mercilessly drove others and within whom 'lurked fierce and passionate fires' (Strachey, 1948). It also becomes evident that what are commonly seen as the glorious events in the Crimea take merely some months out of the life of Florence Nightingale and that her main concerns lie not with the wounded *per se* but rather with the higher levels of administration and with the manipulation of the Cabinet at home in England. Nor is she heedful only of nursing, but her greater efforts are directed to political ends and encompass such divergent interests as social welfare, army reform, sanitation in India, hospital administration and the instituting of favoured figures into office for her own designs (Woodham-Smith, 1951). It also becomes obvious that to some she could be no 'ministering angel' but rather an interfering nuisance. Furthermore, she was in no way a simple woman as the legend prefers to picture her, but had a high station in life and far-reaching intellectual interests as her writings show. Her discourses, for example, include works on biostatistics, translations of Plato, analysis of religious matters, selections of Bible stories for children, as well as writings in nursing and hospital administration.[1] Facts as depicted in history and biography, therefore, tend to deny the saintly woman with a lamp, which the legend has perpetuated. It is interesting also that the face presented by the legend emerged during her own lifetime (Woodham-Smith, 1951) and is still the prevalent popular image.

Upon further examination of the popular face of Florence Nightingale, however, it becomes clear that it represents those aspects of femininity which are deemed culturally desirable. The historical face, on the other hand, presents her with the characteristics tinged with masculinity, aggression and a divorcement from the home and family aspects of femininity. These latter tendencies are not entirely acceptable for women in our society, and hence appear to remain in the province of history rather than become part of the popular image.

Florence Nightingale as occupational status enhancer

To appreciate the function of the Florence Nightingale legend as status-elevator for the occupation of nursing, and as a means whereby nursing became integrated into 19th century English society, it is useful to outline the nature of the field at that time.

It is popular among writers of nursing history to depict the role of nurse as going back into pre-history to the times when men aided an ailing fellow. Since then the history of the occupation has been a colourful one, as the responsibility for nursing the sick passed through the hands of goddesses of healing, priestesses, virgins, sisters of religious orders, penitent sinners, criminals, and lay women of doubtful repute. At the time of the Crimean War the world of nursing in Europe was straining to evolve from the province of the sacred on the one hand, and from the profane on the other. Sisterhoods, often considering the nursing of the sick a distasteful duty which it was their lot in life to perform, controlled schools for nurses and hospitals for the sick. When not in the hands of religious orders, nursing was in the hands of women of the lower classes, women of questionable character, of inordinate thirst for alcoholic beverages and other unmentionable vices (Woodham-Smith, 1951).[2] It was from the latter category of nursing, in particular, that the image of Florence Nightingale rescued the occupation. Nursing, through the medium of the legend, became invested with hues of respectability. Furthermore, the legend, in pointing out the virtues of a relatively safe sacrifice, made nursing publicly acceptable as an undertaking for virtuous and dedicated women.

It is significant that Florence Nightingale, although widely accepted as the culture-heroine of the occupational sub-culture, was not the first recognized nurse, nor the founder of the first school of nursing, nor even the first trained nurse.[3] The key to her adoption, therefore, must lie in other virtues.

Firstly, the deeds of Florence Nightingale represent in a spectacular way the cultural values of humanitarianism and romanticism. This alone brought her, and nursing, wide popular acclaim.

Secondly, however, a further theme pervades the Nightingale legend, namely that of the 'safe sacrifice'. This sacrifice is one wherein the individual expects to relinquish neither life nor limb, nor even perhaps the more cherished aspects of existence, but those portions less valued, such as comfort and security.[4] The end for which this sacrifice is made, must be deemed of course culturally worthy. Of this order are the sacrifices that society can, and does, demand of all its members. The truly heroic sacrifice, in the full sense of the term, is too costly as it involves the relinquishing of life. In Florence Nightingale's case, her sacrifice was one of temporarily forgoing the comforts and creature delights of moneyed upper-class English existence (which bored her anyway). Furthermore, the very role she was defying by becoming a nurse and going far into the male territory of war, namely the role of upper-class femininity, was also her protector. She was able to achieve her sacrifice because she was still granted the traditional accord allowed to females of her status, even though she stretched the very boundaries of 19th century womanhood to encompass feats hitherto unknown for genteel females. In effect, it was a breach of respectable femininity to go to the battlefield, but the men surrounding her there permitted her presence, and even revered it, because she was a lady. Florence Nightingale does represent, therefore, in a manner dramatic and clearly explicit, the 'safe sacrifice', a demand nursing must make of its recruits if it is to survive and flourish. She reflects admirably the safeness of the sacrifice. Although exposed to blood, sweat and toil, she remains ever sweet, dainty and eternally feminine.

Thirdly, her adoption as culture-heroine must have some basis in the status she enjoyed in Victorian England. Being from the upper echelons of English society, the untitled aristocracy, she is a powerful figure and can invest nursing with the social approval it so sorely lacked. Here was an upper-class woman, one who associated with prime ministers and dukes and yet one who did the work of a nurse and could be labelled as such.

Above all, she was culturally defined as a heroine and thus conferred on nursing some of the positive values she had accrued. In short, she was a perfect vehicle whereby nursing could lever itself into acceptable occupational status and integrate itself into society as a respectable work role.

Florence Nightingale in two schools of nursing

Once established as a 'respectable' occupation, nursing has continued to change. As is the nature of change, it seeps in slowly and affects some segments of the field before others, and hence it is that at the same point in time older ideologies exist with newer and more progressive ones. This is the case with nursing education where schools structured much on the lines of the 19th century exist along with faculties of nursing education in universities. Admittedly there are many variations of both traditional and university schools. This discourse, however, will limit itself to the clearly defined polarities.

The former schools are, on the whole, hospital-controlled. The emphasis tends to be on ward practice and the students receive an education somewhat analogous to an apprenticeship where the hospital maintains the students throughout their 3 years of training and shoulders the expense of their education in exchange for the student devoting much of her time to staffing the hospital wards. The teachers at these schools tend to be concerned with the accurate performance of procedures, with having students respect those higher on the nursing hierarchy, and with having nurses remember that their duty is to follow the doctor's orders.

The university schools, on the other hand, are more analogous to other professional schools within the university framework. They have left far behind them the floor scrubbing and linen washing of the youth of nursing and have adopted values such as intellectual abstraction, a liberal outlook and a broad general education. The task-orientation is supplanted by an emphasis on intellectual curiosity, on solid theoretical knowledge and on ideas that the nurse is one of the 'professional team' of which the doctor is but another member.

The differences between these two schools are perhaps most clearly indicated by the semantic reflections of their various ideologies and most markedly in the terms they use to refer to the process by which a student becomes a nurse. To the hospital school it is 'training', but to the university school it is 'education'. This difference is further noticeable in the rhetoric of referring to ward practice and caring for patients. The hospital school defines it as 'duty', the university school as 'lab'.

Despite differing ideologies on the process of making nurses, both schools make reference to the person of Florence Nightingale. It is not the same Florence Nightingale, however, who appears in these schools, but one who displays markedly different faces.

Traditional school

As was stated earlier the traditional school could be described as retaining many of the task orientations of the 19th century, as emphasizing ward practice for students and as advocating submission to authority. At the same time the traditional school is very concerned with professionalism and devotes much of its time to issues such as professional ethics, professional adjustments, professional behaviour and professional appearance. The bedside image is a strong one, and there are vague notions among faculty members that even though a student may do poorly academically, she may have the more desirable attributes and that is the potential to be a good nurse, namely one who is nurturant and comforting at the bedside. Conversely, there are also vague suspicions about the nursing abilities of a student who does remarkably well academically. Introduction of new recruits to the school often includes allusions to the sacrifices that will be required from them as members of the profession, the long hours, the heartbreaks, the dedication to the patient. Such sacrifices themselves imply the prestige that a Puritan society will afford the nurse, but the recruits are also promised the rewards of seeing patients improve and go home. It is interesting that this is one lecture of indoctrination that is widely acclaimed among the students.

Usually in courses in nursing history designed to give the recruit a professional heritage, the story of Florence Nightingale is discussed. It must be remembered that these recruits bring with them to the nursing school the public, or popular, image of the Nightingale legend. From the possible elements within the Nightingale story, the traditional school selects those relevant to the heroism and sacrifice during the Crimean War. Students are told of the hardships Florence Nightingale underwent in order to go to the Crimea, the hours of endless toil she undertook to reach her goals in nursing care for the wounded, and the many nursing measures she introduced to better the lot of the ill.

University school

The schools of nursing on university campuses tend to separate themselves from the traditional world of nursing and to ally themselves with other professional schools within the structure of the university. This separation takes the form of movement away from the world of tasks. Although the latter receives begrudging recognition as being some part of the realm of the nurse's duties, the university schools have submerged tasks by extensive curriculum revisions, a wider theoretical education in the sciences, an espousement of the social sciences and an emphasis on a good general education. While the traditional school is sensitive to the superior position and ability of the doctor, the university school impresses the student with the belief that his superiority lies in the area of traditional medical science, whereas the nurse must take responsibility for the socioemotional aspects of the patient's care. While the traditional school is concerned with professionalism, the university school is more concerned with instilling scholarship and intellectual curiosity into the student. The image of the widely educated woman is a favoured one, and is often supported by a curriculum which permits students to take courses of a liberal arts nature. Professionalism appears not to be an issue and even the very word is used very loosely and without stress. The problems lie rather around the making of a nurse and an academic woman. This person has to be proficient in such things as essay writing, analytical thinking, library scholarship and so on.

As befits the age of science this school goes to the factual recording of the life of Florence Nightingale to formulate its story. It draws upon her status and work in England. Recruits who, like their sisters in the hospital school, have a popular image of the legend are surprised to learn that Florence Nightingale's work in the Crimea was not her main contribution to humanity. They are told of her endeavours in social reform, in bio-statistics, and of her perusal of knowledge generally. They are told that she was responsible for the first authoritative work in bio-statistics, that she was a woman of high social class and remarkable political power and that she was liberally educated and ever active in matters intellectual. She is shown as a woman who retired from the trivialities of Victorian social life so that she could maintain an immense correspondence and be exceptionally productive in the writing of reports and papers, designed to manipulate those in formal power to bring about change. The traditional nursing aspects of the Florence Nightingale image are negated with statements which maintain that she had not practised nursing before her sojourn in the Crimea, and that any training she had taken had been very meagre, encompassing only three months with the Deaconesses at Kaiserwerth and a short period with the Sisters of Charity in Paris. So broad had been the interests of this woman that 'We can't claim her all for ourselves'. This face of Florence Nightingale also shows her as an innovator, a person who was able to project images of the nursing role into the future, which the school hopes it will be able to educate and encourage its students to do.

The progressive university school, therefore, selects those portions of the Nightingale story which are salient for the emergence of nursing into the academic community. This version is indeed an adaptation to the changed, and changing, institutional sub-culture which it must serve. No longer is the traditional expressive value of sacrifice sufficient, but rather the instrumental values of intellectuality and academic leadership become dominant. This new face of Florence Nightingale does not express only the prevalent concerns of the university school. It also trades on the inherent sanctity of the culture-heroine, as well as the popular acclaim given her, to make the new concerns more acceptable to the traditionally oriented novice. In this way institutional unity is enhanced and a common goal is clearly defined.

The legend of Florence Nightingale has many faces and many functions. To a questioning society cold towards the emergence of nursing, the story is a romantic, humanitarian and honourable one. To female sub-culture, it is a story of womanhood and sacrificing safely. To novices in nursing it is the face of the school in which they are enrolled. To those asked to accept and incorporate change it shows a face which reflects the very change desired. To some women it projects the face of traditional womanhood, to others it shows how traditional femininity could be combined with a career. In short, the image of Florence Nightingale is so elastic that it is able to reflect a large range of values and concerns, both in society and in the occupational sub-culture.

Notes

1. A perusal of the writings of Florence Nightingale reveals the following: *A Contribution to the Sanitary History of the British Army During the Late War with Russia*, Harrison and Sons, 1859; *Suggestions for Thought to the Searchers after Truth among the Artisans of England*, privately printed for Miss Nightingale, three volumes, Eyre and Spottiswoode, 1860; *The Zeminder, the Sun, and the Watering Pot as Affecting Life and Death in India*, unpublished, proof copies among the Nightingale papers, 1873–76; *A Sub-Note of Interrogation: What will our Religion be in 1999?*, Frasers Magazine, July 1973. See also Woodham-Smith, 1951, p. 329.
2. The figure of Charles Dickens' 'Sairey Gamp' (*Martin Chuzzlewit*) exemplifies this kind of nurse well.
3. Histories of nursing show the existence of schools of nursing such as at Paris and Kaiserwerth, established about 1836 and 1617 respectively (*sic*), and in Ireland in 1816. In addition there were organizations in England, such as The Protestant Sisters of Charity inspired by Elizabeth Fry. (*Editors' Note*: Kaiserwerth school of nursing was founded in 1836 but we have been unable to check the date given for the Paris school of nursing.)
4. This is not intended to imply that nursing does not have its dangers. On the contrary, nurses have run heavy risks in war and peace and especially in earlier stages of medical knowledge when contagion was an ever-present enemy. Safe sacrifice here means partial, but not full, sacrifice.

References

Strachey, L. (1948) *Eminent Victorians*, Chatto & Windus, London
Woodham-Smith, C. (1951) *Florence Nightingale*, McGraw-Hill, New York

Reprinted by permission of Churchill Livingstone, Edinburgh. Elvi Whittaker and Virginia Olesen (1978) The faces of Florence Nightingale: functions of the heroine legend in an occupational sub-culture. In *Readings in the Sociology of Nursing* (Dingwall, R. and McIntosh, J., eds), Churchill Livingstone, Edinburgh, pp. 22–31, 34. (This article was originally reproduced by permission of the Society for Applied Anthropology from *Human Organization*, 1964, **23**, 123–130.)

Chapter 36

The functioning of social systems as a defence against anxiety[2]

I. Menzies

...The trained nursing staff are entirely deployed in administrative teaching, and supervisory roles, although those who are deployed in operational units working with patients also carry out a certain amount of direct patient-care. Student nurses are, in effect, the nursing staff of the hospital at the operational level with patients, and carry out most of the relevant tasks. From this point of view, it is necessary that student nurses be deployed so as to meet the nurse-staffing requirements of the hospital. The student nurse spends comparatively little time undergoing formal instruction. She spends three months in the Preliminary Training School before she starts nursing practice, and six weeks in the nursing school in each of the second and third years of training. For the rest of the time she is in 'practical training', i.e. acquiring and practising nursing skills by carrying out full-time nursing duties within the limits of her competence. The practical training must be so arranged that the student has the minimal experience of different types of nursing prescribed by the General Nursing Council.[1] The hospital offers, and likes nurses to have, certain additional experience available in specialist units in the hospital. The hospital's training policy is that the student nurse has approximately three months continuous duty in each of the different types of nursing. Each student nurse must be deployed in a way that fulfils these training requirements.

The possibilities of conflict in this situation are many. The nursing establishment of the hospital is not primarily determined by training needs, which take second place to patient-centred needs and the needs of the medical school. For some considerable time before the start of the study, the senior nursing staff had been finding it increasingly difficult to reconcile effectively staffing needs and training needs. Pressures from patient-care demanded that priority be given to staffing, and constant training crises developed. The policy of three-month training tours had in effect been abandoned and many tours were very short;[2] some nurses came almost to the end of their training without having had all the necessary experience, and others had a serious imbalance owing to too much of the same kind of practice. These crises created the more acute distress because senior staff wished to give increasing priority to training and to raise the status of the nurse as a student.

The senior staff began to feel that there was a danger of complete breakdown in the system of allocation to practical work and sought our help in revising their methods. My purpose in writing this paper is not, however, to follow the ramifications of this problem. I will make some reference to it at relevant points, and will consider later why the existing method persisted so long without effective modification in spite of its inefficiency.

The therapeutic relationship with the hospital was to some extent based on the belief that we would be wise to regard the problem of student-nurse allocation as a 'presenting symptom' and to reserve judgement on the real nature of the difficulties and the best form of treatment until we had done further diagnostic work. We began, therefore, with a fairly intensive interviewing programme. We held formal interviews with about 70 nurses, individually and in small groups, and with senior medical and lay staff; we carried out some observational studies of operational units; and we had many informal contacts with nurses and other staff. Respondents knew the problem we were formally studying, but were invited to raise in interview any other issue that they considered central to their occupational experience. Much further research material was collected in the later meetings with senior staff as we worked together on the findings from the interviewing programme.[3]

As our diagnostic work went on, our attention was repeatedly drawn to the high level of tension, distress, and anxiety among the nurses. We found it hard to understand how nurses could tolerate so much anxiety, and, indeed, we found much evidence that they could not. In one form or another, withdrawal from duty was common. About one-third of student nurses did not complete their training. The majority of these left at their own request, and not because of failure in examinations or practical training. Senior staff changed their jobs appreciably more frequently than workers at similar levels in other professions and were unusually prone to seek postgraduate training. Sickness rates were high, especially for minor illnesses requiring only a few days' absence from duty.[4]

As the study proceeded we came to attach increasing importance to understanding the nature of the anxiety and the reasons for its intensity. The relief of the anxiety seemed to us an important therapeutic task and, moreover, proved to have a close connection with the development of more effective techniques of student-nurse allocation.

Defensive techniques in the nursing service

In developing a structure, culture, and mode of functioning, a social organization is influenced by a number of interacting factors, crucial among which are its primary task, including such environmental relationships and press-ures as that involves; the technologies available for performing the task; and the needs of the members of the organization for social and psychological satisfaction, and, above all, for support in the task of dealing with anxiety.[5-7] In my opinion, the influence of the primary task and technology can easily be exaggerated. Indeed, I would prefer to regard them as limiting factors, i.e. the need to ensure viability through the efficient performance of the primary task and the types of technology available to do this set limits to possible organization. Within these limits, the culture, structure, and mode of functioning are determined by the psychological needs of the members.[8]

The needs of the members of the organization to use it in the struggle against anxiety leads to the development of socially structured defence mechanisms, which appear as elements in the structure, culture and mode of functioning of the organization.[9] An important aspect of such socially structured defence mechanisms is an attempt by individuals to externalize and give substance in objective reality to their characteristic psychic defence mechanisms. A social defence system develops over time as the result of collusive interaction and agreement, often unconscious, between members of the organization as to what form it shall take. The socially structured defence mechanisms then tend to become an aspect of external reality with which old and new members of the institution must come to terms.

In what follows I shall discuss some of the social defences that the nursing service has developed in the long course of the hospital's history and currently operates. It is impossible here to describe the social system fully, so I shall illustrate only a few of the more striking and typical examples of the operation of the service as a social defence. I shall confine myself mainly to techniques used within the nursing service and refer minimally to ways in which the nursing service makes use of other people, notably patients and doctors, in operating socially structured mechanisms of defence. For convenience of exposition, I shall list the defences as if they are separate, although, in operation, they function simultaneously and interact with and support each other.

Splitting up the nurse–patient relationship

The core of the anxiety situation for the nurse lies in her relation with the patient. The closer and more concentrated this relationship, the more the nurse is likely to experience the impact of anxiety. The nursing service attempts to protect her from the anxiety by splitting up her contact with patients. It is hardly too much to say that the nurse does not nurse patients. The total work-load of a ward or department is broken down into lists of tasks, each of which is allocated to a particular nurse. She performs her patient-centred tasks for a large number of patients, perhaps as many as all the patients in the ward, often 30 or more in number. As a corollary, she performs only a few tasks for, and has restricted contact with, any one patient. This prevents her from coming effectively into contact with the totality of any one patient and his illness and offers some protection from the anxiety this arouses.

Depersonalization, categorization, and denial of the significance of the individual

The protection afforded by the task-list system is reinforced by a number of other devices that inhibit the development of a full person-to-person relationship between nurse and patient, with its consequent anxiety. The implicit aim of such devices, which operate both structurally and culturally, may be described as a kind of depersonalization or elimination of individual distinctiveness in both nurse and patient. For example, nurses often talk about patients, not by name, but by bed numbers or by their diseases or a diseased organ, 'the liver in bed 10' or 'the pneumonia in bed 15'. Nurses themselves deprecate this practice, but it persists. Nor should one underestimate the difficulties of remembering the names of say 30 patients on a ward, especially the high-turnover wards.

There is an almost explicit 'ethic' that any patient must be the same as any other patient. It must not matter to the nurse whom she nurses or what illness. Nurses find it extraordinarily difficult to express preferences even for types of patients or for men or women patients. If pressed to do so, they tend to add rather guiltily some remark like 'You can't help it'. Conversely, it should not matter to the patient which nurse attends him or, indeed, how many different nurses do. By implication it is the duty as well as the need and privilege of the patient to be nursed and of the nurse to nurse, regardless of the fact that a patient may greatly need to 'nurse' a distressed nurse and nurses may sometimes need to be 'nursed'. Outside the specific requirements of his physical illness and treatment, the way a patient is nursed is determined largely by his membership of the category patient and minimally by his idiosyncratic wants and needs. For example, there is one way only of bed-making, except when the physical illness requires another; only one time to wash all patients in the morning.

The nurses' uniforms are a symbol of an expected inner and behavioural uniformity; a nurse becomes a kind of agglomeration of nursing skills, without individuality; each is thus perfectly interchangeable with another of the same skill-level. Socially permitted differences between nurses tend to be restricted to a few major categories, outwardly differentiated by minor differences in insignia on the same basic uniform, an arm stripe for a second-year nurse, a slightly different cap for a third-year nurse. This attempts to create an operational identity between all nurses in the same category.[10] To an extent indicating clearly the need for 'blanket' decisions, duties and privileges are accorded to categories of people and not to individuals according to their personal capacities and needs. This also helps to eliminate painful and difficult decisions, e.g. about which duties and privileges should fall to each individual.... Something of the same reduction of individual distinctiveness exists between operational sub-units. Attempts are made to standardize all equipment and layout to the limits allowed by their different nursing tasks, but disregarding the idiosyncratic social and psychological resources and needs of each unit.

Detachment and denial of feelings

A necessary psychological task for the entrant into any profession that works with people is the development of adequate professional detachment. He must learn, for example, to control his feelings, refrain from excessive involvement, avoid disturbing identifications, maintain his professional independence against manipulation and demands for unprofessional behaviour. To some extent the reduction of individual distinctiveness aids detachment by minimizing the mutual interaction of personalities, which might lead to 'attachment'. It is reinforced by an implicit operational policy of 'detachment'. 'A good nurse doesn't mind moving.' A 'good nurse' is willing and able without disturbance to move from ward to ward or even hospital to hospital at a moment's notice. Such moves are frequent and often sudden, particularly for student nurses.

The implicit rationale appears to be that a student nurse will learn to be detached psychologically if she has sufficient experience of being detached literally and physically. Most senior nurses do not subscribe personally to this implicit rationale. They are aware of the personal distress as well as the operational disturbance caused by overfrequent moves. Indeed this was a major factor in the decision to initiate our study. However, in their formal roles in the hierarchy they continue to initiate frequent moves and make little other training provision for developing genuine professional detachment. The pain and distress of breaking relationships and the importance of stable and continuing relationships are implicitly denied by the system, although they are often stressed personally, i.e. non-professionally, by people in the system.

Reducing the weight of responsibility in decision-making by checks and counter-checks

The psychological burden of anxiety arising from a final, committing decision by a single person is dissipated in a number of ways, so that its impact is reduced. The final act of commitment is postponed by a common practice of checking and rechecking decisions for validity and postponing action as long as possible. Executive action following decisions is also checked and rechecked habitually at intervening stages. Individuals spend much time in private rumination over decisions and actions. Whenever possible, they involve other nurses in decision-making and in reviewing actions.

The nursing procedures prescribe considerable checking between individuals, but it is also a strongly developed habit among nurses outside areas of prescribed behaviour. The practice of checking and counter-checking is applied not only to situations where mistakes may have serious consequences, such as in giving dangerous drugs, but to many situations where the implications of a decision are of only the slightest consequence, e.g. on one occasion a decision about which of several rooms, all equally available, should be used for a research interview. Nurses consult not only their immediate seniors but also their juniors and nurses or other staff with whom they have no functional relationship but who just happen to be available.

The nursing services in general have shown a similar resistance to change in the face of great changes in the demands made on them. There can be few professions that have been more studied than nursing, or institutions more studied than hospitals. Nurses have played an active part in initiating and carrying out these studies. Many nurses have an acute and painful awareness that their profession is in a serious state. They eagerly seek solutions, and there have been many changes in the expressed aims and policy of the profession. There have also been many changes in the peripheral areas of nursing, i.e. those which do not impinge very directly or seriously on the essential features of the social defence system. Against that background, one is astonished to find how little basic and dynamic change has taken place. Nurses have tended to receive reports and recommendations with a sense of outrage and to react to them by intensifying current attitudes and reinforcing existing practice.

An example of a general nursing problem that threatens crisis is the recruitment of nurses. Changes in medical practice have increased the number of highly technical tasks for nurses. Consequently, the level of intelligence and competence necessary for a fully trained and efficient nurse is rising. The National Health Service has improved the hospital service and made it necessary to have more nurses. On the other hand, professional opportunities for women are expanding rapidly and the other professions are generally more rewarding than nursing in terms of the opportunity to develop and exercise personal and professional capacities as well as in financial terms. The increasing demand for high-level student nurses is therefore meeting increasing competition from other sources. In fact, recruiting standards are being forced down in order to keep up numbers. This is no real solution, for too many of the recruits will have difficulty in passing the examinations and be unable to deal with the level of the work. Many of them, on the other hand, would make excellent practical nurses on simpler nursing duties. So far, no successful attempt has been made in the general hospitals to deal with this problem, e.g. by splitting the role of nurse into different levels with different training and different professional destinations.

Notes

1. The nursing body that controls nurse-training.
2. A sample check of actual duration showed that 30 per cent of student moves took place less than 3 weeks after the previous move and 44 per cent less than 7 weeks.
3. It is a feature of a therapeutic study of this kind that much of the most significant research

material emerges in its later stages when the emphasis of the work shifts from diagnosis to therapy. Presentation and interpretation of data, and work done on resistances to their acceptance, facilitate the growth of insight into the nature of the problem. This extends the range of information seen to be relevant to its solution, and helps overcome personal resistances to the disclosure of information. An impressive feature of the study here reported was the way in which, after a spell of working on the data, the senior nursing staff themselves were able to produce and execute plans directed towards dealing with their problems.

4. There is much evidence from other fields that such phenomena express a disturbed relation with the work situation and are connected with a high level of tension. See, for example, Hill and Trist (1953).

5. Bion (1955) has put forward a similar concept in distinguishing between the sophisticated or work group concerned with a realistic task and the basic-assumption group dominated by primitive psychological phenomena; the two 'groups' being simultaneously operative aspects of the same aggregation of people.

6. The importance of anxiety and defences against it has been much stressed in psycho-analytical theories of personality development. Freud's earliest works show his interest and he develops his theory in later work (Freud, 1955, 1948). The central developmental role of anxiety and defences has, more recently, been much stressed by Melanie Klein and her colleagues (Klein, 1952, 1948a, 1948b).

7. For a fuller discussion of the primary task and related factors see Rice (1958).

8. The different social systems that have developed under long-wall coal-mining conditions, using the same basic technology, are a good example of how the same primary task may be performed differently using the same technology when social and psychological conditions are different. They have been discussed by Trist and Bamforth (1951).

9. Jaques (1955) has described and illustrated the operation of such socially structured defence mechanisms in an industrial organization. The term is his.

10. In practice it is not possible to carry out these prescriptions literally, since a whole category of nurses may temporarily be absent from practical duties on formal instruction in the nursing school or on leave.

References

Bion, W. R. (1955) Group dynamics: a review. In *New Directions in Psycho-analysis* (Klein, M., Heimann, P. and Money-Kyrle, R. E. eds), Tavistock Publications, London/Basic Books, New York

Freud, S. (1948) *Inhibitions, Symptoms and Anxiety,* Hogarth Press and Institute of Psycho-analysis, London

Freud, S. (1955) *Studies on Hysteria.* Standard Edition, Vol. II, Hogarth Press and Institute of Psycho-analysis, London, pp.1–251

Hill, J. M. M. and Trist, E. L. (1953) A consideration of industrial accidents as a means of withdrawal from the work situation. *Human Relations,* 6, 357–380

Jaques, E. (1955) Social systems as a defence against persecutory and depressive anxiety. In *New Directions in Psycho-analysis* (Klein, M., Heimann, P. and Money-Kyrle, R. E., eds), Tavistock Publications, London/Basic Books, New York

Klein, M. (1948a) The psychogenesis of manic-depressive states. In *Contributions to Psycho-analysis (1921–1945),* Hogarth Press and Institute of Psycho-analysis, London

Klein, M. (1948b) The importance of symbol formation in the development of the ego. In *Contributions to Psycho-analysis (1921–1945),* Hogarth Press and institute of Psycho-analysis, London

Klein, M. (1952) Some theoretical conclusions regarding the emotional life of the infant. In *Developments in Psycho-analysis*, Hogarth Press and Institute of Psycho-analysis, London

Rice, A. K. (1958) *Productivity and Social Organisation: The Ahmedabad Experiment*, Tavistock Publications, London

Trist, E. L. and Bamforth, K. W. (1951) Some social and psychological consequences of the longwall method of coal-getting. *Human Relations*, **4**, 3–38

Chapter 37

The fabrication of nurse–patient relationships

David Armstrong

It is a deeply held assumption that the role of caring, which for so long has been at the heart of nursing, has meant a close relationship between nurse and patient. Certainly the doctor with the technological devices and interests in biochemical pathways has often seemed in danger of relating to the patient only as a biological object; but in contrast the nurse, through being constantly by the patient's side and caring for the patient's basic functions, has of rights a special relationship. The very essence of nursing has been presented as the humane relationship between the sick and the caring.

The body of the patient

In one sense a relationship is simply a term used to denote the relative positions of two objects in time and space or within a classification system – a chair has a certain relationship to a table, abdominal pain has a relationship with appendicitis and so on. But in discussing the nurse–patient the usual assumption is that this relationship is qualitatively different in that it is not between two objects but between two subjects. It is important to emphasize these two meanings of the term 'relationship' because there is evidence that while the word may have remained the same the actual form and nature of the relationship between patient and nurse may have undergone a fundamental reformulation within the last decade. If the nurse–patient relationship had been of the 'subjective' variety and of central importance then its discussion and analysis might be expected to have constituted a core component of the standard textbooks which attempt to distil the essence of nursing for the benefit of the student.

Identification of the particular meaning of the nurse–patient relationship can be illustrated by the discussion in the 21st edition of *Practical Nursing*, published in 1969, in which one chapter on 'elementary psychology' was included because it was felt that nursing should be characterized by the 'right kind of relationship' (Gordon Pugh, 1969). In this chapter it was stated that each patient was an individual human being and not simply a case – a claim which would undoubtedly find contemporary support. Yet when the details of the relationship are examined it is, perhaps, not so familiar.

The nurse–patient relationship was one in which both parties had a role. The nurse's chief role was described as gaining the trust of the patient. Moreover, by being graceful, nicely turned out and looking fit and well she could convey a sense of good health, well-being and happiness to the patient. It is clear that the relationship was not construed as something dynamic, that led to problems of communication, of meanings and misunderstanding, of emotions and feelings. The nurse plays a part; the patient watches and hopefully is impressed. The passivity of both actors in the relationship is confirmed by the role assigned the patient: he 'will abide by instructions and will cooperate in the carrying out of the treatment'.

The rather wooden actors described in the 1969 scenario can be contrasted with the mutual psychological involvement of nurse and patient that Kratz describes in her book *The Nursing Process* some 10 years later (Kratz, 1979): 'The interaction between two people', she observes, 'influences the behaviour of each'. The problem, Kratz suggested, was that the British nursing profession was so much more familiar with physical rather than emotional problems. Indeed it might fairly be claimed that until recently the British nursing profession denied the patient even had emotions (and, by implication, neither did the nurse).

A powerful illustration of these various positions can be found in the nursing care of the dying which by today's standards involves difficult emotional relationships. In her 1969 text Gordon Pugh suggested that the main role of the nurse was to attend to 'physical needs'. The only acknowledgement of the patient's psychological needs was the suggestion that the nurse might be able to relieve the patient's loneliness and that she should take care of what she said in the patient's presence.

Some three years later in the 3rd edition of *Bedside Nursing* the patient's emotional and spiritual needs, which were to be met by listening with sympathy and compassion, were recognized (Darwin *et al.*, 1972). At the same time, despite this listening, it was noted that some people reacted to death in an hysterical and inappropriate way which may be due to immature behaviour and which could cause distress to others. As usual the response to this possible crisis in the relationship was for the nurse to keep out of it, to remain calm and dignified at all times so that other patients might draw comfort from her behaviour.

The mechanistic view of relationships is further illustrated by the analysis of the nurse's own reaction to the dying patient. In its current image a relationship is a two-way affair: acknowledgement therefore of the patient's emotional needs and responses without recognizing that the nurse too has a similar repertoire suggests that the intimate relationship is more of a stance than a reality. Thus, for example in the 1st edition of Darwin *et al.*'s text of

1964 it was noted that nurses might have their own emotional difficulties; by the 3rd edition of 1972 a more sophisticated link was established by the suggestion that the difficulties in dealing with the dying might spring from the nurse's own anxieties. Yet the role of the nurse as a participant in a delicate situation was immediately circumscribed: the nurse ultimately had no need of solutions, she simply followed sister's instructions. In effect the passive relationship between nurse and patient was reproduced between sister and nurse.

In similar vein, *Modern Nursing: Theory and Practice* demanded that the patient had 'courage and humour' while nurses needed a liking for people, physical health, manual dexterity, intelligence, education and integrity (Hector, 1976). Care of the dying required only that the body of the patient was nursed. As late as 1977, in *Basic Nursing*, it was argued that 'basic nursing care of the dying patient is concerned with his comfort and the relief of any distressing symptoms' (Bendall and Raybould, 1977).

Yet by the mid-1970s changes were underway as the relationship between nurse and patient became seen as more problematic. In the 2nd edition of *The Principles of Nursing* published in 1973 Roper expanded her chapter on 'helping the patient to communicate' from 7 to 17 pages and made it the first chapter of the book 'because interaction between (a patient and nurse) is vital to the process of nursing' (Roper, 1973).

In 1978, in *An Outline of Basic Nursing Care*, it was stated that compassion was necessary but on its own was not enough; listening was at least equally important, as communication was a two-way business (Welsh *et al.*, 1978). This approach was reflected in the advice on dealing with the dying patient. Empty reassurance was valueless: the nurse had to establish an atmosphere of trust – not, as in the past, so as to eliminate communication – but so that the patient could voice his or her own anxieties and the nurse could listen with compassion and understanding. It was not enough, Roper observed in *The Elements of Nursing*, for the nurse 'to be a tender loving person, though it helped' (Roper *et al.*, 1980).

Relationships and identities

Michel Foucault has suggested that traditional perceptions of the patient as a discrete, analysable, passive body emerged at the end of the eighteenth century when various techniques arose through which the body could be explored (Foucault, 1963). In effect the body had no independent existence prior to the analysis which established its particular social identity; the body as an object was neither a universal belief nor truth but was the product of ways of perceiving and examining it; the body, for all its apparent invariate biological reality, was a fabrication of certain social practices and of particular techniques of analysis.

The body achieved an objective and individual status in a variety of institutional settings such as the school, the prison, the barracks and the workshop which were contemporaneous with the emergence of the modern hospital and theories of localized pathology (Foucault, 1977). In so far as medicine was concerned the surveillance techniques were embodied in the techniques of clinical examination, the process of diagnosis and the cognitive base of pathological anatomy. Together these new medical practices established as a reality the outline of a passive body and an objectified patient. It is, perhaps, not until Nightingale's *Notes on Nursing* later in the nineteenth century, which in their emphasis on the physical environment of the patient (ventilation, noise, food, bedding, cleanliness, etc.) together with the importance of accurate observation succeeded in formalizing an analogous physical context and reality for the patient, that the discipline of nursing established parallel techniques of objectification.

It was only in the 1950s and early 1960s that medical writers began to find the patient's personality (as against the patient's body) of importance in response to treatment: they found compliance an unrecognized problem and identified doctor–patient communication as a neglected area. The result was a massive literature on the doctor–patient relationship which served principally to render that relationship problematic and to establish its protagonists as 'real' people (Armstrong, 1982, 1983).

A way of illustrating this argument is to take a fairly mechanical unproblematic relationship between two people, say that between the customer and a cashier in a supermarket. Both parties have well defined roles, their interaction is usually minimal and neither party expects to have to negotiate differences of meaning or mutual anxieties. Imagine now a large research grant being awarded to investigate the relationship. Both parties would have to start examining their relationship so they could relate their feelings to the research team: the confession of silent thoughts would be encouraged and new problems of misunderstandings would be identified. Gradually a mechanistic relationship – virtually between a bag of shopping and a cash till – becomes problematic in that as the customer comes to look for and respond to the personal meanings of the cashier so the cashier becomes more than an extension of the till but a 'whole person' in her own right.

From the nursing literature outlined above it is probably fair to say that until recently the relationship between patient and nurse was similar in its mechanistic passivity to that between customer and cashier. Certainly there was a relationship but it was extremely limited in the identity it provided for its participants. Patients had to obey and show respect, nurses had to follow sister's instructions and walk in a dignified way. The patient was a biological object whose body was observed: the nurse was part of the machinery of surveillance which described and thereby objectified the body it monitored.

In the last decade or so however the nursing task has been redefined (the 'nursing process' being an important part of that reconstruction) and its object, the patient, has commensurately changed its nature.[1] The nurse is now instructed to communicate with the patient as a subjective being: the patient must confess and the nurse must listen. The nursing process, for example, offers a pervasive analysis and constant awareness of the patient's (and nurse's) personal worlds. The nursing process as observed in 1981 in *Systematic Nursing Care* is 'a tool of integrity and of human rights' (Long, 1981). It involves the provision of care according to the patient's particular needs; it requires the nursing staff 'to communicate more with each other in giving care'. From a simple concern with the care of the patient's bodily functions, nursing has started to become a surveillance apparatus which both monitors and evinces the patient's personal identity: in so doing it helps fabricate and sustain that very identity.

Political reconstruction

It might be argued that despite the recent recognition of the problem of subjectivity and its formalization in nursing textbooks there always has been a nursing tradition which implicitly handled the patient as a 'whole-person'. The argument for this tradition is both historical and biographical.

First, the historical case: various 'histories' of nursing have celebrated the close connection between nurse and patient, though most of these, as Davies' recent volume points out, simply amount to self-congratulatory propaganda (Davies, 1980). However, in terms of the thesis of this paper such histories, whatever their historiographic faults, are admissible evidence so long as their date of authorship is taken into account: histories written before about 1960 will reveal an essentially biological body for the patient in the past while those written since will discover a subjective body in the same historical sources. In short these histories belong to the same analysis which provoked the emergence of the subjective patient.

Woodham-Smith's classic biography of Florence Nightingale of 1951 (which Versluysen suggests is one of the few writings to avoid picturing 'a stereotype of a stereotype' (Versluysen, 1980)) can be used by way of illustration (Woodham-Smith, 1951). Woodham-Smith concludes from a reading of *Notes on Nursing* that 'It is impossible to doubt, after reading it, that Miss Nightingale was a gentle and sympathetic nurse' (Woodham-Smith, 1951). To modern ears that might sound like praise but, in context, their meaning refers to an earlier nursing paradigm. Nightingale's view (which her biographer mentions) was that the nurse was there 'to spare (the patient) from taking thought for himself' (Nightingale, 1859). In other words the role of the nurse was not to incite subjectivity but to repress it: 'In the hospital it is the relief from all anxiety afforded by the rules of a well-regulated institution which has often such beneficial effect on the patient' (Nightingale, 1859). Whereas the essence of the modern relationship is communication that of Nightingale's is silence; indeed whispered anxieties are not therapeutic so much as pathological: 'in general patients who are really ill, do not want to talk about themselves. Hypochondriacs do, but ... we are not on the subject of hypochondriacs' (Nightingale, 1859).

Second, there is the biographical case: nurses today can remember that in the past nurses already implicitly had modern communication skills or developed them through less formalized methods than that of the textbook. Yet it is strange that what is now held retrospectively to have been a vital component of nursing seemingly left no impression on historiographic material; but there is another explanation.

In the claim for an historically constant 'meaningful' nurse–patient relationship it is possible to recognize a solution to a political problem. The thesis of this paper is that subjectivity is invented: yet according to its supposed nature, subjectivity transcends invention. Whole people, communication, idiosyncratic meanings, etc., are not held to be fabrications but are, according to the newest nursing psychology, an inviolate part of everyone. In effect to sustain the contemporary meaning of subjectivity, history has to be rewritten, memories jolted and in the process an elaborate myth constructed around the historical constancy of the nurse–patient relationship. The image of the caring nurse has existed for perhaps a hundred years, but behind the myth is only an ephemeral crystallization of various lines of social analysis.

Note

1. It was only in the last decade that this formal task redefinition seems to have affected general nursing. There is however an earlier literature from the 1960s informed by psychoanalytic principles which emerged from the changes in psychiatric care and nursing in the late 1950s. I am grateful to Gill Chapman for bringing this to my attention. See for example, Martin, D. and Allen, D. (1969) A week's learning experience in the psychology of nursing. *Nursing Times*, 137–140.

References

Armstrong, D. (1982) The doctor-patient relationship: 1930–1980. In *The Problem of Medical Knowledge: Towards A Social Constructivist View of Medicine* (Wright, P. and Treacher, A., eds), Edinburgh University Press, Edinburgh

Armstrong, D. (1983) *Political Anatomy of the Body: Medical Knowledge in Britain in the 20th Century*, Chap. 11, Cambridge University Press, Cambridge

Bendall, E. R. D. and Raybould, E. (1977) *Basic Nursing*, 4th edn, Lewis, London

Darwin, J. *et al.* (1964) *Bedside Nursing: An Introduction*, 1st edn; 3rd edn, 1972, Heinemann, London

Davies, C. (ed.) (1980) *Rewriting Nursing History*, Croom Helm, London

Foucault, M. (1963) *Birth of the Clinic: An Archeology of Medical Perception*, Tavistock, London

Foucault, M. (1977) *Discipline and Punish: The Birth of the Prison*, Allen Lane, London

Gordon Pugh, W. T. (1969) *Practical Nursing*, 21st edn, Allen Lane, London

Hector, W. (1976) *Modern Nursing: Theory and Practice*, 6th edn, Heinemann, London

Kratz, C. R. (ed.) (1979) *The Nursing Process*, Baillière Tindall, London

Long, R. (1981) *Systematic Nursing Care*, Faber and Faber, London

Nightingale, F. (1859) *Notes on Nursing: What It Is and What It Is Not*, Harrison, London; reprinted, p. 63, Duckworth, London, 1970

Nightingale, F. (1859) *Ibid.*, p.63

Nightingale, F. (1859) *Ibid.*, p.55

Roper, N. (1973) *The Principles of Nursing*, 2nd edn, Livingstone, Edinburgh

Roper, N. *et al.* (1980) *The Elements of Nursing*, Churchill Livingstone, London

Versluysen, M. C. (1980) Old wives' tales? Women healers in English history, In *Rewriting Nursing History* (Davies, C., ed.), Croom Helm, London

Welsh, E. M. *et al.* (1978) *An Outline of Basic Nursing Care*, 2nd edn, Heinemann, London

Woodham-Smith, C. (1951) *Florence Nightingale 1820–1910*, London

Reprinted from *Social Science and Medicine*, **17**(8), David Armstrong, The fabrication of nurse–patient relationships, 457–460, © 1983, with kind permission from Elsevier Science Ltd, The Boulevard, Langford Lane, Kidlington OX5 1GB, UK.

Chapter 38

Emotional labour: skill and work in the social regulation of feelings

N. James

In recent empirical sociology studies of women are the richest source of reference on feelings. Where emotion is mentioned in other studies, it is mentioned tangentially in debates on family, organizations and paid work – for instance Strauss *et al.* detail 'comfort work' and 'sentimental work' as part of 'The social organization of medical work' (1985). In referring to such studies it needs to be borne in mind that they too are shaped by historical developments which separate rationality from emotion, and are especially influenced by the sexual division of labour (Dex, 1985; Davies and Rosser, 1986; Hearn and Parkin, 1987).

Evidence that emotion and feelings are part of everday life are most easily verified by self-examination. Arguments that the social expression of emotion is not the unpredictable, illogical behaviour which directly contrasts with 'rationality' are persuasive. Russell Hochschild in an article on 'emotion work' sees the 'emotive experience of normal adults in daily life' as 'orderly' and gives examples of individuals managing their emotions. In an interactive account of emotion which she describes as being 'between' Goffman and Freud, she emphasizes that emotion work is regulated by social exchange (Russell Hochschild, 1979).

The embodiment of extremes of emotion in rites and rituals is an indication that social regulation of feelings is universal, but I suggest that these elements of the management of emotion are the tip of the iceberg. For the most part management of emotion is a routine, predictable process, less reliant on personality than Russell Hochschild suggests, and rather more reliant on the 'emotional labour' of others.

The management of emotions has many of the connotations associated with labour – the relatively modern definition of labour as productive work, in addition to older senses with labour meaning any kind of difficult effort, and labour as pain (Williams, 1981). Emotional labour is hard work and can be sorrowful and difficult. It demands that the labourer gives personal attention which means they must give something of themselves, not just a formulaic response. Its value lies in its contribution to the social reproduction of labour power and the social relations of production, with the divide between home and work and the gender division of labour influencing the forms in which it is carried out. The contribution of emotional labourers is explored in more detail below but my argument is that it is a form of skilled, regulatory labour which is carried out in the 'public' domain of the workplace as well as in the 'privacy' of home.

The social structures affecting the forms emotional expression takes make it a suitable subject for core sociological study, but the more specific notion of emotional labour connects it with ideas of paid work. From a study of nursing the dying (James, 1986), the 'labour' element of emotional labour became apparent not only because it connects the management of emotions with the workplace, but also because it denotes the association with a process which can be demanding and exhausting, and subject to different forms of organization.

At a hospice where I spent five months as a participating observer the guiding ideology, as it is in most hospices, was of 'total care'. This is defined as 'social, spiritual, emotional and physical' care and thus encompasses elements of care which are usually obscured in medical settings. In particular it highlights the point that social, spiritual and psychological difficulties require management and attention in the same way that physical symptoms do. It was not that the emotions were 'irrational', far from it. A period of grief, anger, loss, despair and frustration were anticipated and entirely appropriate responses in coming to terms with death, the final 'life event'. However the expression of such emotions can be painful to watch, and awkward to respond to. In particular such expressions are fraught with contradiction as they do not fit in with standard ideas of what should occur at the workplace nor with standard ideas of workplace skills.

Emotion at home

Emotional labour is most easily recognized as part of the caring role of women in the home. Although the social regulation of emotions is brought about through emotional labour, as a form of labour it appears to be insulated from other forms of labour, and is poorly recorded and under-explored. It is my contention that this is precisely because it involves both women and 'emotion' with their negative connotations. Because emotional labour is seen as 'natural', unskilled women's work, because it is unpaid and because it is obscured by the privacy of the domestic domain where much of it takes place, the significance of its contribution and value in social repro-duction is ignored.

One of the results of the gender division of labour is that women carry the prime responsibility for working with emotions. More than that though 'emotional' becomes part of a major cluster of other adjectives by which 'masculine' and 'feminine' are differentiated and through which the emotional/rational divide of female/male is perpetuated.

... Emotional labour does not exist in isolation from the conditions under which it is carried out, rather the circumstances under which it takes place influence the content and form of emotional labour. Since the early work of regulating emotion is carried out in the privacy of the 'home' the emotional labour is shaped by the responsibilities and status that go with 'caring work'.

Caring, which often includes routine maintenance of the household, could be described as having emotional labour, physical labour and organization as its component parts (James, 1987), so that the emotional labour is carried out within the context of the organization and physical labour which must also be carried out.

In the home emotional labour is fitted in as part of the range of maintenance requirements of children to be put to bed, clothes to be washed and ironed, shopping that needs to be bought, meals to be planned, husband coming in from work, and cleaning that takes the cleaner from room to room. Although 'being available' is a key factor in emotional labour, the flexibility of place and circumstances in which it can be carried out can be made to have advantages. For example intimate conversations are more likely to take place in the bedroom or the bathroom than at the shops.

Emotional labour is flexibly organized so that it can be responsive to the needs of others. To be effective the 'labourer's' skills must include firstly, being able to understand and interpret the needs of others, secondly being able to provide a personal response to these needs, thirdly being able to juggle the delicate balance of each individual and of that individual within the group, and fourthly being able to pace the work, taking into account other responsibilities.

Emotional labour requires learned skills in the same way that physical labour does. Access to the skills is open to anyone who has the interest or who has an obligation to learn them, but some practitioners are better than others. Like physical labour, there are certain techniques which, if adeptly applied, give a better outcome to emotional labour, both for the person caring and for the person being cared for. In some circumstances advice is sought, in others action is required, and in others a sense of perspective, of 'rightness' is to be established.

Thus this aspect of 'care' involves hard practicalities, as well as its symbolic value of personal attention, warmth, involvement and empathic understanding but as Shirley Dex notes, the nature of skill, far from being clear and unambiguously defined, is integrally bound up in the sexual division of labour. She goes on to point out that the caring occupations like child-care, nursery nurses, and a whole array of social servicing jobs done by women are also thought to be generally fairly unskilled. In practice what this means is that the skills involved are not recognized as skills, either by employers or society or often the women themselves.

Dealing with other people's feelings is labour not only because it contributes to social reproduction but also because it is hard work. Emotional labour can be as exhausting as physical labour. Sitting with a distressed person (child, friend, relative), listening to someone when they are angry, courageous, resentful or sad, and acquiring the ability just to 'be' with someone who is lonely, frightened or in pain, is taxing and requires an appropriate response. Comfort, confrontation, humour, empathy or action may each be appropriate in different circumstances. As with physical labour, after a sustained period of emotional labour, an alternative or a rest are necessary; for coping with a friend whose wife has just left is as tiring as comforting a child whose best friend has abandoned them and both demand close attention from the listener.

When emotions are thought to be 'irrational' it is hard to associate them with organization, yet managing them requires anticipation, planning, timetabling and trouble-shooting as does other 'work', paid and unpaid.

Emotional labour is organized and managed both in the private domain of home and the public domain of the workplace. The forms it takes are affected by the dominant organization so that the form of emotional labour within the relatively pliable routines in the home differs from that which is possible within the rigidity of workplace organization, where principles of timetabling and control are vital. Emotional labour requires a flexibility of response to different circumstances and different people's needs and requests that cannot be timetabled and routinized as easily as physical tasks are.

In practice, both males and females regulate and repress feelings. But the distinction between home being the primary place for 'personal feelings' and associated with women, and the workplace being for 'economic production' and associated with men may have implications for the extent to which emotion is expected to be regulated at home, but repressed in the workplace. The repression of feeling which is sanctioned at work as a condition of efficient production does not mean that the feelings disappear. Rather the feelings are temporarily banished, but will eventually be expressed elsewhere – at home, or possibly in leisure pursuits. Thus, by making the expression of feelings in the workplace unacceptable, labour processes affect not only how feelings are expressed in the workplace, but also the emotional labour which is likely to be necessary at home.

Emotional labour is a commodity in the sense that it is expedient for industry, commerce and services to make use of it. Although it is an area that needs futher exploration, I am not the first to suggest that emotional labour is a commodity (Russell Hochschild, 1983).

Russell Hochschild's analysis of 'flight attendants' in *The Managed Heart* illustrates one way in which a specific, highly public form of emotional labour is directly appropriated for the purpose of maximizing airline company profits. I use the concept of emotional labour in a broader sense than Russell Hochschild, to cover the processes through which emotional labour are carried out in the public and the domestic domain, and I suggest that the more common form of emotional labour is that where its centrality and value are not recognized. In the workplace the employment of emotional labourers is widespread in tasks where close personal attention is required, though the value of what they do is often unrecognized. Instead low-paid, low-status women are employed to manage the emotions of others, thereby facilitating the labour of others. Usually incorporated as part of another job or task, the work of dealing with other people's emotions is moulded by a more dominant role. However the hidden component of the work does not stop it from being vital to the work.

Davies and Rosser observed the skills required of Higher Clerical Officers, a branch of managerial officer working in the health services. They noted a particular form of this job where the skills involved were those of 'mature women'. They show that the HCO's job draws on the women's:

> organizational skills developed ... in household management and on their experience in the home handling emotions and creating an appropriate atmosphere for the task in hand (Davies and Rosser, 1986, p.105).

Emotional labour in the workplace

Hearn proffers the male dominated professions such as medicine, the law and the church as examples of 'emotional managers', 'characteristically involved in the selective control of the emotions of themselves and others' (Hearn, 1987). But he notes that although they may define the limits and action of emotion for other workers and clients, the problems of dealing with the emotional control are primarily located through others. Thus male professionals set the parameters while others, usually female 'semi-professionals', do the work.

The hospice referred to earlier is a good example of this. At hospices, unlike the HCO job, emotional 'care' is recognized as part of the job. Nevertheless, though the male Medical Director was in charge of coordinating the 'total care', much of the difficult work of emotional labour, for instance telling people they are going to die, fell to the female physician first quoted. More significant though is the aftermath of such disclosure, which may go on over days and weeks, and is largely managed by the female nursing staff.

In terms of the organization of emotional labour the hospice staff took it as part of their work, and integrated it to the extent that they felt they had not completed their work properly if that type of caring work had not been part of their day.. . .

────────

It has been my argument that emotional labour carried out in the public domain is subject to the same key forces as emotional labour in the domestic domain, leaving it unrecognized, unrecorded and unrewarded in both. Though emotional labour is shaped by the conditions under which it is carried out, the flexibility of emotional labour means that it can be at least partially adapted to specific circumstances, including those of the workplace. Though the significance of their emotional labour is as invisible in the workplace as it is in the domestic domain, women may be employed specifically to make use of these 'natural' skills.

The material, political and social consequences of emotional labour are obscured. Though emotional labour is a core part of the maintenance and continuity of labour power and the social relations of production in the workplace and in the domestic domain it remains unrecognized as a form of labour. This is both the result of and contributes to the gender division of labour through which women's skills and labour are undervalued, because they are women's not men's. There exists a distorting, divisive conceit through which men are associated positively with rational thought and action while women are negatively associated with emotional reaction. This false distinction faciliates a gender division of labour through which men's labour is understood to be central to the creation of value, while women's work is considered peripheral, subordinated as merely 'support' work, equally marginalized in private and public domains. Though the imperatives of patriarchy and capitalism need emotional labour, it is the dominance of those imperatives which hide and deride both the labour and the labourers.

References

Davies, C. and Rosser, J. (1986) Gendered jobs in the health service: a problem for labour process analysis. In *Gender and the Labour Process* (Knight, D. and Wilmott, H., eds), Gower, Hampshire

Dex, S. (1985) *The Sexual Division of Work*, Wheatsheaf, Brighton

Hearn, J. (1987) *The Gender of Oppression*, Wheatsheaf, Brighton

Hearn, J. and Parkin, W. (1987) *'Sex' at 'Work': The Power and Paradox of Organization Sexuality*, Wheatsheaf, Brighton

Heller, A. (1979) *A Theory of Feelings*, Van Gorcum, Assen, The Netherlands

James, V. (1986) *Care and work in nursing the dying*. Unpublished PhD thesis, University of Aberdeen

James, V. (1987) Care = emotional labour + physical labour + organization. Unpublished IHCS paper, University College of Swansea

Russell Hochschild, A. (1979) Emotion work, feeling rules and social structure. *American Journal of Sociology*, 85, 551–575

Russell Hochschild, A. (1983) *The Managed Heart*, University of California Press, Berkeley

Strauss, A., Fagerhaugh, S., Suczek, B. and Wiener, C. (1985) *Social Organization of Medical Work*, University of Chicago Press, Chicago

Williams, R. (1981) *Keywords*, Fontana, London

Reprinted by permission of Blackwell Publishers, Oxford. N. James (1989) Emotional labour: skill and work in the social regulation of feelings. *Sociological Review*, 37(1), 18–20, 22, 23, 26, 27, 29, 31, 33.

The emotional labour of nursing: its impact on interpersonal relations, management and the educational environment in nursing

Pam Smith

The emotional labour of care

But is emotional labour as a concept the same as care? What are the similarities and differences and the inherent contradictions of treating emotional labour as a commodity?

I apply the concept of emotional labour to nursing because nurses are expected to be emotionally caring and display emotional styles similar to those of flight attendants.

I first experienced caring as labour during interviews with students and patients when the language that they used and the feelings that they expressed conveyed a sense of the sheer emotional work required to sustain the traditional image of smiling nurses, holding patients' hands. During one such interview a student described the following incident. 'I've had times when I've been with another nurse and we've been changing a patient's bed and he's shouted at her or been rude or something. Well the procedure goes on as if nothing has happened. And when we've finished she just drifts off. And I actually go after her and say "Are you alright? I would have been very unhappy if he'd said that to me". I think it's so important that we notice each other's distress so that we don't have to cry alone in a corner.'

As this account demonstrates, nurses not only laboured emotionally for patients, but also for each other. The ward sister was the key person who set the tone for the caring climate on her ward. As one student explained 'if sister cares then I don't need to take the whole caring attitude of the whole ward on my shoulders'.

Nursing and care

It is interesting to examine the way nursing leaders and educationalists conceptualize care. A look at the literature shows an increasing emphasis on the emotional aspects of caring and its promotion as distinctly nursing work since the influential Briggs report (DHSS, 1972).

Jean (now Baroness) McFarlane, a prominent nurse academic, in a keynote address to the Royal College of Nursing maintained that the words 'nursing' and 'caring' have similar roots. She says: 'Caring signifies a feeling of concern, of interest, of oversight, with a view to protection. Nursing means ... to nourish and cherish (McFarlane, 1976, p.189).

McFarlane wanted to see an end to the nurse as the doctor's handmaiden and the emergence of a new role in which caring was pre-eminent. By describing nursing in terms of 'helping, assisting, serving, caring for' patients, McFarlane was seeking to raise the status of so-called basic tasks to the level of unique nursing skills. In a subsequent paper, she provided a philosophy and work method called the nursing process, to do this (McFarlane, 1977). The nursing process, regarded by many as an American import, promotes a people- rather than task-orientated approach to patients and raises the profile of emotional care at the same time that, as Hochschild notes, the growth of the service sector and 'people jobs' has made communication and encounter the central work relationship.[1]

The body–mind dichotomy

Concepts of care are fraught with contrasts and contradictions. Is it labour or is it love? Is it natural or is it a skill? Is it about feelings or tasks? Does it come from the heart, the head or the hand? Is it guided by mind or body? Or should caring be seen as an integrated whole?

Hochschild's work is sometimes criticized because it is seen as perpetuating the body–mind dichotomy which has its origins in positivism, western dualism and what Mary O'Brien calls 'male-stream' thought.[2] Pat Benner, an American Professor of Nursing, applies a philosophical approach to the concept of care, which she says transcends the body–mind split and enables connection and concern between nurse and patient. Emotions are seen as the key to this connection because 'they allow the person to be engaged or involved in the situation. ... The alienated, detached view of emotions, as unruly bodily responses that must be controlled actually cuts the person off from being involved in the situation in a complete way' (Benner and Wrubel, 1989).

Views such as these represent a trend over the past decade amongst nurses in the USA and Europe to move to a more holistic approach to care and away from 'a nation's blind embrace of high tech medicine' (Gordon, 1988).

Concepts of care and emotional labour

Care as a concept is complex. It is referred to on a number of different levels. Nursing leaders exhort nurses to care, but their definitions are limited because they fail to take into account the emotional complexity of caring. Neither do they consider the way in which care is stereotyped as women's 'natural' work nor the gender division of labour and the power relations between doctors (predominantly men) and nurses (predominantly women) within the health service which marginalize care to 'the little things'.

Care is an important notion for nurses and patients. They see it as the essential ingredient of the 'good' nurse and use it to refer to the emotional component of nursing which underpins her technical and physical activities. Student nurses felt better able to care for patients when they felt cared for themselves by the trained ward staff and their teachers. Because care was such a marginalized activity and conceptually ill-defined, I wanted to use the data to re-define it. The accounts of caring from both students and patients suggest that 'caring' does not come naturally. Nurses have to work emotionally on themselves in order to appear to care, irrespective of how they personally feel about themselves, individual patients, their conditions and circumstances. They can also be taught to manage their feelings more effectively.

These data fitted the definition of emotional labour elaborated by Arlie Hochschild (1983), whose work I discovered well into my data collection. I had not started out with the notion of care as emotional labour, but my data led me to select an appropriate framework. I then put Arlie's definition and analysis of emotional labour to the test each time I asked questions of my data. In this way I was able to assess its theoretical viability in the context of nursing. I was interested to find therefore that James (1986) had chosen to combine the two terms in her research, by referring to nursing the dying as 'carework'. The importance of defining care as work cannot be under-estimated if this most essential ingredient of what nurses do is to be recognized and valued. But recognition and value are not enough. Care must be supported educationally and organizationally in the institutions where nurses work and learn and by the political and economic structures within society (Tronto, 1987).

The gendered nature of nursing work and the perpetuation and predominance of the Nightingale image are examined in Chapter 2. These findings are of particular interest to recruitment officers at national and institutional level. With a falling population of 18-year-old women from which student nurses were traditionally recruited and a declining interest in nursing as a career, the nurses in my study may fast be disappearing as a distinct group. One important question is whether the predominant image of nursing as women's traditional work will have to change. Evidence from current recruitment literature and posters suggests recruiters recognize that it does. The technical aspects of nursing are given a higher profile and men and older women are targeted as potential recruits (Department of Health, 1990).

=========

... I suggest that the emotional components of caring require formal and systematic training to manage feelings, grounded in a theoretical base such as psychology, sociology and the acquisition of complex interpersonal skills. In this way emotion work will be made visible and valued in its own right and not viewed as *just* part of the package of women's work.

Nurse academics are also proposing nursing theories that go beyond the conceptual limitations of the nursing process. These developments hold possibilities for using research findings from studies such as mine to build an empirically tested knowledge base rooted in practice.

The UKCC's Project 2000 is committed to preparing practitioners who are 'knowledgeable doers' and to teach students 'how to learn and how to analyse, to give them confidence and the motivation and facilities to develop themselves in relation to a changing environment' (UKCC, 1985, p.21). These recommendations encourage nurses to re-examine traditional definitions of nursing knowledge, teaching and learning based on notions of tacit knowledge which is uncodified and transmitted through tone, feel and expression (Collins, 1974; Eraut 1985, p.119). These approaches are more appropriate to recognizing emotional labour as a key component of nursing, requiring the acquisition of a set of hitherto uncodified skills.

Notes

1. The nursing process has two components: the underlying philosophy that promotes a people-orientated approach to patients based on models of care such as Henderson's (1960), and Roper's (1976) living activities and a problem-solving work method. The nursing process as work method recommends the organization of nursing into four stages defined as assessment, planning, implementation and evaluation of patient care.

   McFarlane (1977) in her keynote address clearly spelt out the skills that nurses would require to practise the 'process' effectively. The observational and interviewing skills spelt out by McFarlane were clearly 'people' skills, the acquisition of which was necessary if the nursing process was to become part of the nurse's 'approach and repertoire'. In the same year (1977), the nursing process appeared for the first time in the syllabus of the national nurse training curriculum (General Nursing Council, 1977). Armstrong (1983) noted that once the nursing process had become officialized in this way, the textbook presentation of the nurse's role changed. Patients were no longer described in strictly biological terms. Psychology and communication skills were emphasized and 'subjectivity' and emotions were encouraged as part of the nurse–patient relationship.

   The introduction of the nursing process, with its emphasis on emotional care, has seen a rapid increase of nursing textbooks and videotapes dealing with the teaching of interpersonal and communication skills. The development of good nurse–patient relationships was hailed as therapeutic and central to the healing process.

   For comprehensive reviews of the nursing process, see De la Cuesta (1979, 1983); Brooking (1986).

   Theoretical limitations of the nursing process have been exposed by a number of writers (Roper *et al.*, 1985). A variety of nursing theories and models are being offered to create an

informed base for the use of the nursing process (Aggleton and Chalmers, 1986; see also Salvage and Kershaw, 1990).
2. Mary O'Brien (1989) defines 'male-stream' thought as 'the massive dense intellectual current of male intellectual history' as opposed to the relatively short public history of feminist understanding (p.3) which allows women to reproduce the world in their own terms. Male-stream thought and the belief that knowledge is 'objective' and 'abstract', promotes dualism and the setting up of opposites in a systematic way. Hence mind is described as abstract, body as material; science as abstract, common sense as material; intellectual work as abstract, manual and domestic labour as material; male as abstract, female as material and so on (p.7).

References

Aggleton, P. and Chalmers, H. (1986) *Nursing Models and the Nursing Process*, Macmillan, London

Armstrong, D. (1983) The fabrication of nurse–patient relationships. *Social Science and Medicine*, **14B**, 3–13

Benner, P. and Wrubel, R. (1989) *The Primacy of Caring: Stress and Coping in Health and Illness*, Addison-Wesley, Menlo Park, CA

Brooking, J. I. (1986) *Patient and family participation in nursing care: the development of a nursing process measuring Scale*. PhD thesis, University of London, King's College

Collins, H. M. (1974) The TEA set: tacit knowledge and scientific networks. *Science Studies*, **4**, 165–186

De la Cuesta, C. (1979) *Nursing process: from theory to implementation*. MSc thesis, London University

De la Cuesta, C. (1983) The nursing process: from development to implementation. *Journal of Advanced Nursing*, **8**, 365–371

Department of Health (1990) *Nurse Recruitment*, HMSO, London

Department of Health and Social Security (1972) *Report of the Committee on Nursing* (Chair: A. Briggs), HMSO, London

Eraut, M. (1985) Knowledge creation and knowledge use in professional contexts. *Studies in Higher Education*, **10**(2), 117–133

General Nursing Council for England and Wales (GNC) (1977) *Training Syllabus. Register of Nurses: General Nursing*, General Nursing Council for England and Wales, London

Gordon, S. (1988) Giving nurses time to care. *Washington Post*, 6 September

Henderson, V. (1960) *Basic Principles of Nursing Care*, International Council of Nurses, Geneva

Hochschild, A. R. (1983) *The Managed Heart: Commercialization of Human Feeling*, University of California Press, Berkeley

James, V. (1986) *Care and work in nursing the dying*. PhD thesis, University of Aberdeen

McFarlane, J. K. (1976) A charter for caring. *Journal of Advanced Nursing*, **1**, 187–196

McFarlane, J. K. (1977) Developing a theory of nursing: the relation of theory to practice, education and research. *Journal of Advanced Nursing*, **2**, 261–270

O'Brien, M. (1989) Reproducing the world. In *Reproducing the World: Essays in Feminist Theory*, Westview Press, USA

Roper, N. (1976), A model for nursing and nursology. *Journal of Advanced Nursing*, **1**, 219–227

Roper, N., Logan, W. and Tierney, A. (1985) The Roper/Logan/Tierney model. *Senior Nurse*, 3(2), 20–26

Salvage, J. and Kershaw, B. (eds) (1990) *Models for Nursing 2*, Scutari Press, London

Tronto, J. C. (1987) Beyond gender difference to a theory of care. *Signs: Journal of Women in Culture and Society*, **12**(4), 644–663

United Kingdom Central Council for Nursing, Midwifery and Health Visiting Educational Policy Advisory Committee (UKCC) (1985) *Project 2000: Facing the Future*. Project Paper 6, UKCC, London

Reprinted by permission of Macmillan Press Ltd, Basingstoke. Pam Smith (1992) *The Emotional Labour of Nursing: Its Impact on Interpersonal Relations, Management and the Educational Environment in Nursing*, Macmillan, London, pp.8–9, 10, 11, 135, 136, 140, 195–196.

The nursing process: from development to implementation[1]

Carmen de la Cuesta

The nursing process is a popular approach to nursing that has gained re-markably rapid acceptance both in the US and the UK. Nowadays, in the US it is synonymous with the practice of modern nursing. This approach forms part of a new direction that is currently taking place within the nursing profession. It has at least attracted the attention of the World Health Organization and gained the support of national professional orga-nizations both in the US and the UK. The nursing process has important consequences in the areas of nursing education and clinical practice which would imply, if it were fully implemented, a radical change in nursing.

The study intends to bring understanding into the practicalities and development of the nursing process. Thus, it has two purposes: to analyse, in sociological terms, its development and to understand whether it can make a practical contribution to nursing.

My sociological interest in the nursing process was aroused because of its sudden arrival in the UK. Why did certain nurses become interested in it and disseminate it? Why was it in 1975 and not before? The study began without any presumption that the nursing process is good or bad, but rather with many questions that rapidly multiplied. Thus, I took it as a fact and I examined the different issues that it evoked. What is the nursing process? A method? A philosophy? An ideology? When did it start? How and why did it develop? Who diffuses it? What are the practical outcomes? What are the problems in its implementation?

Since the nursing process began in the US and was disseminated to the UK, the study of nursing practice and sociological context in both countries has been necessary.

There is a great amount of American literature on this subject, more than any one person could read. Therefore I made a selection of the books and articles written. The selection aimed to identify those writings that had greatest influence on the theory's development, those writings which had the most significant impact and which nurses are most likely to encounter. To identify these works I used four types of sources: three bibliographical lists on the subject previously compiled in the UK by the Department of Health and Social Security, the Royal College of Nursing (RCN), and the Nursing Department of the University of Manchester; a random selection of books and articles from the US and the UK on the nursing process in order to identify authors who were most frequently quoted as sources; a list of those books at the RCN library in greatest demand; and the stock of works held in the library of a hospital nursing school where the nursing process was being implemented. With all the data collected from these sources, I elaborated a list of those authors most frequently encountered. This gave me a total selection of 14 books and four journal articles. In addition to the systematic analysis of these works, I read 23 other US journal articles and two more texts.

Since the UK literature was limited, I was able to analyse all the works included in the RCN bibliographical series up to March 1978 plus other later articles known from different sources. This involved the analysis of 27 articles, two unpublished papers, and one chapter from a book.

I made biographies of 13 of the principal people who had been or still are diffusers of the concept in the UK. The purpose of this was to study the diffusion process. The selection was made through an approximation to a snowball sampling technique.

I interviewed 29 nurses in a UK hospital where in some wards the nursing process was implemented. The purpose of this was to study the implementation as seen by practitioners. Since a complete sampling frame of the staff was not available, I used a two stage sampling design. First I selected the wards at random and then the staff involved. Furthermore, I interviewed 22 US nurses to study the genesis of the nursing process, the social context in which it developed, its diffusion and the current state of the issue. There were neither time nor opportunity for rigorous sampling of these nurses but they were all known in advance to be actively involved with the nursing process.

Development and diffusion of the nursing process

The idea that nursing is a process rather than a set of separate actions, started to emerge in the US in [the] 1950s. The earliest evidence I could find was in a lecture by Lydia Hall entitled 'The quality of nursing care' and given before a meeting of the Department of Baccalaureate and Higher Degree Programs of the New Jersey League for Nursing held on 7 February 1955 at Seaton Hall University. However, it was not until the 1960s that the nursing process was described in detail. Orlando (1961) reintroduced the concept in her book. From this time on, interest in the nursing process grew rapidly. Articles appeared in the nursing press focusing on specific aspects of the general concept (Francis, 1967; McCain, 1965; Durand and Prince, 1966; Peplau, 1960; Hewitt and Pesznecker, 1964; Kelly, 1966; Little and Carnevali, 1967; Phaneuf, 1966). Simultaneously, the nursing process began to be taught in institutions of higher education. At this stage it was seen primarily as a teaching tool. However, there is some evidence in the literature of the decade suggesting that in a few hospitals it was implemented in an experimental way, but its use was not common throughout the country. It was in the 1970s when the bulk of what we know today was developed and published. It also began to be implemented in hospitals. The majority of the authors who were developing the nursing process were from the educational sector.

Sociologically, the most remarkable aspect of the nursing process was the rapidity of its transference from the educational setting to clinical practice. The key to this transference was the American Nurses' Association (ANA) (1965) position paper in education that implied a reform in education; through it the nursing process was able to achieve a mass resocialization of large number of practising nurses. Already qualified nurses were impelled to undertake post-experience training just at the time when the nursing process was becoming the prevailing concept in the institutions of higher education. Thus, the large number of nurses who wanted to upgrade their qualifications learned about the nursing process and its application to the hospital. However, it was also disseminated by the more traditional and slower routes: articles in the nursing press, the entry into work of students educated in the new ideas and through in-service education. Although the idea of the nursing process became widespread, this did not mean that it was accepted as standard practice in nursing. This further stage came during the 1970s. At that time it was recommended by the ANA in order to achieve quality nursing practice, and the Joint Commission on the Accreditation of Hospitals (JCAH), the body in the US that legally certifies hospital services, made the preparation of care plans a prerequisite for the accreditation of nursing services. Thus, in the mid-1970s, the nursing process was not only a popular idea, but well on the way to institution.

The analysis of the sociological context in which it emerged shows that it appeared in a period in which there were major structural changes in the American society and medicine. These included the expansion of tertiary education, the emergence of the women's liberation movement, the growth of knowledge in the medical and social sciences, the increase of other health occupations, the rise in the costs of health services and the rise in the public expectations towards them. But it also emerged at a time where there was in nursing a discontented feeling both with the general status of the profession and with the quality of patient care. These led to a broad movement toward professional status which included the classical traits: the quest for autonomy, knowledge based practice, personalized services and the rise of educational qualifications; as well as other policies designed to gain public acceptance, e.g. the emphasis on total patient care, and the evaluation of benefits to patients.

The analysis of the literature shows that the content of the nursing process was shaped by the American context. Its theory incorporated the trends at that time, articulated them and facilitated their realization. It acted both as a coping mechanism for the discontent among nurses, and at the same time reinforced them. Thus, the content of the nursing process was not accidental. It involved more than a consideration of better nursing practice: it was also a professional strategy. It was the product of a particular place at a particular time and it is in the integration into contemporary American society which explains its success in the US.

In the UK the nursing process did not grow autonomously: it was taken from the US in [the] 1970s and then disseminated. However, it was not something completely new; it had precursors which prepared the grounds for its diffusion. Before it emerged there was a time of considerable discontent and internal debate within the British nursing. Nurses were unhappy with the existing system of delivering care and were seeking more satisfactory methods of nursing. The review of the nursing press during this period revealed a number of persistent critiques and reform proposals. The principal themes of discontent were: a rejection of a task orientated approach to nursing, the lack of individualized care, the low level of nurses' job satisfaction and the superficial nature of the nurse–patient relationship. As an antidote to these problems a number of approaches to nursing emerged; patient-centred care, patient assignment, total patient care, team nursing, progressive patient care. These approaches were all partial reforms that did not completely cope with the difficulties. It was in this context that the nursing process arrived. The content analysis shows that it amalgamated these criticisms into one comprehensive approach that offered apparent remedy to discontent long felt by practitioners.

In 1973 the very first discussions of the nursing process took place, the first articles were published in 1975 and by 1977 it was being implemented at hospital level. It first attracted nurses from the educational sector; of manifest appeal was the fact that it represented a device to understand and teach nursing. Then, it appealed to nurses in hospitals because it promised to reform the practice of nursing. The diffusion of the nursing process was extremely rapid: it emerged around 1973, by 1977 was included in the training syllabus for general nursing and begun to be implemented, and by 1979 the first British book was published.

... The nursing process is not just a theoretical and practical concept but an ideology in the technical sense as well, that is a body of ideas that did not arise spontaneously from pure reflection, but as a response to emerging problems and trends in a particular society at a particular time. Therefore, it is vulnerable to interpretations across cultures. Indeed, it was demonstrated that the nursing process has a different content in the UK and US.

Note

1. This paper is based on a presentation made at the First Open Conference 'Research – a challenge for nursing practice'. Uppsala, Sweden, 11–14 August 1982.

References

American Nurses' Association (1965) American Nurses Association first position on education for nursing. *American Journal of Nursing*, **65**, 106–111

Durand, M. and Prince, R. (1966) Nursing diagnosis: process and decision. *Nursing Forum*, **5**, 50–64

Francis, G. M. (1967) This thing called problem solving. *Journal of Nursing Education*, **6**, 27–29

Hewitt, H. E. and Pesznecker, B. L. (1964) Blocks to communication with patients. *American Journal of Nursing*, **64**, 101–103

Kelly, N. C. (1966) Nursing care plans. *Nursing Outlook*, **14**, 61–64

Little, D. E. and Carnevali, D. C. (1967) Nursing care plans: let's be practical about them. *Nursing Forum*, **6**, 61–67

McCain, R. F. (1965) Nursing by assessment – not intuition. *American Journal of Nursing*, **65**, 82–83

Orlando, I. J. (1961) *The Dynamic Nurse–Patient Relationship*, Putnams, New York

Peplau, H. E. (1960) Talking with patients. *American Journal of Nursing*, **60**, 960–964

Phaneuf, M. C. (1966) The nursing audit for evaluation of patient care. *Nursing Outlook*, **14**, 51–54

Reprinted by permission of Blackwell Science, Oxford. Carmen de la Cuesta (1983) The nursing process: from development to implementation. *Journal of Advanced Nursing*, **8**, 365–371.

Chapter 41

Medicine as an institution of social control

Irving Kenneth Zola

The theme of this essay is that medicine is becoming a major institution of social control, nudging aside, if not incorporating, the more traditional institutions of religion and law. It is becoming the new repository of truth, the place where absolute and often final judgments are made by supposedly morally neutral and objective experts. And these judgments are made, not in the name of virtue or legitimacy, but in the name of health. Moreover, this is not occurring through the political power physicians hold or can influence, but is largely an insidious and often undramatic phenomenon accomplished by 'medicalizing' much of daily living, by making medicine and the labels 'healthy' and 'ill' *relevant* to an ever increasing part of human existence.

Although many have noted aspects of this process, by confining their concern to the field of psychiatry, these criticisms have been misplaced.[1] For psychiatry has by no means distorted the mandate of medicine, but indeed, though perhaps at a pace faster than other medical specialities, is following instead some of the basic claims and directions of that profession. Nor is this extension into society the result of any professional 'imperialism', for this leads us to think of the issue in terms of misguided human efforts or motives. If we search for the 'why' of this phenomenon, we will see instead that it is rooted in our increasingly complex technological and bureaucratic system – a system which has led us down the path of the reluctant reliance on the expert.[2]

An historical perspective

The involvement of medicine in the management of society is not new. It did not appear full-blown one day in the mid-twentieth century. As Sigerist (1943) has aptly claimed, medicine at base was always not only a social science but an occupation whose very practice was inextricably interwoven into society. This interdependence is perhaps best seen in two branches of medicine which have had a built-in social emphasis from the very start – psychiatry[3] and public health/preventive medicine.[4] Public health was always committed to changing social aspects of life – from sanitary to housing to working conditions – and often used the arm of the state (i.e. through laws and legal power) to gain its ends (e.g. quarantines, vaccinations). Psychiatry's involvement in society is a bit more difficult to trace, but taking the histories of psychiatry as data, then one notes the almost universal reference to one of the early pioneers, a physician named Johan Weyer. His, and thus psychiatry's involvement in social problems lay in the objection that witches ought not to be burned; for they were not possessed by the devil, but rather bedeviled by their problems – namely they were insane. From its early concern with the issue of insanity as a defence in criminal proceedings, psychiatry has grown to become the most dominant rehabilitative perspective in dealing with society's 'legal' deviants. Psychiatry, like public health, has also used the legal powers of the state in the accomplishment of its goals (i.e. the cure of the patient) through the legal proceedings of involuntary comitment and its concomitant removal of certain rights and privileges.

The potential and consequences of medical control

The list of daily activities to which health can be related is ever growing and with the current operating perspective of medicine it seems infinitely expandable. The reasons are manifold. It is not merely that medicine has extended its jurisdiction to cover new problems,[5] or that doctors are professionally committed to finding disease,[6] nor even that society keeps creating disease.[7] For if none of these obtained today we would still find medicine exerting an enormous influence on society. The most powerful empirical stimulus for this is the realization of how much everyone has or believes he has something organically wrong with him, or put more positively, how much can be done to make one feel, look or function better.

Conclusion

C. S. Lewis warned us more than a quarter of a century ago that 'man's power over Nature is really the power of some men over other men, with Nature as their instrument'. The same could be said regarding man's power over health and illness, for the labels health and illness are remarkable 'depoliticizers' of an issue. By locating the source and the treatment of problems in an individual, other levels of intervention are effectively closed. By the very acceptance of a specific behaviour as an 'illness' and the definition of illness as an undesirable state, the issue becomes not whether to deal with a particular problem, but *how* and *when*.[8] Thus the debate over homosexuality, drugs or abortion becomes focused on the degree of sickness attached to the phenomenon in question or the extent of the health risk involved. And the more principled, more perplexing, or even moral issue, of *what* freedom should an individual have over his or her own body is shunted aside.

As stated in the very beginning this 'medicalizing of society' is as much a result of medicine's potential as it is of society's wish for medicine to use that potential. Why then has the focus been more on the medical potential than on the social desire? In part it is a function of space, but also of political expediency. For the time rapidly may be approaching when recourse to the populace's wishes may be impossible.

To return to our opening caution, this paper is not an attack on medicine so much as on a situation in which we find ourselves in the latter part of the twentieth century; for the medical area is the arena or the example *par excellence* of today's identity crisis – what is or will become of man. It is the battleground, not because there are visible threats and oppressors, but because they are almost invisible; not because the perspective, tools and practitioners of medicine and the other helping professions are evil, but because they are not. It is so frightening because there are elements here of the banality of evil so uncomfortably written about by Hannah Arendt (1963). But here the danger is greater, for not only is the process masked as a technical, scientific, objective one, but one done for our own good. A few years ago a physician speculated on what, based on current knowledge, would be the composite picture of an individual with a low risk of developing atherosclerosis or coronary-artery disease. He would be:

> . . . an effeminate municipal worker or embalmer completely lacking in physical or mental alertness and without drive, ambition, or competitive spirit; who has never attempted to meet a deadline of any kind; a man with poor appetite, subsisting on fruits and vegetables laced with corn and whale oil, detesting tobacco, spurning ownership of radio, television, or motorcar, with full head of hair but scrawny and unathletic appearance, yet constantly straining his puny muscles by exercise. Low in income, blood pressure, blood sugar, uric acid and cholesterol, he has been taking nicotinic acid, pyridoxine, and long term anti-coagulant therapy ever since his prophylactic castration.[9]

Thus I fear with Freidson:

> A profession and a society which are so concerned with physical and functional wellbeing as to sacrifice civil liberty and moral integrity must inevitably press for a 'scientific' environment similar to that provided laying hens on progressive chicken farms – hens who produce eggs industriously and have no disease or other cares.[10]

Nor does it really matter that if, instead of the above depressing picture, we were guaranteed six more inches in height, thirty more years of life, or drugs to expand our potentialities and potencies; we should still be able to ask: what do six more inches matter, in what kind of environment will the thirty additional years be spent, or who will decide what potentialities and potencies will be expanded and what curbed.

Notes

1. Szasz, T. (1961) *The Myth of Mental Illness*, Harper and Row, New York; and Leifer, R. (1969) *In the Name of Mental Health*, Science House, New York.
2. E.g. Toffler, A. (1970) *Future Shock*, Random House, New York; and Slater, P. E. (1970) *The Pursuit of Loneliness*, Beacon Press, Boston.
3. Foucault, M. (1965) *Madness and Civilization*, Pantheon, New York; and Szasz, *op. cit.*
4. Rosen, G. (1955) *A History of Public Health*, MD Publications, New York; and Rosen, G. (1963) The evolution of social medicine. In *Handbook of Medical Sociology* (Freeman, H. E., Levine, S. and Reeder, L. G., eds), Prentice-Hall, Englewood Cliffs, N.J., pp. 17–61.
5. Szasz, *op. cit.*; and Leifer, *op. cit.*
6. Freidson, E. (1970) *Profession of Medicine*, Dodd, Mead & Co., New York; Scheff, T. (1964) Preferred errors in diagnoses. *Medical Care*, 2, 166–172.
7. Dubos, A. (1959) *The Mirage of Health*, Doubleday, Garden City, N.Y.; and Dubos, R. (1965) *Man Adapting*, Yale University Press.
8. This general case is argued more specifically in Zola, I. K. (1968) *Medicine, Morality, and Social Problems – Some Implications of the Label Mental Illness*. Paper presented at the Amer. Ortho-Psychiat. Ass., March 20– 23.
9. Myers, G. S., quoted in Lasagna, L. (1968) *Life, Death and the Doctor*, Alfred Knouf, New York, 1968, pp. 215– 216.
10. Freidson: *op. cit.*, p. 354.

References

Arendt, H. (1963) *Eichmann in Jerusalem – A Report on the Banality of Evil*, Viking Press, New York
Sigerist, H. (1943) *Civilization and Disease*, Cornell University Press, New York

Reprinted by permission of Blackwell Science, Oxford. Irving Kenneth Zola (1972) Medicine as an institution of social control. *Sociological Review*, 20, 487, 488, 497, 500, 502–504.

Chapter 42

Professions and patriarchy

Anne Witz

Professions and patriarchy

The spectre of the 'semi-profession' has haunted discussion of gender and professionalisation. Indeed, gender was integral to the very definition of a 'semi-profession' which according to Etzioni (1969) has two defining features. It is an occupation located within a bureaucratic organisation and one in which women predominate. The sheer preponderance of women places a brake on the extent to which these occupations can professionalise (Etzioni, 1969; Simpson and Simpson, 1969) ... it was claimed that 'semi-professions' are not professions because women lack occupational motivation, ambition and any drive toward intellectual mastery (sic), are incapable of exercising authority over men (due to their own belief in male superiority), or of forming occupational communities and maintaining constructive colleague relations because they are 'less able than men to disagree impersonally, without emotional involvement ... think in value terms rather than intellectualising a problem' and tend to spend their time comparing notes on clothing styles and child-rearing which 'does not have the same professionalizing effect as the task-related contacts of professionally dedicated workers' (Simpson and Simpson, 1969, p. 241). Consequently, the subordinate position of the (female) semi-profession in relation to the (male) profession is due to the fact that women are willingly compliant and tractable subordinates, ideally suited to the role of 'hand-maidens of a male occupation that has authority over them' (Simpson and Simpson, 1969, p. 231).

In short, because women are not men, 'semi-professions' are not professions. It is paradoxical that the functionalist paradigm of profession within which the semi-professions thesis is located has been largely displaced, but the semi-professions thesis lingers on. Very recently Rueschemeyer (1986, p. 137) is able to casually suggest that the 'high devotion/low power syndrome' of the social service professions 'articulates well with traditional conceptions of women's role'. The 'semi-profession' thesis is based on an androcentric model of profession, which takes what are in fact the successful professional projects of man at a particular point in history to be the paradigm of profession.

Gender and medical professionalisation

The 1858 Medical (Registration) Act had set up a male monopoly and had effectively excluded women from access to the ranks of the medical profession. The act's parliamentary sponsor, William Cowper-Temple, had never intended this, and indeed there was nothing in the wording of the act to legally exclude women from becoming registered medical practitioners. In fact, gendered exclusionary mechanisms did not operate at the institutional level of the state, but in the institutions of civil society: the university medical faculties, the various Royal Colleges of Physicians and of Surgeons and other medical corporations, as well as teaching hospitals. Women were excluded from medical education and examination in all of the institutions which made up the nineteen portals of entry onto the medical register.

Medical professionalisation is perhaps one of the best examples of a male professional project. But medicine was not to remain an exclusive male preserve for long. The male monopoly over legitimate medical practice was quickly challenged by aspiring women doctors ... the following case study of men, women and medical practice in the nineteenth century provides the terrain on which to demonstrate the utility of two of the closure concepts set out in the previous chapter. Professional closure in medicine was historically constructed as a mode of patriarchal closure, and was sustained by gendered strategies of exclusion. Women's challenge to the exclusive male prerogative over medical practice provides an example of a gendered strategy of inclusion, which I have defined as a countervailing, usurpationary response on the part of an excluded group.

First, though, before detailing the elaborate twists and turns of women's struggle to enter the medical profession and medical men's staunch defence of their male monopoly, it is necessary to set the scene for this episode by surveying the relationship between gender and healing activities in the pre-modern era and identifying broader structural and historical shifts in the transition from pre-modern to modern medical practice.

Gender and medical professionalisation: from the pre-modern to the modern era

The 1858 Medical (Registration) Act was the lynchpin of the formation of the modern medical profession. It gave legal definition to the term 'qualified medical practitioner' by setting up a state-sponsored register of qualified practitioners and delineating the legal as well as the institutional parameters of the modern medical profession (Waddington, 1984, pp. 136–137). Drawing on Larson's distinction between heteronomous and autonomous means of closure, the 1858 Medical Act represented the use of heteronomous means, in the form of a monopoly secured through legislative tactics within the institutional arena of the state. Thereafter, the General Medical

Council, the statutory body set up under the terms of the 1858 Act, focussed its energies on credentialist tactics by mobilising autonomous means of closure and attempting to consolidate and impose some uniformity on existing, diverse systems of medical education and examination. There were nineteen routes of entry onto the medical register; systems of medical education and examination institutionally located in civil society, in the medical colleges and university medical faculties (cf. Stevens, 1966). Professional closure in medicine was secured in the twin arenas of the state and civil society and it was this process, together with processes linked to the institutional relocation of medical practice from the domestic to the market arena, that sounded the death knell for women's participation in healing practices.

In previous centuries, health care had been provided by a range of itinerant and community-based healers, many of whom were women, and it was the elimination of these types of healers, together with the control of newly emergent ones, which were processes at the core of medicine's modern evolution (Larkin, 1983). By the mid-nineteenth century, however, medical diagnosis and treatment had become the exclusive prerogative of medical men, and women had become restricted to the care of the sick, as nurses, and to the attendance of women during natural labour, as midwives. When the profession formally unified in 1858, male groups of physicians, surgeons and apothecaries were included whilst the female group of midwives was not (Verluysen, 1980).

So the history of the transition from the pre-modern to the modern practice of medicine is also the history of the restructuring of gender divisions in health care as women were excluded from certain spheres of competence and confined to others. The twin concepts of gendered exclusion and demarcation, set out in the previous chapter, therefore become crucial in charting the complex restructuring of gender divisions in the emerging modern medical division of labour in the nineteenth century. Generally, however, sociological analyses of the rise of the modern medical profession (Waddington, 1984; Larson, 1977; Freidson, 1970; Berlant, 1975; Elliott, 1972) have neglected to examine the twin processes of professionalisation and masculinisation that marked the transition from pre-modern to modern medical practice. This has been left to a small body of feminist analyses (Ehrenreich and English, 1973a, b, 1979; Oakley, 1976; Verluysen, 1980; Chamberlain, 1981; Doyal, 1986; Pinchbeck, 1981; Clark, 1919).

The overall task confronting women who wished to practise medicine in Britain was to establish the means whereby the link between education and occupation could be made by women as well as by men. The key to the maintenance of professional closure as patriarchal closure in medicine lay in the exclusion of women from the institutional arenas of medical education and examination that made up the nineteen state-approved routes of access to registered medical practice under the terms and conditions of the 1858 Medical Act. Exclusionary mechanisms were embedded in the sphere of civil society, in the medical corporations and modern university. They were only indirectly reinforced within the institutional arena of the state. This suggests that, although legalistic tactics in the form of state sponsored registration have been central to modern professional projects, including that of medicine, patriarchal closure has been primarily sustained through credentialist tactics by controlling access to education and accreditation.

Aspiring women doctors' inclusionary strategy initial concentrated on gaining access to university medical education and examination, through countervailing credentialist tactics. But the universities proved remarkably resilient to women's usurpationary claims, so priority was eventually given to countervailing legalistic tactics of usurpation and the attempt to gain access to medical education and examination by lobbying parliament for an amendment of the 1858 act. But women's struggle to enter the medical profession was not simply a form of occupational politics, but was also a form of gender politics. It is possible to distinguish between credentialist and legalistic tactics of occupational politics, and the equal rights and separatist tactics of gender politics. These four tactics may combine in various ways, as Table [1] illustrates.

Women, then, used credentialist and legalistic tactics. They challenged mechanisms of gendered exclusion embedded within credentialism and operating within the autonomous means of professional closure, namely the institutional locations of the modern university and medical corporations. This element of women's usurpationary strategy is described as a counter-vailing credentialist tactic. Women also challenged the mechanisms of gendered exclusion ... at the institutional level of the state ... by seeking state sponsorship of their usurpationary project (just as medical men had sought state sponsorship for their professional project) in the form of parliamentary bills that sought to amend the 1858 Medical Act. This facet of women's usurpationary strategy is described as a countervailing legalistic tactic.

Along the dimension of gender politics a distinction may be made between an equal rights and a separatist tactic as the specifically gendered tactics of usurpationary struggle. The equal rights tactic describes women's attempts to break the male prerogative over the system of medical education and examination by gaining access to existing, male-dominated systems of medical education and examination, namely the modern universities and medical corporations. In addition, separatist tactics were resorted to, as

Table 3.1 Tactics of usurpation

Equal rights	The University of Edinburgh, 1869–74	1. Universities (Scotland) (Degrees to Women) Bill, 1875 2. Medical (Qualifications) Bill, 1876
Separatist	The London School of Medicine for Women, established 1874	Medical Act Amendment (Foreign Universities) Bill, 1874 and 1876

women attempted to open up separate, gender-specific routes of access to the system of medical education and registration.

The following analysis of women's usurpationary struggle in the 1860s and 1870s examines, first, credentialist tactics pursued on the terrain of civil society and, second, legalistic tactics pursued in the institutional arena of the state legislature.

Credentialist tactics

Between 1869 and 1873 a group of women led by Sophia Jex-Blake struggled to receive medical education and present themselves for medical degrees at the University of Edinburgh. This episode has been well documented (cf. Jex-Blake, 1886; Thorne, 1915; Bell, 1953) ... In 1869 Sophia Jex-Blake was refused admission to medical classes by the Senate of Edinburgh University, not on grounds of principle but of expediency. It was not worth making concessions for the convenience of one lady (Jex-Blake, 1886, pp. 71–75; Bell, 1953). Then four other women – Edith Pechey, Isabel Thorne, Matilda Chaplin and Mrs Evans – joined her and, as there were then five, the university could no longer exclude them on the grounds of expediency alone. The five women were admitted to be matriculated and study medicine, although in separate classes from male students. The women paid medical lecturers three times the fee that the male students did for the privilege.

However, in 1870 the opponents of medical women attempted to prevent them from completing their medical education by putting pressure on medical lecturers who were providing separate classes. The women switched to the Edinburgh Extra-Mural School, where three doctors admitted them to classes. The gathering opposition to the women students was led by Professor Christison of the Medical Faculty, a manager of the Royal Edinburgh Infirmary, which had accepted the women for clinical instruction. Christison then managed to reverse this decision on constitutional grounds. Male undergraduates then began to take an active part in the struggle against the women ... fuelled, suggests Bell (1953) by the glowing academic achievements of the women at the end of the winter session (1869–70) when four of them gained honours and one of them, Edith Pechey, came first in the chemistry examination, an achievement which merited a Hope Scholarship. However, this was awarded to the man immediately below her on the class list (Jex-Blake, 1886; pp. 81–83; Bell, 1953, p. 72).

In November 1870 the 'indignities' (Lutzker, 1974) and 'petty annoyances' (Thorne, 1915) to which the women were increasingly subject came to a head in the riot at Surgeon's Hall, where the women were to sit an examination. A dense crowd had gathered outside the hall and the gates were slammed in their faces by a number of young men 'who stood within, smoking and passing about bottles of whisky, while they abused us in the foulest possible language' (Jex-Blake, 1886, p. 92). One of the medical students already in Surgeon's Hall came to their aid and opened the gate for them. During the examination a sheep was pushed in by the rioters. When the examination was over, the women left protected against the rioters by a bodyguard (armed with osteological specimens, recalled Isabel Thorne) of some of their fellow students (Jex-Blake, 1886, p. 93; Thorne, 1915, p. 14).

This incident of public and collective male violence, both physical and verbal, against women who openly transgressed the bounds set for them within patriarchal relations is evocative of the violence and sexual assault meted out to a deputation of suffragettes on 'Black Friday', 18 November 1910 (cf. Morrell, 1981). In 1913 Christabel Pankhurst was to argue that the manners of chivalry can only be maintained while women willingly abide by the restrictive rules men have imposed upon them, but that, once women challenge these rules, chivalry is dead (cf. Spender, 1982; Sarah, 1983). Indeed, Sophia Jex-Blake referred somewhat ironically to the rioters outside Surgeons Hall as 'chivalrous foes' (1886, p. 93).

However, male power in the institutional sphere of civil society is not routinely exercised as force or physical and verbal intimidation, but simply by changing the rules. By July 1873 the University of Edinburgh, by a series of elaborate twists and turns, had succeeded in restoring the patriarchal status quo ante by declaring that, although the women medical students could continue to receive medical instruction in separate classes, this did not imply any right to obtain medical degrees (Jex-Blake, 1886, p. 138). 'The majority of medical men in the University ... were adverse to them; and the doors of the Scotch University were shut against admission of ladies' (*Hansard* CCXXX 1876, p. 998).

The struggle at Edinburgh demonstrated that the modern university system provided a key site for the institutionalisation of gendered credentialist tactics. It was a countervailing credentialist tactic because it sought to replace gendered collectivist criteria of exclusion with non-gendered criteria of inclusion. It was also an equal rights tactic because it sought to secure the admission of women to an existing, traditionally male-dominated institution of medical education.

References

Bell, E. Moberly (1953) *Storming the Citadel: The Rise of the Woman Doctor*, Constable, London

Berlant, J. L. (1975) *Profession and Monopoly*, University of California Press, Berkeley

Chamberlain, M. (1981) *Old Wives' Tales: Their History, Remedies and Spells*, Virago, London

Clark, A. (1919) *Working Life of Women in the Seventeenth Century*, George Routledge, London (Reprinted 1981, Virago, London)

Doyal, L. (1986) Women, health and medicine. In *Women in Britain Today* (Beechey, V. and Whitelegg, E., eds), Open University, Milton Keynes

Ehrenreich, B. and English, D. (1973a) *Complaints and Disorders: The Sexual Politics of Sickness*, Feminist Press, New York

Ehrenreich, B. and English, D. (1973b) *Witches, Midwives and Nurses: A History of Women Healers*, Writers and Readers Publishing Co-operative, London

Ehrenreich, B. and English, D. (1979) *For Her Own Good: 150 Year of the Expert's Advice to Women*, Pluto Press, London

Elliott, P. (1972) *The Soviology of the Professions*, Macmillan, London.

Etzioni, A. (1969) *The Semi-Professions and their Organization*, Free Press, New York.

Freidson, E. (1970) *Professional Dominance: The Social Structure of Medical Care*, Atherton Press, New York

Jex-Blake, S. (1886) *Medical Women: A Thesis and a History*, Oliphant, Andersen & Ferrier, Edinburgh

Larkin, G. (1983) *Occupational Monopoly and Modern Medicine*, Tavistock, London

Larson, M. (1977) *The Rise of Professionalism*, University of California Press, California

Lutzker, E. (1974) The London School of Medicine for Women: origin and important contributions to medicine by a few graduates. *Proceedings of the XXIII Congress of the History of Medicine*, 1, 357–366

Morrell, C. (1981) *'Black Friday' and Violence Against Women in the Suffragette Movement*, Women's Research and Resources Centre, London

Oakley, A. (1976) Wisewomen and medicine men: changes in the management of childbirth. In *The Rights and Wrongs of Women* (Mitchell, J. and Oakley, A., eds), Penguin, Harmondsworth

Pinchbeck, I. (1930) *Women Workers and the Industrial Revolution* (Reprinted 1981, Virago, London)

Rueschemeyer, D. (1986) *Power and the Division of Labour*, Polity Press, Cambridge

Sarah, E. (1983) Christabel Pankhurst: reclaiming her power (1880–1958). In *Feminist Theorists: Three Centuries of Women's Intellectual Traditions* (Spender, D., ed.), The Women's Press, London

Simpson, R. L. and Simpson, I. H. (1969) Women and bureaucracy in the semi-professions. In *The Semi-Professions and their Organization* (Etzioni, A., ed.). Free Press, New York

Spender, D. (1982) *Women of Ideas – And What Men Have Done to Them*, Routledge & Kegan Paul, London

Stevens, R. (1966) *Medical Practice in Modern England*, Yale University Press, New Haven and London

Thorne, I. (1915) *Sketch of the Foundation and Development of the London School of Medicine for Women*, Women's Printing Society, London

Verluysen, M. (1980) Old wives' tales? Women healers in English history. In *Rewriting Nursing History* (Davies, C., ed.), Croom Helm, London

Waddington, I. (1984) *The Medical Profession in the Industrial Revolution*, Gill & MacMillan, Ireland

Reprinted by permission of Anne Witz (1992) *Professions and Patriarchy*, Routledge, London, pp. 60, 61, 73–75, 88–91.

Chapter 43

The hospital and its negotiated order

A. L. Strauss, D. Ehrlich, R. Bucher and M. Sabshin

A professionalized locale

A hospital can be visualized as a professionalized locale – a geographical site where persons drawn from different professions come together to carry out their respective purposes. At our specific hospital, the professionals consisted of numerous practicing psychiatrists and psychiatric residents, nurses and nursing students, psychologists, occupational therapists, and one lone social worker. Each professional echelon has received noticeably different kinds of training and, speaking conventionally, each occupies some differential hierarchical position at the hospital while playing a different part in its total division of labor.

But that last sentence requires elaboration and amendment. The persons within each professional group may be, and probably are, at different stages in their respective careers. Furthermore, the career lines of some may be quite different from those of their colleagues: thus some of our psychiatrists were just entering upon psychoanalytic training, but some had entered the medical specialty by way of neurology, and had dual neurological psychiatric practices. Implicit in the preceding statement is that those who belong to the same profession also may differ quite measurably in the training they have received, as well as in the theoretical (or ideological) positions they take toward important issues like etiology and treatment. Finally, the hospital itself may possess differential significance for colleagues: for instance, some psychiatrists were engaged in hospital practice only until such time as their office practices had been sufficiently well established; while other, usually older, psychiatrists were committed wholeheartedly to working with hospitalized patients.

Looking next at the division of labor shared by the professionals: never do all persons of each echelon work closely with all others from other echelons. At our hospital it was notable that considerable variability characterized who worked closely with whom – and how – depending upon such matters as idealogical and hierarchical position. Thus the services of the social worker were used not at all by some psychiatrists, while each man who utilized her services did so somewhat differently. Similarly some men utilized 'psychologicals' more than did others. Similarly, some psychiatrists were successful in housing their patients almost exclusively upon certain wards, which meant that, wittingly or not, they worked only with certain nurses. As in other institutions, the various echelons possessed differential status and power, but again there were marked internal differences concerning status and power, as well as knowledgeability about 'getting things done'. Nor must it be overlooked that not only did the different professions hold measurably different views – derived both from professional and status positions – about the proper division of labor; but different views also obtained within echelon. (The views were most discrepant among the psychiatrists.) All in all, the division of labor is a complex concept, and at hospitals must be seen in relation to the professionalized milieu.

The grounds for negotiation

Negotiation and the division of labor are rendered all the more complex because personnel in our hospital – we assume that the generalization, with some modification, holds elsewhere – share only a single, vaguely ambiguous goal. The goal is to return patients to the outside world in better shape. This goal is the symbolic cement that, metaphorically speaking, holds the organization together: the symbol to which all personnel can comfortably, and frequently point – with the assurance that at *least* about this matter everyone can agree! Although this symbol, as will be seen later, masks a considerable measure of disagreement and discrepant purpose, it represents a generalized mandate under which the hospital can be run – the public flag under which all may work in concert. Let us term it the institution's constitutional grounds or basic compact. These grounds, this compact, are never openly challenged; nor are any other goals given explicit verbal precedence. (This is so when a hospital, such as ours, also is a training institution.) In addition, these constitutional grounds can be used by any and all personnel as a justificatory rationale for actions that are under attack. In short, although personnel may disagree to the point of apoplexy about how to implement patients' getting better, they do share the common institutional value.

The problem, of course, is that when the personnel confront a specific patient and attempt to make him recover then the disagreements flare up – the generalized mandate helps not at all to handle the specific issue – and a complicated process of negotiation, of bargaining, of give-and-take necessarily begins. The disagreements that necessitate negotiation do not occur by chance but are patterned. Here are several illustrations of the grounds that lead to negotiation. Thus, the personnel may disagree over what is the proper placement within the hospital for some patient: believing that, at any given time, he is more likely improve when placed upon one ward rather than upon another. This issue is the source of considerable tension between physicians and ward personnel. Again, what is meant by 'getting better' is itself open to differential judgment when applied to the progress – or retrogression – of a particular patient. This judgment is influenced not only by professional experience and acquaintance with the patient but is also influenced by the very concept of getting better as held by the different echelons. Thus the aides – who are laymen – have quite different notions about these matters than do the physicians, and on the whole those notions are not quite equivalent to those held by nurses. But both the nurses and the aides see patients getting better according to signs visible from the patient's daily behavior while the psychiatrist tends to relate these signs, if apprehended at all, to deeper layers of personality; with the consequence that frequently the staff thinks one way about the patient's 'movement' while the physician thinks quite otherwise, and must argue his case, set them right, or even keep his peace.

If negotiation is called for because a generalized mandate requires implementation, it is also called for because of the multiplicity of purpose found in the hospital. It is incontestable that each professional group has a different set of reasons for working at this hospital (to begin with, most nurses are women, most physicians are men); and of course colleagues inevitably differ among themselves on certain of their purposes for working there. In addition, each professional develops there his own specific and temporally limited ends that he wishes to attain. All this diversity of purpose affects the institution's division of labor, including not only what tasks each person is expected to accomplish but also how he maneuvers to get them accomplished. Since very little of this can possibly be prefigured by the administrative rule-makers, the attainment of one's purposes requires inevitably the cooperation of fellow workers. This point, once made, scarcely needs illustration.

However, yet another ground of negotiation needs emphasizing: namely, that in this hospital, as doubtless elsewhere, the patient as an 'individual case' is taken as a virtual article of faith. By this we mean that the element of medical uncertainty is so great, and each patient is taken as – in some sense – so unique, that action round and about him must be tailor-made, must be suited to his precise therapeutic requirements. This kind of assumption abets what would occur anyhow: that only a minimum of rules can be laid down for running a hospital, since a huge area of contingency necessarily lies outside those rules. The rules can provide guidance and command for only a small amount of the total concerted action that must go on around the patient. It follows, as already noted, that where action is not ruled it must be agreed upon.

One important further condition for negotiation should be mentioned. Changes are forced upon the hospital and its staff not only by forces external to the hospital but also by unforeseen consequences of internal policies and negotiations carried on within the hospital. In short, negotiations breed further negotiations.

Chapter 44

Professional powers: a study of the institutionalization of formal knowledge

Eliot Freidson

The problem is how to identify professions as a group, and there I noted the scholarly controversies surrounding definition and specification and argued that resolution is unlikely to occur. Taking only the traditional status professions, the differences between medicine and law are very great, and they are in turn quite different from university teaching, the ministry, and the military. Add architecture, dentistry, accounting, and engineering, among the older occupational professions, and one can argue that the differences among them are too great to allow generalization. Indeed, part of the course of disagreement among scholars about the attributes to be used in defining *profession* arose from the fact of those differences. Scholarly controversy, however, has not succeeded in discouraging others from the use of *profession* as a social category or folk concept. Indeed, controversy among scholars specializing in the study of the professions has either not penetrated to or, if it has, not discouraged other scholars concerned with broader issues like the class system of modern society. Some have seen higher education (if not necessarily the formal knowledge one might assume is its product) as the key to the formation of a 'new class' that has a special position in the class system of advanced societies.

Professions and the new class

There are a number of different orientations underlying the idea of a new class. The first to become concerned with the possibility that a new kind of middle class was developing was Emil Lederer early in this century (for sketch of Lederer's work, see Bell, 1976, pp.69–72). Subsequent development of the idea involved the notion that the old middle class of the nineteenth century, which was composed largely of small businessmen and members of traditional status professions like law and medicine, was being supplanted, or at least pushed aside, by a rising new middle class composed of salaried members of the administrative or managerial staff, the specialized professions, and, depending on the writer, the clerical and technical staffs of large public and private organizations (for historical sketches of the development of the notion, see Mills, 1951; Crozier, 1971, pp.21–40; and Giddens, 1973, pp.177–97).

At its broadest the new class is an undifferentiated, broad white-collar class, its members sharing only its ostensibly 'clean' work. That is essentially the way Mills (1951) conceived of it. At its narrowest in present-day writings it is conceived of as composed solely of intellectuals who are professionals in the arts, journalism, and academia and of others involved in government regulatory and welfare activities (for a delineation of how major notions of the new class vary in their inclusiveness, see Brint, 1984). Historians who have used the idea have similarly differed in their conceptions of the class, Lasch (1979) apparently including only some academics and the personal service professions and Bledstein (1976) including everyone, including baseball players, who may be said to hold a 'culture of professionalism' that is oriented toward careerism and mobility (cf. Lederer's discussion of the 'life rhythms' of the civil servant in Bell, 1976, p.70; and for a cogent critique of historians' use the idea of profession, see Veysey, 1975). On the whole, as Bell put it, it is a 'muddled concept' (Bell, 1979).

How is it possible to speak of the professions collectively, as a category if not a class? Scholars are in sufficient disagreement about definition that they differ in the occupations they would include as professions and those they would exclude. However, the official category of the US census does exist as a social reality and, what is more, forms the framework for the collection of comprehensive empirical information about the labor force in the United States and the delineation of those occupations that taken together are classified as professions. By its decision to include some occupations as professions and to exclude others it presents us with an official categorical portrait of professions. For those new class theorists who are concerned with determining who are members of the new class and how they are distributed through the labor force, the census provides an official collation and classification for the nation. Can it be used to represent the professions productively? Obviously, since it *is* used, we should know more about it in any case. But by examining what some new class theorists postulate to be important about a class in which professions are prominent we can also generate some criteria by which to evaluate the intellectual usefulness of the category. Let me sketch two interesting and related new class theories, show what issues they are concerned with in considering professions an important part of the new class, and then go on to examine the relevant census categories in sufficient detail to appraise their usefulness in representing the issues. This will lead me to conclude by suggesting the criteria by which I shall identify the social category *professions* in the chapters to follow.

Two theories

Two related versions of new class theory employ the US census as a source for identifying the members of that class and estimating their number in the labor force. I refer to the notion of the 'Professional-Managerial Class' created by the Ehrenreichs (Ehrenreich and Ehrenreich, 1977a, 1977b) and the notion of the 'New Class' of intellectuals and technical intelligentsia created by the late Alvin Gouldner (1979). First the Ehrenreichs.

After reviewing some of the efforts at defining the new middle class by previous Marxian writers, the Ehrenreichs advance the notion of the Professional-Managerial Class, so named in order to signal the exclusion of sales and clerical workers, who are classified by them with the working class, and in order to avoid confusion with the old middle class of self-employed professionals, tradesmen, farmers, and the like. The Professional-Managerial Class is seen to have been created by a process that began in the last half of the nineteenth century. According to the Ehrenreichs' theory, the capitalist class sought to quell working-class unrest by improving its methods of control of workers in both the workplace and the community. It supported the development of science, engineering, education, and health and welfare services toward that end. This meant encouraging the growth of occupations to staff the activities of such services. Thus the extraordinary growth in number and importance of such workers as teachers, social workers, engineers, nurses, lower- and middle-level managers, journalists, advertising personnel, experts in child rearing, truant officers, city planners, writers, accountants, lawyers, and physicians, who, among others, compose the Professional-Managerial Class.

That class cannot be considered part of the working class because, even though it is salaried by the capitalists, as is the working class, and thus in an objective position of antagonism to them, it can exist 'only by virtue of the expropriation of the skills and culture once indigenous to the working class' (Ehrenreich and Ehrenreich, 1977a, p.17) and by exercising control over the working class in the interest of the status quo. It is neither working nor capitalist class, those professionals and managers in it having in common both their structural position between capital and labor and their common function of organizing the means of production and reproducing the class relations of capitalism.

The typical way in which the occupations of the Professional-Managerial Class are organized is as professions that claim commitment to public service and possession of an esoteric body of specialized formal knowledge and that seek freedom from evaluation and control by others. But since specialization is divisive, the occupations of the class are not unified by their class position and do not act as a class. The deepest division is between managers and administrators who are tied to business and industry and professionals providing personal services. That division is easy to over-emphasize, however, for both managers and professionals partake of higher education, and their children tend to go to college together and to intermarry. Members of the class have a common life-style, part of which is rooted in anxiety about assuring that their children gain 'decent' jobs under circumstances in which jobs can no longer be directly inherited.

Delineating the professional category

If we cannot find a reasonably homogeneous set of occupations in the official census category, and if we cannot find consensus among scholars' methods of discriminating professions that employ easily available and reasonably reliable information, how can we identify that group of occupations we can call collectively *professions*? Let us agree, first, with new class theorists and students of intellectuals and the intelligentsia that a critical criterion lies in some degree of exposure to higher education and the formal knowledge it transmits. But remembering the importance to potential understanding of the professions' capacity to exercise power and of the problem of gaining a living, let us add the criterion that they are occupations for which education is a prerequisite to employment in particular positions. Formal education creates qualification for particular jobs, from which others who lack such qualification are routinely excluded (Collins, 1979). Such a circumstance is likely to mean that those occupations have developed a coherent organization that effectively undertakes a 'market project' (Larson, 1977) that succeeds in carving out a labor-market shelter, a social closure, or a sinecure for its members in the labor market.

In the occupations listed in the census category bearing on professions we have already seen the amount of variation in that criterion. Among the traditional professions, medicine, but not law, the clergy, or university teaching, comes close to complete social closure, but so does a profession of considerably lesser prestige, income, and education – schoolteaching. Engineering is close in a *de facto* fashion, but hiring on the basis of credentials is discretionary for employers, and there is the constant likelihood that some jobs held by engineers can be given instead to drafters and lower-level technologists. There is nothing to prevent employers from doing that. The vast majority of all nurses, librarians, accountants, and, depending on how they are defined, social workers do not have to have any specific number of years of specialized training in institutions of higher education for their jobs. In this book I shall include them, however, because the leadership and upper tier of those occupations do have higher education and specialized training and are pressing for 'higher' standards. For that reason, too, as well as for their history, I would include architects. Furthermore, by this criterion we must also include some managers as professionals – namely, those managers and administrators for whose jobs specific educational credentials are required. It is no accident that Wright *et al.* (1982, p.719) found that, by their 'class location' criteria, conventionally classified 'professionals' were 'managerial' in 52 per cent of the cases. Among those managers listed separately in the census it might be appropriate to include health administrators as members of the professions and certainly necessary to include school principals and superintendents among the *administrators, primary and secondary schools.*

References

Bell, D. (1976) *The Coming of Post-Industrial Society*, Basic Books, New York
Bell, D. (1979) The new class: a muddled concept. *Society*, **16** (January-February), 15–23
Bledstein, B. J. (1976) *The Culture of Professionalism*, W. W. Norton, New York
Brint, S. G. (1984) 'New class' and cumulative trend explanations of the liberal attitudes of professionals. *American Journal of Sociology*, **90** (July), 30–71
Collins, R. (1979) *The Credential Society*, Academic Press, New York
Crozier, M. (1971) *The World of the Office Worker*, University of Chicago Press, Chicago
Ehrenreich, B. and Ehrenreich, J. (1977a) The professional-managerial class. Part 1. *Radical America*, **11** (March-April), 7–31
Ehrenreich, B. (1977b) The professional-managerial class. Part 2. *Radical America*, **11** (May-June), 7–22
Giddens, A. (1973) *The Class Structure of the Advanced Societies*, Harper and Row, New York
Gouldner, A. W. (1979) *The Future of the Intellectuals and the Rise of the New Class*, Macmillan Press, London
Larson, M. S. (1977) *The Rise of Professionalism: A Sociological Analysis*, University of California Press, Berkeley
Lasch, C. (1979) *Haven in a Heartless World.* Basic Books, New York
Mills, C. W. (1951) *White Collar*, Oxford University Press, New York
Veysey, L. R. (1975) Who's a professional? Who cares? *Reviews in American History*, **December**, 419–423
Wright, E. O., Hachen, D., Costello, C. and Sprague, J. (1982) The American class structure. *American Sociological Review*, **47** (December), 709–726

Reprinted by permission of The University of Chicago Press, Chicago. E. Freidson (1986) *Professional Powers: A Study of the Institutionalization of Formal Knowledge*, The University of Chicago Press, Chicago, pp.41–46, 59–60.

Chapter 45

Uncertainty in medical prognosis: clinical and functional[1]

Fred Davis

Medical sociology is indebted to Talcott Parsons (1951) for having called attention to the important influence of uncertainty on the relationship between doctor and patient in the treatment of illness and disease. This is decribed as a primary source of strain in the physician's role, not only because clinically it so often obscures and vitiates definitive diagnoses and prognoses, but also because in an optimistic and solution-demanding culture such as ours it poses serious and delicate problems in the communicating of the unknown and the problematic to the patient and his family. In line with this view, Renée Fox (1957) has recently made an insightful analysis of the curriculum of a medical school, showing how, both from a formal and an informal standpoint, one of its functions is to socialize the student to cope more successfully with uncertainty.

Granting the self-evident plausibility of the hypothesis, sociological studies of medical practice thus far have neglected to assess empirically its scope and significance in the actual treatment of specific illnesses or diseases.[2] As a ready-made explanation of a disturbing element in the relationship between doctor and patient, the concept – uncertainty – stands in danger of being applied in a catch-all fashion whenever, for example, the sociologist notes that communication from doctor to patient is characterized by duplicity, evasion, or other forms of strain. That other factors, having relatively little to do with uncertainty, can also systematically generate strain in the relationship may unfortunately be ignored because of the disposition to subsume phenomena under pre-existent categories.

The present paper examines the scope and significance of uncertainty as evidenced in the treatment of a particular disease. Specifically, it seeks to distinguish between 'real' uncertainty as a clinical and scientific phenomenon and the uses to which uncertainty – real or pretended, 'functional' uncertainty – lends itself in the management of patients and their families by hospital physicians and other treatment personnel.

The disease in question is paralytic poliomyelitis, and the subjects are fourteen Baltimore families, in each of which a young child had contracted the disease. These were studied longitudinally over a two-year period by an interdisciplinary team of social scientists and research physicians whose broad interest was in assessing the total impact of the experience on child and family. Except for one family that dropped out midway in the study, in each case the child with polio and his parents were interviewed at intervals from the time of the child's admission to a pediatrics ward in the acute stage of the disease to approximately a year and a half following his discharge from a convalescent hospital.

From the very first interview with the parents, held within a week or so following the child's admission to the hospital, to the fourteenth and final interview with them some two years later, the research was aimed at determining at every stage what the parents knew and understood about polio in general and their child's condition in particular and through whom and how they came to acquire such knowledge and understanding as they had on these matters. In addition to being interviewed in home and office, the parents were also observed from time to time in the hospital on visiting days – this being their only regular opportunity to discuss their child's condition with the physician-in-charge as he made his round of the ward. It might be noted here that, with few exceptions, the parents soon came to regard these encounters as especially frustrating and of little value in getting information on questions which were troubling them. Although the situation on visiting day did not permit the observers to come away with word-for-word records of what went on, their perfunctory character was sufficiently evident to substantiate the descriptions later given by the parents in interview. As one mother remarked:

> Well, they [the doctors] don't tell you anything, hardly. They don't seem to want to. I mean, you start asking questions and they say, 'Well, I only have about three minutes to talk to you'. And the things that you ask, they don't seem to want to answer you. So I don't ask them anything any more.

By bringing together the interview and observational data gathered from these several sources, it was possible to compare and contrast, at successive stages of the disease and its treatment, what the parents knew and understood of the child's condition with what the doctors knew and understood. One must assume that the doctor's knowledge of the disease and its physical effects is more accurate, comprehensive, and profound than that of the parents. The problem, then, could be stated: How much information was communicated to the parents? How was it communicated? And what consequences did this communication have on the parents' expectations of the child's illness and prospects for recovery?[3] And, since in paralytic poliomyelitis (as in many other diseases and illnesses) uncertainty does affect the making of diagnoses and prognoses, an attempt was made to assess the scope, significance, and duration of uncertainty for the doctor.

But what is of special interest here is the way in which uncertainty, a *real* factor in the early diagnosis and treatment of the paralyzed child, came more and more to serve the purely managerial ends of the treatment personnel in their interaction with parents. Long after the doctor himself was no longer in doubt about the outcome, the perpetuation of uncertainty in doctor-to-family communication, although perhaps neither premeditated nor intended, can nonetheless best be understood in terms of its functions in the treatment system. These are several, and closely connected.

Foremost is the way in which the pretense of uncertainty as to outcome serves to reduce materially the expenditure of additional time, effort, and involvement which a frank and straightforward prognosis to the family might entail. The doctor implicitly recognizes that, were he to tell the family that the child would remain crippled or otherwise impaired to some significant extent, he would easily become embroiled in much more than a simple, factual medical prognosis. Presenting so unwelcome a prospect is bound to meet with a strong – and, according to many of the treatment personnel, 'unmanageable' – emotional reaction from parents; among other things, it so threatens basic life-values which they cherish for the child, such as physical attractiveness, vocational achievement, a good marriage, and, perhaps most of all, his being perceived and responded to in society as 'normal, like everyone else'. Moreover, to the extent to which the doctor feels some professional compunction to so inform the parents, the bustling time-conscious work milieu of the hospital supports him in the convenient rationalization that, even were he to take the trouble, the family could not or would not understand what he had to tell them anyway.[4] Therefore, in hedging, being evasive, equivocating, and cutting short his contact with the parents, the doctor was able to avoid 'scenes' with them and having to explain to and comfort them, tasks, at least in the hospital, often viewed as onerous and time-consuming.

Second, since the parents had been told repeatedly during the first weeks of the child's illness that the outcome was subject to great uncertainty, it was not difficult for them, once having accepted the idea, to maintain and even to exaggerate it, particularly in those cases in which the child's progress fell short of full recovery. For, equivocally, uncertainty can be grounds for hope as well as despair; and when, for example, after six months of convalescence the child returned home crippled, the parents could and characteristically did interpret uncertainty to mean that he still stood a good chance of making a full and natural recovery in the indefinite future. The belief in a recuperative moratorium was held long after there was any real possibility of the child's making a full recovery, and with a number of families it had the unfortunate effect of diverting them from taking full advantage of available rehabilitation procedures and therapies. In fact, with few exceptions the parents typically mistook rehabilitation for cure, and, because little was done to correct this misapprehension, they often passively consented to a regimen prescribed for the child which they might have rejected had they known that it had nothing to do with effecting a cure.[5]

Last, it must be noted that in the art (as opposed to the science and technique) of medicine, a sociologically inescapable facet of treatment – often irrespective of how much is clinically known or unknown – is frequently that of somehow getting the patient and his family to accept, 'put up with', or 'make the best of' the socially and physically disadvantageous consequences of illness. Both patient and family are understandably reluctant to do this at first, if for no other reason than that it usually entails a dramatic revaluation in identity and self-conception.

Notes

1. Revised version of a paper read at the annual meeting of the American Sociological Society, Chicago, September, 1959. I wish to thank Anselm Strauss, Julius A. Roth, and Stephen A. Richardson for their valuable criticisms. Acknowledgment is also due my former colleagues, Harvey A. Robinson, Joseph S. Bierman, Toba Tahl, Arthur Silverstein, and Martin Gorten, of the Polio Project, Psychiatric Institute, University of Maryland Medical School, with whom I collaborated in research. The project was aided by a grant from the National Foundation.
2. Partial exception must be made for the as yet largely unpublished works of Julius A. Roth (Community Studies, Inc., Kansas City, Missouri) on treatment procedures in the tuberculosis hospital. Several of the points to be discussed here are treated from a somewhat different vantage point by Roth under such headings as 'Control of Information' and 'Negotiation and Bargaining between Staff and Patients'.
3. See Davis, F. (1956) Definitions of time and recovery in paralytic polio convalescence. *American Journal of Sociology*, LXI (May), 582–587.
4. Cf. Kutner, B. (1958) Surgeons and their patients. In *Patients, Physicians and Illness* (Gartly Jaco, E., ed.), Free Press, Glencoe, Ill. Particularly with working-class families, of which there were ten out of fourteen in the study, the propensity of doctors (and other professionals, for that matter) to resort to this particular rationalization is accentuated accordingly. However, the barriers toward giving any parent this kind of information appeared so pervasive that the four lower-middle-class and middle-class families fared hardly any better.
5. See Moore, W. E. and Tumin, M. N. (1949) Some social functions of ignorance. *American Sociological Review*, XIV (December), 787–795.

References

Fox, R. (1957) Training for uncertainty. In *The Student Physician* (Merton, R. K., Reader, G. and Kendall, P. L., eds), Harvard University Press, Cambridge, Mass., pp. 207–241.
Parsons, T. (1951) *The Social System*, Free Press, Glencoe, Ill., pp. 466–469.

Reprinted by permission of The University of Chicago Press. Fred Davis (1961) Uncertainty in medical prognosis: clinical and functional. *The American Journal of Sociology*, LXVI (July 1960–May 1961), 41–42, 44–45.

Chapter 46

The doctor–nurse game

Leonard I. Stein

The relationship between the doctor and the nurse is a very special one. There are few professions where the degree of mutual respect and cooperation between co-workers is as intense as that between the doctor and nurse. Superficially, the stereotype of this relationship has been dramatized in many novels and television serials. When, however, it is observed carefully in an interactional framework, the relationship takes on a new dimension and has a special quality which fits a game model. The underlying attitudes which demand that this game be played are unfortunate. These attitudes create serious obstacles in the path of meaningful communications between physicians and nonmedical professional groups.

The physician traditionally and appropriately has total responsibility for making the decisions regarding the management of his patients' treatment. To guide his decisions he considers data gleaned from several sources. He acquires a complete medical history, performs a thorough physical examination, interprets laboratory findings, and at times, obtains recommendations from physician-consultants. Another important factor in his decision-making are the recommendations he receives from the nurse. The interaction between doctor and nurse through which these recommendations are communicated and received is unique and interesting.

The game

One rarely hears a nurse say, 'Doctor I would recommend that you order a retention enema for Mrs. Brown'. A physician, upon hearing a recommendation of that nature, would gape in amazement at the effrontery of the nurse. The nurse, upon hearing the statement, would look over her shoulder to see who said it, hardly believing the words actually came from her own mouth. Nevertheless, if one observes closely, nurses make recommendations of more import every hour and physicians willingly and respectfully consider them. If the nurse is to make a suggestion without appearing insolent and the doctor is to seriously consider that suggestion, their interaction must not violate the rules of the game.

Rules of the game

The cardinal rule of the game is that open disagreement between the players must be avoided at all costs. Thus, the nurse must communicate her recommendations without appearing to be making a recommendation statement. The physician, in requesting a recommendation from a nurse, must do so without appearing to be asking for it. Utilization of this technique keeps anyone from committing themselves to a position before a sub rosa agreement on that position has already been established. In that way open disagreement is avoided. The greater the significance of the recommendation, the more subtly the game must be played.

The scoring system

Inherent in any game are penalties and rewards for the players. In game theory, the doctor–nurse game fits the nonzero sum game model. It is not like chess, where the players compete with each other and whatever one player loses the other wins. Rather, it is the kind of game in which the rewards and punishments are shared by both players. If they play the game successfully they both win rewards, and if they are unskilled and the game is played badly, they both suffer the penalty.

The most obvious reward from the well-played game is a doctor–nurse team that operates efficiently. The physician is able to utilize the nurse as a valuable consultant, and the nurse gains self-esteem and professional satisfaction from her job. The less obvious rewards are no less important. A successful game creates a doctor–nurse alliance; through this alliance the physician gains the respect and admiration of the nursing service. He can be confident that his nursing staff will smooth the path for getting his work done. His charts will be organized and waiting for him when he arrives, the ruffled feathers of patients and relatives will have been smoothed down, his pet routines will be happily followed, and he will be helped in a thousand and one other ways.

The doctor–nurse alliance sheds its light on the nurse as well. She gains a reputation for being a 'damn good nurse'. She is respected by everyone and appropriately enjoys her position. When physicians discuss the nursing staff it would not be unusual for her name to be mentioned with respect and admiration. Their esteem for a good nurse is no less than their esteem for a good doctor.

The penalties for a game failure, on the other hand, can be severe. The physician who is an unskilled gamesman and fails to recognize the nurses' subtle recommendation messages is tolerated as a 'clod'. If, however, he interprets these messages as insolence and strongly indicates he does not wish to tolerate suggestions from nurses, he creates a rocky path for his travels. The old truism 'If the nurse is your ally you've got it made, and if she has it in for you, be prepared for misery', takes on life-sized proportions. He receives three times as many phone calls after midnight than his colleagues. Nurses will not accept his telephone orders because 'telephone orders are against the rules'. Somehow, this rule gets suspended for the skilled players. Soon he becomes like Joe Bfstplk in the 'Li'l Abner' comic strip. No matter where he goes, a black cloud constantly hovers over his head.

The unskilled gamesman nurse also pays heavily. The nurse who does not view her role as that of a consultant, and therefore does not attempt to communicate recommendations, is perceived as a dullard and is mercifully allowed to fade into the woodwork.

Genesis of the game

To understand how the game evolved, we must comprehend the nature of the doctors' and nurses' training which shaped the attitudes necessary for the game.

Medical student training

The medical student in his freshman year studies as if possessed. In the anatomy class he learns every groove and prominence on the bones of the skeleton as if life depended on it. As a matter of fact, he literally believes just that. He not infrequently says, 'I've got to learn it exactly, a life may depend on me knowing that'. A consequence of this attitude, which is carefully nurtured throughout medical school, is the development of a phobia: the overdetermined fear of making a mistake. The development of this fear is quite understandable. The burden the physician must carry is at times almost unbearable. He feels responsible in a very personal way for the lives of his patients. When a man dies leaving young children and a widow, the doctor carries some of her grief and despair inside himself; and when a child dies, some of him dies too. He sees himself as a warrior against death and disease. When he loses a battle, through no fault of his own, he nevertheless feels pangs of guilt, and he relentlessly searches himself to see if there might have been a way to alter the outcome. For the physician a mistake leading to a serious consequence is intolerable, and any mistake reminds him of his vulnerability. There is little wonder that he becomes phobic. The classical way in which phobias are managed is to avoid the source of the fear. Since it is impossible to avoid making some mistakes in an active practice of medicine, a substitute defensive maneuver is employed. The physician develops the belief that he is omnipotent and omniscient, and therefore incapable of making mistakes. This belief allows the phobic physician to actively engage in his practice rather than avoid it. The fear of committing an error in a critical field like medicine is unavoidable and appropriately realistic. The physician, however, must learn to live with the fear rather than handle it defensively through a posture of omnipotence. This defense markedly interferes with his interpersonal professional relationships.

═════════

Nursing student training

Unlike the medical student, who usually learns to play the game after he finishes medical school, the nursing student begins to learn it early in her training. Throughout her education she is trained to play the doctor–nurse game.

═════════

The student, however, is also given messages quite contrary to the ones described above. She is continually told that she is an invaluable aid to the physician in the treatment of the patient. She is told that she must help him in every way possible, and she is imbued with a strong sense of responsibility for the care of her patient. Thus she, like the physician, is caught in a paradox.

The first set of messages implies that the physician is omniscient and that any recommendation she might make would be insulting to him and leave her open to ridicule. The second set of messages implies that she is an important asset to him, has much to contribute, and is duty-bound to make those contributions. Thus, when her good sense tells her a recommendation would be helpful to him she is not allowed to communicate it directly, nor is she allowed not to communicate it. The way out of the bind is to use the doctor–nurse game and communicate the recommendation without appearing to do so.

═════════

Comment

The doctor and nurse have a shared history and thus have been able to work out their game so that it operates more efficiently than one would expect in an indirect system. Major difficulty arises, however, when the physician works closely with other disciplines which are not normally considered part of the medical sphere. With expanding medical horizons encompassing cooperation with sociologists, engineers, anthropologists, computer analysts etc., continued expectation of a doctor–nurselike interaction by the physician is disastrous. The sociologist, for example, is not willing to play that kind of game. When his direct communications are rebuffed the relationship breaks down.

The major disadvantage of a doctor–nurselike game is its inhibitory effect on open dialogue which is stifling and anti-intellectual. The game is basically a transactional neurosis, and both professions would enhance themselves by taking steps to change the attitudes which breed the game.

Reprinted by permission of the American Medical Association. Leonard I. Stein (1967) The doctor–nurse game. *Archives of General Psychiatry*, **16**, 699–703. © 1967, American Medical Association.

Chapter 47

When nurse knows best: some aspects of nurse/doctor interaction in a casualty department

David Hughes

Introduction

The character of everyday interactions between nurses and doctors in the various settings of hospital life has received surprisingly little attention in the literature of the behavioural sciences. Many sociologists, possibly taking a cue from Freidson's (1968, 1970, Chapter 3) seminal writings on the position of the 'paramedical' professions,[1] have chosen to view the relationship in terms of a fairly unproblematic subordination of nursing staff to physician control. Among other things they note that the medical profession exercises considerable control over the knowledge base of the nursing profession; that typically nurses assist in, rather than initiate the focal tasks of diagnosis and treatment; and that much nursing work tends to be performed at the request of, or under the supervision of the doctor.

Stein's (1967) account of the 'doctor–nurse game' is perhaps the most influential qualification or extension of the traditional perspective (see, for example, Dingwall and McIntosh, 1978, pp.107–108; Keddy *et al.*, 1986). Drawing on his personal experience as a physician, Stein describes how nurses learn to show initiative and offer significant advice, while appearing to defer passively to the doctor's authority. Nurses use subtle non-verbal and cryptic verbal cues to communicate recommendations, which in retrospect appear to have been initiated by the doctor. The 'game' ensures that open disagreement is avoided and carries advantages for both parties: the doctor gains from the nurse's knowledge and experience, while the nurse gains increased self-esteem and professional satisfaction from her more demanding role.

The model that emerges from these writings provides a useful overview of the doctor–nurse relationship, but it is not clear that it holds equally in all medical settings or for all doctors and nurses, even in the UK context. To the extent that it has gained unqualified acceptance, sociologists may have been guilty of assuming a homogeneity in the division of labour that is simply not justified by empirical evidence. A number of studies show that middle or lower participants in complex organizations frequently exercise more influence than their formal position would suggest (Mechanic, 1962), but accounts of analogous informal arrangements in the medical care sphere are few.

―――――――

This paper aims to describe certain central features of doctor–nurse interaction in a hospital casualty department. It focuses on areas where nurses' work does appear to move closer to the focal tasks of diagnosis and treatment, and on instances where observed patterns of doctor–nurse interaction appear to be at odds with the traditional dominant–subservient model.

Nurses and patient categorization

The nature of nursing work in the Casualty setting is shaped by the need to process large numbers of acute cases with limited Departmental resources, and often against the background of considerable clinical uncertainty. Most casualty work involves the categorization and early treatment of patients, rather than continuing patient care. The 'sorting' function of the Department brings staff into contact with a patient population which includes both those suffering from life-threatening conditions, and those who turn out to have no determinable illness or pathology. Patient processing is made all the more difficult because in certain circumstances attenders with serious illness conditions may be almost indistinguishable at first sight from various categories of 'problem' patients – drunks, malingerers, and psychologically disturbed persons who will in most cases not be admitted to hospital (see Bagley, 1971; Dingwall and Murray, 1983; Jeffery, 1979; Mannon, 1976; Roth, 1972a, 1972b.)

The formal responsibility of the Casualty Officer (CO) for diagnosis is set out in a Hospital Memorandum (H.M. (62) 83) which states that:

> The responsibility for sorting patients who present themselves at a hospital into those who do not need hospital and those who do cannot properly be carried out by other than a registered medical practitioner. It should not be placed on the nursing staff.

In practice, however, the line between diagnosis and the more general process of patient categorization is rarely a clear one. Inevitably, given the heavy demands on the time of medical staff, much of the responsibility for the early processing and triaging of patients falls on nurses. Each patient's passage through the Department occasions a series of practical judgements regarding the courses of action to be taken at a particular stage. COs would face an impossible workload if such decision-making were not shared

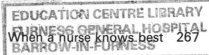

with other staff. In fact, not infrequently nurses find themselves moving close to areas of judgement for which the doctor takes legal responsibility.

One significant though unobtrusive source of nurse influence on patient categorization arises from the nurse's central role in the organization of patient throughput (compare Mauksch, 1965, 1966). In the Department studied, the degree of control exercised by senior nursing staff over the pace of work, the movement of patients, and the allocation of patients to doctors, varies according to the personnel on duty and the time of day (it is strongest when junior doctors are on duty, and particularly at night), but is almost always discernible to some degree. Patients arriving by ambulance or coming through from reception are typically met by a senior nurse who directs them to wait outside one of three doctor's consulting rooms or sends them to the various specialist treatment and recovery rooms that lie off a central corridor. Different types of patients typically take different routes through the Department, and the decision to direct patients to one room rather than another usually itself signals that a provisional categorization has been made. Thus, for example, patients 'coming in' as 'collapses' typically take one of two routes following arrival. Those suspected of having serious medical conditions such as head injury, CVA, cardiac problems, and the like would normally be moved directly to the resuscitation room for attention. Those thought to involve non-serious or disvalued conditions on the other hand – drunks, known epileptics, and 'regulars' known to feign or exaggerate illness conditions – would usually be placed in the recovery room, and might not see a doctor for some time. In many cases it is only after lengthy investigation and with the passage of time that the accuracy or inaccuracy of initial judgements is determined. In the meantime the path taken by the patient is likely to affect such matters as the length of time elapsing before examination by a doctor, the extent of monitoring of the patient's condition by other casualty staff, and the physical facilities immediately at hand if treatment becomes necessary.

Of course, the early processing of patients frequently involves far more than allocation to different rooms. Patient categorization can be a complex and extended process: almost all patients are filtered by other staff before they get to see a doctor. Ambulance crews (Hughes, 1980b; Hutchinson, 1983), receptionists (Gibson, 1977; Prottas, 1979, Chapter 4), and even porters (Hughes, 1980a) may all become involved in pre-processing work: but the part played by nurses is often central. How far they go in seeking clues to the patient's condition is again likely to vary according to which medical staff are on duty. Minimally, in cases considered serious enough to bypass the receptionist, nurses carry out routine observations (temperature, pulse, blood pressure, respiration), and determine basic patient details. But in very many cases they question patients and their escorts at some length about the circumstances leading up to attendance, and look for indicators of the patient's condition and character in his or her appearance and possessions.

Particularly in less straightforward cases, theorising about the likely condition may involve an interplay of ideas between coworkers, and a collaborative effort to investigate various possibilities. The following case from my field notes[2] illustrates the kind of interaction that occurs between different staff grades during the initial stages of patient processing. In this instance the doctor does see the patient at a relatively early stage, but then moves on to deal with other cases while nursing staff begin the search for clues to condition. It is significant that much of the information that is available to both the CO and MHO in advance of the clinical examinations is passed on by nursing staff. Though in this case the history is thin the nurses act as mediators between the ambulance crew and the CO, and collect together such items of information as are available. Moreover, it is nurses rather than the doctors who are most ready to put into words their ideas regarding matters that should be checked, and even possible diagnoses.

The patient appeared to be comatose and an airway had been placed in his throat. A staff nurse met the stretcher party: 'What happened then? He just collapsed?' Ambulance crewmen: 'On a train'. SRN: 'Oh, he collapsed on a train'. The CO was alerted by a nurse, and followed the group into the resuscitation room. He asked if the man could be roused, but left after a minute or so to look at another patient. Two nurses and two ambulance crewmen around the stretcher were trying to get a response by speaking loudly, and pinching or pushing part of the patient's body. SRN: 'There's no smell is there?' The man was transferred to a trolley and undressed. The nurses began carrying out routine observations, but the only unusual feature that was mentioned was a large bruise on the patient's upper chest and shoulder. The CO came back into the room and the bruise was pointed out to him. A nurse asked if they should put in another airway (the other one had been removed and the patient's breathing seemed rather difficult), and the doctor agreed. The doctor indicated a scar on the patient's abdomen, and began carrying out a chest examination. He asked what the patient's pulse was. 'Eighty', the SRN replied. She asked if she should telephone the local psychiatric hospital to see if a patient was missing. 'Yes'. The doctor examined the patient's eyes, and mentioned that the pupils were slightly dilated. SRN: 'He doesn't smell as though he's been drinking.' CO: 'No, I don't think he has'. The doctor left and an SEN began inserting an airway. The patient choked slightly and she had to use a suction device to clear his throat: 'I'm sure he's had a fit'. I asked what indicated that. 'Well they breathe irregularly and the tongue tends to go back into the throat. I don't think he's an overdose'. The patient was taken to X-ray.

Shortly afterwards the MHO arrived in the department, and one of the nurses told him about the case. I had the opportunity to speak to him as he waited for the patient to return from X-ray, and he told me that he knew little about the case. (...) The CO came across and outlined the circumstances of the man's arrival. The MHO had briefly looked in on the man in X-ray. He remarked that his pupils 'seem alright'. CO: 'They're slightly dilated'. MHO: 'They looked alright down in X-ray'. CO: 'Somebody thought he might be from the local mental hospital'. MHO: 'Why, did they know him?' CO: 'No, they just thought he might be.' The MHO said he thought the patient looked like an overdose. The CO said that in fact an overdose case had just come in, and the MHO went to look at that patient.

A few minutes later the MHO returned to look at the first patient. He examined the man's chest and eyes, and checked his response to pain by squeezing his earlobe. He looked at the X-ray plate and indicated the clavicle area: 'We're very short of room, you know. Do you think we could call this a trauma case? It is a trauma case really isn't it?' SEN: 'Yes look at the X-ray.' The doctor pushed his ballpoint pen into various points on the patient's arms and legs, observing his responses. The patient did not seem to react much to pressure on the sole of his right foot, but when the doctor changed the spot slightly the response was more apparent, and he did not comment. He had a further look at the man's eyes with the aid of an electric torch: 'This guy needs looking after. We'll put him in ward ... oh, ward eleven. The only thing is the shoulder.' SEN: 'Do you want trauma to look at him?' MHO: 'Yes, will you refer him to them?' SEN: 'You have to refer him to them.' MHO: 'I thought you did that on "cas".' SEN: 'Well, we can call the House Officer down.'

The 'trauma man' was called, but I did not witness his examination of the patient. However, in a subsequent conversation with a nurse he said that he would admit the patient as a trauma case if the 'medical people' had 'finished with him'. A fractured clavicle showed on the X-ray and he also suspected a head injury because of the patient's unconsciousness. The MHO subsequently agreed to the patient's admission as a trauma case.

Although the above case presents somewhat unusual problems of diagnosis nurses frequently take the lead in the search for information in the way that occurs in the early stages of the processing of this patient. Thus they often undertake relatively detailed physical examinations. Handbags and pockets are searched for medication, drugs, cards detailing illness conditions, information on identity and the like. Attempts are made to trace past record cards. In cases where patients present bizarre or irrational behaviour telephone calls may be made to the local psychiatric hospital. Such detective work very often leads nurses to make a provisional diagnosis of their own (or at least an assessment of relative priority), and is often the source of much of the information later passed on to the doctor. Where nurses are reasonably sure that certain investigations such as ECGs will be required, they may themselves carry them out so that results are available by the time the doctor arrives. Similarly where nurses believe certain treatments such as stomach washouts or suturing to be required they may prepare the equipment and get the patient ready, even though the doctor has not yet become involved in the processing of the case.

Many of these activities are highly consequential in themselves, but they often take on added significance by suggesting a framework of expectation for doctors when they encounter the patient for the first time. Talking of the difficulties of diagnosis presented in the case of the patient taken off the train described above, the MHO told me: 'It's the kind of excitement I don't want. I like to have a story. What was he doing on the train? Where's he come from? How did he collapse?' I said that I supposed in such a case that the physical signs would be crucial. 'Yes', he replied, 'but I'm afraid that you need a story to be able to interpret the physical signs'. Very often it will be nursing staff who collect the available facts and fit them together to amount to some understandable course of events, so providing the starting point for subsequent investigation. The doctor may attach more or less credence to this information according to his estimation of the competence of the staff involved, but will rarely be in a position to ignore it completely. Most nurses questioned in the study acknowledged that casualty work often involved making judgements about patients' conditions. But in their view this fell well short of diagnosis:

> SRN: That's not diagnosis though. You might look at a patient and say this is a heart attack or this is a stroke. Sometimes it's obvious what it is. But you don't tell them, you leave that up to the doctor.

In essence these nurses do not count themselves as taking part in diagnosis because they do not inform the patient of the nature of his condition or indeed make any firm pronouncements about it. From my observations there are many instances where nurses tell patients who have not yet seen a doctor such things as that a wound will require suturing, a fracture is present, a stomach wash out will have to be done, or that there is no possibility of hospital admission for a presented condition. However, they do so in a way which avoids acknowledgement of any clear personal responsibility for such judgements, and which, if necessary, allows decisions to be presented as the result of collective deliberations.

=====

Where nurses find themselves more openly assuming responsibility for the organization of a doctor's work, the whole tone of the relationship is likely to be affected. The outward show of deference usually taken to accompany an unobtrusive exercise of influence in accounts of the 'doctor–nurse game' will from time to time patently be absent. Frequently sisters or staff nurses suggest (in a way that implies direction rather than advice) that doctors should come and perform a particular task – such as suturing – before they do anything else. Sometimes there are quite brusque exchanges when nurses reprimand junior doctors for such things as not coming when asked, keeping patients waiting for long periods, taking long meal breaks, and being late on duty. Indeed, in a number of instances recorded in my research field notes criticism extended beyond the matter of the pacing of work to the question of the doctor's professional competence or manner.

=====

The present study portrays the nurse–doctor relationship in terms of a gradient of behaviour. Sometimes, in much the way that Stein's (1967) account of the 'doctor–nurse game' suggests, recommendations take the form of subtle cues or cryptic references to information unearthed by the nurse. But for much of the time nurses seem much less preoccupied with concealing their role of advice-givers than the 'game' metaphor suggests. Nurses, even while acknowledging the doctor's clinical authority, frequently offer advice on the many aspects of departmental practice in an open and straightforward way. More rarely, senior nursing staff intervene quite bluntly to point out shortcomings in the work of certain junior doctors, and effectively take control of the processing of particular patients.

In almost all cases involving these breakdowns of deference the doctors involved are junior in rank, relatively inexperienced, and recent Asian immigrants. If we translate Goffman's terms into those of his teacher, Everett Hughes, we can say that the situations involved are, in essence, ones where certain of the expected status-determining characteristics of doctors are absent – where contradictions of status are apparent to nurses. In one of the classic papers of the sociology of work, Hughes (1945) suggested that there grows up about a status, in addition to its specifically defining traits, a complex of expected auxiliary characteristics. In the case of doctors: 'If one takes a series of characteristics, other than medical skill and a license to practice it, which individuals in our society may have, and then thinks of physicians possessing them in various combinations, it becomes apparent that some of the combinations seem more natural and more acceptable than others to the great body of potential patients. Thus a white, male, Protestant physician of old American stock would be acceptable to patients of almost any social category in this country' (Hughes, 1945, p.354). Ethnic membership may be considered a master status-determining trait in most Western societies. But professional standing is also a powerful characteristic, particularly in the specific relationships of professional practice. From this perspective, relations between young, inexperienced, Asian COs and mature, experienced, Anglo-Saxon nurses almost inevitably involve dilemmas of status, and some departure from expected role relationships. Though the language may now appear somewhat dated, Everett Hughes' analysis is capable of marriage to contemporary socio-logical perspectives.[3] Hughes, admittedly, was concerned with contra-dictions of status primarily in terms of combinations of personal characteristics that violate normative expectations regarding occupational incumbency, but such contradictions are also likely to have direct implications in terms of interactional performance. Particularly, where contrasts like experienced nurse/inexperienced doctor, and indigenous nurse/overseas doctor are involved, differential competence in utilizing relevant bodies of social knowledge is perhaps the most salient interactional manifestation of 'status' characteristics. Elsewhere Hughes (1971, p.287) himself argued that: 'An occupation consists in part of the implied or explicit license that some people *claim or are given* to carry out certain activities ...' (my emphasis), and plainly the successful prosecution of such claims depends (for skilled occupations at least) on the display and competent manipulation of specialist knowledge.

Arguably, 'dilemmas of status' emerge and find resolution in the course of accomplishing the various practical activities that comprise casualty work: in the casualty setting they arise most typically when nurses see the need to provide interactional help to doctors so that medical work will get done. Rather unsurprisingly, the research reported here documented numerous instances where inexperienced COs depended on experienced nurses for information on departmental procedures and usual hospital practice even in some cases on correct clinical procedures. Perhaps more interestingly, nurses emerged as the carriers and mediators of social knowledge that remained important to diagnosis even where COs possessed good clinical expertise. Thus where junior doctors were involved, particularly those from overseas, nurses' skill in interpreting the social cues associated with a case, or indicating the significance of social information passed on by ambulance crews or receptionists, was often critical in framing clinical work. Needless to say, that observation is not intended as an aspersion on the professional competence of overseas doctors, but merely reflects their problems in practicing medicine in a strange culture, and the compensatory strategies that nurses adopt.

Notes

1. Freidson's recent statements on the division of labour in medical care are more carefully qualified than his early writings. There is, for example, a much clearer acknowledgement of the importance of discretion in nursing work albeit a discretion that is often severely curtailed: 'While few can doubt that nurses employ considerable discretion routinely in the course of their work, the elaborateness of the occupational division of labour, especially in some of the special diagnostic and treatment facilities of modern hospitals, creates constraints on individual discretion that are greater than appears to be the case for most professions that either are superordinate in the division of labour or function in a fairly simple division of labour. But nurses do work in a complex and not a detailed division of labour' (Freidson, 1986).
2. Staff in the Department came to tolerate my open use of a small note book during my periods of observation. Rough notes made on the spot were later written up more fully, and form the basis of the extracts reproduced in this paper. Some grammatical changes have been made, and interspersed notes on the processing of other patients have been removed for the sake of clarity. Although some of the details of patient management in the Department may have changed since the research was completed, use of the present tense is retained to help preserve the sense of the original field notes.
3. Dingwall and Strong (1985), for example, draw heavily on Hughes' work in their attempt to develop a critique of the negotiated order perspective on organizations which is also influenced by ethnomethodology and the sociology of language.

References

Bagley, C. (1971) The sick role, deviance, and medical care. *Social and Economic Administration*, 5(3), 193–209

Dingwall, R. and McIntosh, J. (eds) (1978) *Readings in the Sociology of Nursing*, Churchill Livingstone, London

Dingwall, R. and Murray, T. (1983) Categorization in accident departments: 'good' patients, 'bad' patients and children. *Sociology of Health and Illness*, 5(2), 127–148

Dingwall, R. and Strong, P. M. (1985) The interactional study of organizations: a critique and reformulation. *Urban Life*, 14(2), 205–231

Freidson, E. (1968) Medical personnel: paramedical personnel. In *International*

Encyclopedia of the Social Sciences (Sills, D. L., ed.), Vol. 10, Collier Macmillan, New York
Freidson, E. (1970) *Profession of Medicine*, Dodd, Mead & Co, New York
Freidson, E. (1986) *Professional Powers: A Study of the Institutionalization of Formal Knowledge*, University of Chicago Press, Chicago
Gibson, H. (1977) *Rules, routines, and records: the work of an A and E department.* Unpublished PhD thesis, University of Aberdeen
Goffman, E. (1956) The nature of deference and demeanour. *American Anthropologist*, 58 (June), 473–502
Hughes, E. C. (1945) Dilemmas and contradictions of status. *American Journal of Sociology*, 50, 353–359
Hughes, E. C. (1971) *The Sociological Eye: Selected Papers on Work, Self, and the Study of Society*, Book II, Aldine/Atherton, Chicago
Hughes, D. (1980a) *Lay assessment of clinical seriousness: practical decision-making by non-medical staff in a hospital casualty department.* Unpublished PhD thesis, University of Wales, U.C. Swansea
Hughes, D. (1980b) The ambulance journey as an information generating process. *Sociology of Health and Illness*, 2(2), 115–132
Hutchinson, S. (1983) *Survival Practices of Rescue Workers: Hidden Dimensions of Watchful Readiness*, University Press of America, Washington D.C.
Jeffery, R. (1979) Normal rubbish: deviant patients in casualty departments. *Sociology of Health and Illness*. 1(1), 90–107
Keddy, B. *et al.* (1986) The doctor–nurse relationship: an historical perspective. *Journal of Advanced Nursing*, 11(6), 745–753
Mannon, J. M. (1976) Defining and treating 'problem patients' in a hospital emergency setting. *Medical Care*, 14(2), 1004–1013
Mauksch, H. O. (1965) The nurse, coordinator of patient care. In *Social Interaction and Patient Care* (Skipper, J. K. and Leonard, R. C., eds), Lippincott, Philadelphia
Mauksch, H. O. (1966) The organisational context of nursing practice. In *The Nursing Profession: Five Sociological Essays* (Davis, F., ed.), Wiley, New York
Mechanic, D. (1962) Sources of power of lower participants in complex organisations. *Administrative Science Quarterly*, 7 (Dec.), 349–364
Prottas, J. M. (1979) *People Processing: The Street-Level Bureaucrat In Public Service Bureaucracies*, Lexington Books, Lexington, Mass.
Roth, J. (1972a) Some contingencies in the moral evaluation and control of clientele: the case of the hospital emergency services. *American Journal of Sociology*, 77(5), 839–855
Roth, J. (1972b) Staff and client control strategies in urban hospital emergency services. *Urban Life and Culture*, 1(1), 39–60
Stein, L. (1967) The doctor–nurse game. *Archives of General Psychiatry*, 16, 699–703.

Reprinted by permission of Blackwell Publishers, Oxford. David Hughes (1988) When nurse knows best: some aspects of nurse/doctor interaction in a casualty department. *Sociology of Health and Illness*, 10(1), 1, 2, 4–9, 15–21

Part III How Far Have We Come? Or Fifty Years of the National Health Service

'Britain was the first country in the world to offer free medical care to the whole population' (Abel-Smith, next chapter). The tremendous achievement of establishing a national health service in which medical treatment and care are made available to rich and poor alike, is one of which the general public is rightly proud. **Abel-Smith** provides a neat pen-portrait of health care before the start of the National Health Service in 1948. He concludes by emphasizing that the priorities within the new service were to be established on the basis of medical need rather than the ability to pay.

However, the visions abounding at the inception of the NHS have not always been realized. Today, there are serious shortcomings in the care that is provided. The well-loved and radical GP, **David Widgery,** working in Tower Hamlets in Inner London before his tragically early death, produced some important work illustrating some of the dissonance between the politics of health and the reality of care. It is salutary to remember what actually happens at 'the sharp end'.

Yet there are clear successes under the umbrella of the NHS, supporting and revivifying it. It is, for instance, to the NHS that blood is donated voluntarily and freely. In a classic text, **Titmuss** explores the 'gift relationship', which he reminds us is 'the gift to the stranger'. Through an examination of the blood donor relationship, Titmuss compares the health care systems of Britain and the USA. The commercialization of blood and donor relationships provides a stunning case study of the dangers of commercialized health.

Nevertheless, there has been continuing disquiet with the functioning of the NHS. The publication of the Black Report in 1980 was an important watershed and opened up some crucial debates. Certainly the evidence suggested that the differences in health care provision for different social classes had not diminished since the introduction of the NHS. In some instances, the sad fact was that these differences had actually increased. **Gray** produced a masterly summary and comment on the Black Report soon after its publication.

Women's issues were comparatively neglected in the Black Report, but

Doyal focuses on some of the ambivalence and contradictions within the NHS in terms of really helping women. The debate is ongoing. Variations by region, by social class, by gender and, more recently, by ethnicity, have all been identified.

The link between poverty and ill-health has, however, been clearly demonstrated. **Peter Townsend**, one of the crucial members of the working group on inequalities in health, under the chairmanship of Sir Douglas Black, continued to provide new evidence in the 1980s of the link between poor health and material deprivation. Townsend, together with **Phillimore** and **Beattie**, found that the areas of highest mortality and morbidity in Britain are overwhelmingly to be found in the North and North-West, in Scotland and in Wales.

Difficult decisions in the allocation of medical resources have to be made. Fifty years after the introduction of the NHS the need to address these issues is particularly pressing as demand for health care becomes ever-greater. **Gillon** usefully addresses the ethical issues relating to the allocation of medical resources and notions of justice.

Despite the fears about the size and nature of the governmental health reforms which started in the late 1980s and which continue apace, the NHS remains the pivot of health care in Britain. Demand for its services remains high, too high, given the belief at the inception of the NHS that, in time, everyone would become more healthy and the demand for health care would correspondingly diminish.

The word 'need' has been prominent in the rhetoric of the NHS yet, **Culyer** argues, the evidence for its success has been less forthcoming. We have, he says, 'muddled through long enough' and failed to address the fundamental issues and questions in the provision of health care which are encompassed by the confusing and vague term 'need'. The call for reform of health care was what **Klein** has called 'one of the international epidemics of the 1990s' and he sets the reforms which have taken place in Britain against the initial aims of the NHS. Despite the many inadequacies and failures of the NHS, support for it remains, as Klein points out, 'rock solid'.

Chapter 48

Health care before the National Health Service

Brian Abel-Smith

The National Health Service started on 5 July 1948. Britain was the first country in the world to offer free medical care to the whole population. Many other countries had developed compulsory health insurance schemes, but under them rights to health care were generally confined to those who had paid contributions and their dependants, and to pensioners. The principle of *universal* coverage for free medical care was entirely new. As Nye Bevan, the Minister who introduced the National Health Service, put it, 'medical treatment and care ... should be made available to rich and poor alike in accordance with medical need and by no other criteria'.

The story of how we came to introduce the service and the prolonged debate about how the service should be organized has often been told. What is remarkable, is that the bold decision to have a national health service was taken in the middle of the Second World War. There was considerable controversy, for example, on such questions as whether it should really cover the whole population including the better off, whether dentistry and spectacles should be included from the start, and who should run the hospitals. But the Act to establish the Service was eventually passed in 1946.

Thirty years later, the older generation can remember from personal experience how health care was provided before the National Health Service opened its doors. The extent of the change can be appreciated by explaining what it was like before 1948.

National health insurance

Nearly half of the population was covered by the Lloyd George compulsory health insurance scheme which started in 1912 (under the 1911 Act). This gave the right to choose and use a general practitioner and to the free drugs he prescribed. By 1948, those covered were manual workers and other employees earning up to £420 a year. The scheme therefore excluded children, wives who did not go out to work, the self-employed, higher paid employees and many old people. Though some people belonged to insurance schemes on a voluntary basis, those who were not insured faced the prospect of paying both the doctor's bill and the cost of the medicines he prescribed.

Free health care was available to schoolchildren and to the poor from a district poor law doctor, or from a poor law institution, but people were very reluctant to face the Relieving Officer and the humiliating family means test which was required before services could be received. Many who could not afford to pay doctors' fees queued, often for several hours, at the so-called 'casualty' departments of the voluntary (charitable) hospitals when what they needed was often the services of a general practitioner rather than a specialist.

Some general practitioners had separate waiting rooms for 'panel' (health insurance) patients and private fee-paying patients, or would only see panel patients at lock-up surgeries while they treated private patients from their own homes. As the major part of the total earnings of general practitioners came from private patients, practitioners were heavily concentrated in the more affluent neighbourhoods. The poorer areas were sparsely served. For example, there were twice as many doctors per head in London as in South Wales. Four times the number of doctors per head lived in Bournemouth than in the industrial Midlands.

Dental and ophthalmic care

Before 1948, those covered by health insurance drew cash benefits for sickness or disablement not from the Government but from 'Approved Societies' – most of them friendly societies. If, after paying out the statutory cash benefits, a friendly society had a financial surplus at its actuarial valuation, it could use it to provide its members with additional benefits. The main benefits provided were dental treatment and spectacles. About half the insured members were probably eligible for spectacles either free or with the member paying part of the cost. Spectacles were also provided by school ophthalmic clinics to children up to school-leaving age. The rest of the population had to buy their own. It was common for patients needing spectacles to go not to the optician but to a cheap chain store where they could try on spectacles until they found a pair which seemed to improve their sight.

In the case of dental care, the whole or much more often only a part of the approved cost of treatment was paid by those friendly societies which provided this additional benefit. Out of the 13 million people eligible for dental benefit only about 6–7 per cent claimed it in any given year. Dental care consisted to a large extent of removing teeth rather than filling them. Indeed, often teeth were extracted and full dentures provided instead. There was, moreover, a major shortage of dentists. There were few in rural areas and the time and expense of travelling to a dentist and the cost falling on the patient were major barriers to use. Apart from a few special units set up during the war, the dental services provided by hospitals were, except in the case of the teaching hospitals, very limited indeed. A survey of three Royal Ordnance factories in 1942 found that only 1 per cent of employees were dentally fit.

Local authorities provided limited dental treatment for expectant and nursing mothers and children under five, but the service could only reach a small proportion of those who needed it. Most authorities required the mother to pay towards the cost of dentures if she could reasonably be expected to do so. For every 100 mothers treated in 1945, there were 36 teeth filled and 316 extracted.

The School Dental Service had been set up in 1907 to give treatment to those children who could not obtain it in any other way, but its development had been slow and erratic. The service was administered by nearly 200 different local authorities and the extent of what they provided varied widely. The Education Act 1944 required local education authorities to provide dental inspections at appropriate intervals, and this was an important contribution to the dental health of children. But standards of dental care were generally low and most people attached little importance to caring for their teeth.

The hospitals

Before the Second World War, the bulk of acute care in hospital and consultations with specialists were provided by the independent voluntary (charitable) hospitals which competed vigorously for charitable donations. Patients were expected to pay what they could afford unless they could show that they made regular contributions to one of the contributory schemes which helped to support the local hospitals or could obtain a 'ticket' from a contributor.

The number, and the quality, of voluntary hospitals varied widely over the country. What could be provided in any particular area depended mainly on the donations of the living and the legacies of the dead rather than on any ascertained need for hospital services. The wealthier cities particularly London had hospitals, many of which were good by the standards of the time. But the smaller industrial towns were much less well provided and most of the hospitals were small. Few peripheral hospitals had proper facilities for X-rays, pathology or even surgery. The voluntary hospitals tended to pay low wages and salaries to staff – particularly to nursing staff. The nurses were expected to work long hours for their low pay.

The consultants and specialists were 'honorary' and did their charitable work in the hospitals without payment for it. They depended for most of their incomes on payments for services to private patients. Thus doctors who limited their work to their specialty could only be found to work in hospitals if there was locally enough private practice to support them in their specialist work. Outside the main centres the hospitals were staffed by general practitioners or by doctors who were part specialist and part general practitioners. In the poorer parts of the country, particularly in Wales and the North of England, there were extremely few specialists because there were so few private patients. Those who were poor could only get good specialist care if they happened to be employed by or live near enough those who could afford to buy it.

With the outbreak of the Second World War, the Emergency Medical Service was established. The Government paid the voluntary hospitals to provide services – originally to air raid casualties but later to a wider category of people whose need for hospital care could be attributed to special war circumstances. Further financial support was given to the voluntary hospitals in the translational period before the National Health Service was established.

To some extent gaps in the acute hospital services were filled by local authority hospitals. They provided the major part of the hospital obstetric services. Some counties and county boroughs had begun to develop acute hospital services after they took over the Poor Law Hospitals from the Poor Law Guardians under an Act of 1929. But the extent to which they did so varied according to the wealth and interest of the authority, the rates it was prepared to raise, and the priority it gave to this particular service. Patients who could afford to pay were charged on a means-tested basis, except in hospitals for infectious diseases, where charges could be waived. Local authority hospitals would normally only serve their own residents. Patients living on the wrong side of a county border would be refused admission even when there were empty beds. While some authorities, such as Birmingham City, Surrey, Middlesex and the London County Council made substantial progress in building up a good hospital system with specialists of high skill, other authorities made little use of their powers to do so. Their hospitals remained just as they had been under the Poor Law, according to a distinguished doctor – 'ill-designed, deficient in sanitation, often isolated, bare, bleak and soulless'.

The local authorities also provided the vast majority of hospital care for the chronic sick, for infectious diseases, mental illness and mental handicap. Over a tenth of the beds were for tuberculosis and other infectious diseases. They were also increasingly being made responsible for securing that arrangements were made for treating such conditions as cancer, venereal diseases and tuberculosis and for supplementing what the voluntary hospitals provided. The concentration of the voluntary hospitals on acute care meant that patients who did not respond to treatment were, after a period, transferred to a Poor Law infirmary for the chronic sick. The contrast in levels of staffing, in food, in the quality of the accommodation, and in the standard of nursing was often very great indeed. Local authorities were faced with a chronic shortage of trained nurses. Patients who were transferred inevitably felt that hope of recovery had been abandoned and that they had been put away to die.

In total, the local authorities provided about four-fifths of the hospital beds of all kinds in Britain but most of them provided types of health care which gave the doctors who worked in them on a whole-time or part-time salaried basis little prestige. Nationally there was a great shortage of hospital beds – particularly for certain cases. Cottage hospitals were often empty while large general hospitals had long waiting lists. Wales was particularly poorly served with hospitals. In South Wales, about half the hospital beds were in buildings which were judged, when they were taken over, to be too small or ill-equipped for their purpose. No general hospital of the requisite size and quality served the thinly-populated areas of North Wales.

Community services

Several hundred different local authorities had the power but not the duty to care for expectant and nursing mothers and children under the age of five. To a widely varying extent, they provided ante-natal and post-natal clinics and welfare centres and employed health visitors to give advice in the home. Local authorities also either employed midwives or arranged for them to be provided by voluntary organizations. The majority of births took place at home usually with a midwife in charge, who would call a doctor if she thought it necessary. Although local authorities had the power to provide home nurses, this was limited to patients suffering from infectious diseases, expectant or nursing mothers or children under five suffering from various conditions. The majority of home nursing services were provided by voluntary district nursing associations financed by donations, payments from patients and grants from the local authorities. Domestic help services could until 1944 only be provided to maternity cases; from that year they could be provided to the sick and infirm. Schoolchildren were inspected in schools and given dental, ophthalmic and orthopaedic treatment as well as treatment for minor ailments at school clinics. Before 1944 local authorities had to recover the cost from the parents unless they could not reasonably be expected to pay. From 1944, local authorities had a duty to see that free treatment was provided including in-patient treatment for schoolchildren and often for under-fives.

Ambulances were operated by a great variety of different agencies – individual hospitals, local authorities, the Red Cross, St John's Ambulance Brigade, police, factories and private operators. Payment had often to be made when the service was used. There was no co-ordinated system until the wartime civil defence service was established, and no guarantee that when an ambulance was desperately needed, one could be found.

The money barrier

Thus while free or partly free services of varying quality were available, there were serious shortages in many parts of the country. There was also a deep-seated reluctance to use the poor law services. The wives of working men in particular would often postpone going to the doctor or taking a child to a doctor because of the fear of a bill which could not be afforded and because of reluctance to ask for charity from the voluntary hospital. Often the compromise was to 'ask the chemist'. Many conditions got worse because of delay in seeking treatment.

Serious illness could also create financial catastrophes for middle-class patients. They might have to pay doctors' bills (both general practitioner and specialist), the cost of medicines and the cost of a nurse to look after them at home or the full cost of care in a nursing home. Private insurance schemes for middle-class patients were only just beginning to be developed. Moreover there was in most of the country a shortage of suitable hospital and nursing home facilities for paying patients.

The introduction of the national health services therefore relieved millions of the financial worry so often associated with illness. No longer did anyone need to delay in seeking health care because of the fear of running up bills they could not afford to pay. The main beneficiaries were housewives, children, the aged, middle-class patients and the self-employed.

But the service was created not just to make services free at point of use but to make them available wherever they were needed. It was designed to secure a much better geographical distribution of general practitioners, of specialists, of dentists and opticians. Last but not least it was established to weld together an unco-ordinated series of hospitals of varying size, function and quality into an integrated and co-ordinated system designed to provide all needed forms of specialist care. The aim as stated in the original Act was 'to secure improvement in the physical and mental health' of the nation's population 'and the prevention, diagnosis and treatment of illness'. According to one highly respected historian it was 'the most unsordid act of British Social policy'.

To enact a noble purpose was only a first step. The hard work of establishing the service had still to be begun. The buildings and trained manpower taken over on 5 July 1948 were far from adequate to realize the ambitious intentions of the legislation. Moreover the continuous advances in medical techniques and technology and the growing expectations of the public were to produce a continuing struggle to establish priorities for the use of limited resources. But what was important was that priorities within the Service were to be established on the basis of medical need rather than ability to pay.

Reprinted by permission of HMSO. Brian Abel-Smith (1978) Health care before the National Health Service. In *National Health Service: The First Thirty Years*, DHSS, London. Crown copyright is reproduced with permission of the Controller of HMSO.

Chapter 49

The National Health: a radical perspective

David Widgery

Introduction

A typical day in the life of a Tower Hamlets GP, I suppose. Forty patients
seen in a day that starts at nine a.m. and doesn't finish till seven, a dozen
referral letters (three trying to get patients moved up outpatient waiting lists
and two about housing problems), two delegations of relatives worried
about elderly relatives, a near-row with a hospital registrar who will 'look
at' an ill patient but can't guarantee admission, one asthma attack averted
with a nebulizer and a wrestling match to fit an IUD for a Somalian mother
of five who nearly bites through her blouse in fear but who can't understand
a word of my attempted reassurance.

Well, at least there were no drunks in the waiting room or manic
depressives trying to climb through the carpark window. Down the
corridor, the health visitors (30 per cent annual turnover in Tower Hamlets)
dash in and out of the local estates supporting isolated mothers and in the
afternoon a Community Psychiatric Nurse (with over a decade's training
and experience but paid less than a City PA) tries to sort out the psychiatric
crises. And back in reception, they're chasing ambulances which haven't
turned up and patient names from ninety national origins which are
perpetually going astray. We all work under constant pressure with
inadequate resources, so it's impossible to get the work in perspective.

And when you watch a blow-dried Tory Minister of Health and Social
Security telling you that the NHS has never had it so good, you know you're
going a bit crazy. 'We are building a better health service and providing
more care for those in need', boasted the Conservative election manifesto in
June 1987. Well, the daily evidence under my professional nose was quite
the reverse. Our health district has the highest birth rate in Britain, mainly
due to the high fertility of recent immigrants from Bangladesh and Vietnam,
an exceptionally high proportion of poorly maintained council housing,
record teenage and adult unemployment, and a large percentage of the single
elderly. The District Psychologist describes the 'degrees of isolation,

depression and child behavioural problems' as 'the worst I have seen anywhere'. Certainly the proportion of young children registered 'at risk' is unusually high. And yet the district has been subjected to a successive loss of revenue and beds which have forced hospital care into fewer and fewer centres which are under siege by the demands of routine clinical work.

The service cuts which the Government require get more horrific each financial year. In 1987/88, the closure of a vital paediatric unit, an Accident and Emergency Department which sees 50,000 East Enders a year, and the loss of 120 acute beds, has only been staved off by an interim saving plan on hospital prescribing devised by the consultants and inconvenient to both patients and GPs. Next year, it looks like total collapse for us and probably another fifty health districts in similar straits.

If the service and the care is better, and, amazingly, in some areas it is, that reflects the determination of the staff and the considerable patience and good-humoured co-operation of their patients rather than central Government policies. These pay lip service to the problems but continue to decant medical money out of the city centres in an 'equalization process' which in reality robs a bankrupt Peter in an effort to aid a penniless Paul.

The gap I experience between Government rhetoric and my working reality is not particular to an inner city GP. Later in the same week an obstetrician in the neighbourhood health district reports to a medical committee on which I sit that the new Homerton Hospital, which only opened this year, has had to transfer two women in established labour across London. One first-time mother, Valerie Brasington, said, 'After three hours I was transferred to a completely different hospital which I had never seen before. By the time I arrived at the Westminster, contractions were coming every two minutes. I was very tense and upset'. In some ways the new Homerton Hospital is a tremendous improvement on the dank, dingy Salvationist maternity hospital it replaced. The problem is, as community and local medical bodies have warned all along, that it is far too small: instead of the needed increase in maternity beds, the newly opened hospital has twenty-two fewer beds than the units it replaced. And Part 2 of the project, the promise on which the closures were sold, has now been mysteriously cancelled. Meanwhile a bed, a midwife and time to recover from labour can no longer be guaranteed in one of the most recently opened hospitals in Britain. Patient 'turnover' (the statistic so beloved of government health statisticians) is so high and job satisfaction so correspondingly low that 33 per cent of midwifery vacancies are unfilled.

And so it goes on. A newly appointed consultant psychiatrist struggling to build community services is, unexpectedly, found relaxing in the local. 'It's crazy', he says, 'the District Manager has instructed us to reduce our clinical workload. They want to pay us to twiddle our thumbs.' And in the *British Medical Journal* a London renal physician whose kidney ward has just been closed, temporarily-but-probably-for-good, reflects on the destinations of his demoralized nurses (two to the private sector, two emigrating) and his own changed life: 'I have adapted to less work, spend less time in the hospital, am often home by six p.m., and read an increasing number of novels.' As for British researchers, who once led the world in medical advances, morale is exceptionally low: the most honourable advice a teaching hospital consultant can now give an aspiring Crick or Fleming is 'emigrate'. And on television I watch nurses on salaries which are a monthly insult painfully deciding to leave the RCN and join the magnificent 3 February protest strike because, as one said, 'We've tried petitions, marches and protests and they just don't take a bit of notice.'

This book comes out of such experiences. It has been written – sometimes in anger, sometimes in sorrow – in the gaps between my full-time work as an East London GP. It is an attempt to unravel just what is happening to our health service and to explain the implications to the public who rely on it. It is also an attempt to restate the socialist case for comprehensive and democratic health care. And in the process it is an attack on the public spending cuts which, in the late eighties, threaten the existence of the NHS.

Reprinted by permission of Chatto & Windus, London. David Widgery (1988) *The National Health: A Radical Perspective*, Chatto & Windus, London, pp. xi–xiii.

Chapter 50

The gift relationship: from human blood to social policy

Richard M. Titmuss

Practically all the voluntary donors whose answers we set down in their own words employed a moral vocabulary to explain their reasons for giving blood. Their view of the external world and their conception of man's biological need for social relations could not be expressed in morally neutral terms. They acknowledged that they could not and should not live entirely as they may have liked if they had paid regard solely to their own immediate gratifications. To the philosopher's question 'what kind of actions ought we to perform?' they replied, in effect, 'those which will cause more good to exist in the universe than there would otherwise be if we did not so act'.

=====

None of the donors' answers was purely altruistic. They could not be for, as we concluded in Chapter 5, no donor type can be depicted in terms of complete, disinterested, spontaneous altruism. There must be some sense of obligation, approval and interest; some feeling of 'inclusion' in society; some awareness of need and the purposes of the gift. What was seen by these donors as a good for strangers in the here-and-now could be (they said or implied) a good for themselves – indeterminately one day. But it was not a good which they positively desired for themselves either immediately or ultimately.

In certain undesired circumstances in the future – situations in which death or disability might be postponable – then the performance by a stranger of a similar action would constitute for them or their families a desired good. But they had no assurance of such action nor any guarantee of the continued existence of the National Health Service. Unlike gift-exchange in traditional societies, there is in the free gift of blood to unnamed strangers no contract of custom, no legal bond, no functional determinism, no situations of discriminatory power, domination, constraint or compulsion, no sense of shame or guilt, no gratitude imperative and no need for the penitence of a Chrysostom.

In not asking for or expecting any payment of money these donors signified their belief in the willingness to other men to act altruistically in the future, and to combine together to make a gift freely available should they have a need for it. By expressing confidence in the behaviour of future unknown strangers they were thus denying the Hobbesian thesis that men are devoid of any distinctively moral sense.

As individuals they were, it may be said, taking part in the creation of a greater good transcending the good of self-love. To 'love' themselves they recognized the need to 'love' strangers. By contrast, one of the functions of atomistic private market systems is to 'free' men from any sense of obligation to or for other men regardless of the consequences to others who cannot reciprocate, and to release some men (who are eligible to give) from a sense of inclusion in society at the cost of excluding other men (who are not eligible to give).

These donors to the National Service we have described in much detail were free not to give. They could have behaved differently; that is to say, they need not have acted as they did. Their decisions were not determined by structure or by function or controlled by ineluctable historical forces. They were not compelled, coerced, bribed or paid to give. To coerce a man is to deprive him of freedom.

The paid seller of blood is confronted and, moreover, usually knows that he is confronted with a personal conflict of interests. To tell the truth about himself, his way of life and his relationships may limit his freedom to sell his blood in the market. Because he desires money and is not seeking in this particular act to affirm a sense of belonging he thinks primarily of his own freedom; he separates his freedom from other people's freedoms. It may be of course that he will not be placed or may not fully realize that he has been placed (as we have suggested in Chapter 8) in such situations of conflicting interests. If so, it can only be because medicine in the person of the doctor has failed to fulfil its scientific basis; it is not seeking to know what is true. In this as in increasingly large areas of medical care today the rationality of applying scientific knowledge now imposes on medicine new obligations to make explicit (where they are concealed) and to eliminate situations of conflicting interests. These obligations are logical consequences of the transformation of folk medicine into scientific medicine. They raise in scientific forms the question of 'truth maximization'. The social costs of untruthfulness are now clear and, as we showed in Chapter 8, they fall randomly on rich and poor alike. The dishonesty of donors can result in the death of strangers.

The unethical consequences of not seeking to know what is true in one sector of medical care spreads corrosively into other sectors and begins to envelop broader areas of social life and non-market institutions; some evidence of the growth of unethical practices affecting prisons, homes for retarded children, hospitals and clinical laboratories was provided in earlier chapters. It seems that more people have less protection against new forms of exploitation as market considerations and the conformities of market behaviour invade the territory of social policy.

—————

From our study of the private market in blood in the United States we have concluded that the commercialization of blood and donor relationships represses the expression of altruism, erodes the sense of community, lowers scientific standards, limits both personal and professional freedoms, sanctions the making of profits in hospitals and clinical laboratories, legalizes hostility between doctor and patient, subjects critical areas of medicine to the laws of the marketplace, places immense social costs on those least able to bear them – the poor, the sick and the inept – increases the danger of unethical behaviour in various sectors of medical science and practice, and results in situations in which proportionately more and more blood is supplied by the poor, the unskilled, the unemployed, Negroes and other low income groups and categories of exploited human populations of high blood yielders. Redistribution in terms of blood and blood products from the poor to the rich appears to be one of the dominant effects of the American blood banking systems.

Moreover, on four testable non-ethical criteria the commercialized blood market is bad. In terms of economic efficiency it is highly wasteful of blood; shortages, chronic and acute, characterize the demand and supply position and make illusory the concept of equilibrium. It is administratively inefficient and results in more bureaucratization and much greater administrative, accounting and computer overheads. In terms of price per unit of blood to the patient (or consumer) it is a system which is five to fifteen times more costly than the voluntary system in Britain. And, finally, in terms of quality, commercial markets are much more likely to distribute contaminated blood; the risks for the patient of disease and death are substantially greater. Freedom from disability is inseparable from altruism.

Reprinted by permission of HarperCollins, London. Richard M. Titmuss (1973) *The Gift Relationship: From Human Blood to Social Policy*, George Allen & Unwin Ltd, London, pp. 237–241, 245–246.

Chapter 51

Inequalities in health – the Black Report: a summary and comment

Alastair McIntosh Gray

The pursuit of equality is a principle that has been deeply embedded in the British National Health Service (NHS) ever since the 1946 NHS Bill (HMSO, 1946) promised comprehensive health care 'available to everyone regardless of financial means, age, sex, employment or vocation, area of residence or insurance qualification'. Despite this intention, and despite almost three decades of health care provided through the NHS, there was by the mid-1970s a widespread concern that inequalities in health in Britain showed no sign of diminishing and had become, perhaps, even more pronounced.

In consequence, a Working Group was appointed in April 1977 at the request of the then Secretary of State for Social Services (Mr. David Ennals), with the task of reviewing information about differences in health status between the social classes, considering possible causes and the implications for policy, and suggesting further research.

The Working Group contained two medical and two sociological members: Sir Douglas Black (Chairman), President of the Royal College of Physicians and the Chief Scientist at the Department of Health and Social Security (DHSS); Professor J. N. Morris, Professor of Community Health at the London School of Hygiene and Tropical Medicine; Dr. Cyril Smith, Secretary of the Social Science Research Council; and Professor Peter Townsend, Professor of Sociology at the University of Essex.

A critical assessment

It was noted earlier that the Report was not well received by the Government on its publication in August 1980. The *Lancet* referred to a 'frosty reception' (Lancet, 1980) from the Secretary of State, to 'publicity in the lowest possible key' (Deitch, 1980), and to the impression 'that Ministers and officials are keen to reduce the Report's impact to a minimum' (Deitch, 1980, p. 545). The *British Medical Journal* spoke of the 'waste of time and effort' in Mr. Jenkin's 'flat rejection of the recommendations' (BMJ, 1980a) and suggested it 'should be examined more closely than Patrick Jenkin's foreword suggests that it has been' (BMJ, 1980b).

By 1981 concern had switched to a 'sustained campaign of demolition against its findings' (Deitch, 1981a) on the part of the Social Services Secretary and doubts whether research commissioned by the DHSS 'is being conducted in a genuinely objective fashion or whether it is being selectively used to bolster a predetermined ideological position taken by the administration' (Deitch, 1981b).

Comments such as these stand as testimony to the importance many observers of health policies and politics attach to the subject of inequalities in health. It is unfortunate, therefore, that the goverment's initial responses to the Report have largely deflected attention from detailed examination and assessment of what the Report actually says. This concluding section is intended as a contribution to that task. It proceeds by considering some aspects of the analysis the Report presents, and then examines the Report's policy recommendations. The issues raised are of necessity selective, and some of the basic tenets of the Report have simply been accepted from the outset. For instance, no one reading the Report could easily contradict the conclusion from the weight of evidence it assembles that systematic class-related differences in health experience do exist; that these are associated with the structure and operation of the socioeconomic system within which people are born, live, and die; and that a way out of these inequalities will involve very much more than individual responses: the Government is inextricably involved.

As the Report itself makes clear, studies of patterns of ill-health are handicapped by the difficulty of obtaining information on morbidity. As a consequence, mortality rates continue to be the main focus of attention. These do give indications of inequalities, and some age- or cause-related mortality rates (e.g. the infant mortality rates) are more sensitive than others in suggesting links with wider socioeconomic factors. Nevertheless, the historical decline of infectious diseases and tuberculosis, and the increased incidence of chronic and degenerative diseases, suggest that the relationship between mortality and morbidity has changed and may be fairly weak. Consequently, the study of mortality rates may not provide an accurate picture of patterns of ill-health: inequalities in death may not be similar to inequalities in health. This problem may be particularly severe in the case of mental illnesses, which rarely result in death yet account at any time for around one in four NHS inpatients. Given also that the recording of mental illnesses may be more prone to measurement errors in the self-assessment used by the GHS than that for physical ailments, it is unfortunate that the Report was unable to explicitly consider this area of morbidity.

A second point to note in the analysis conducted by the Working Group is the portrayal of inequalities in the form of a gradient across social or occupational classes. In fact, ... for many diseases cause-specific mortality rates for men in social class III-M (manual) are lower than those for social class III-N (nonmanual), while the very limited number of women in social class I (around 1 per cent of the female working population) must make the standardized mortality ratios for this class less meaningful than those for classes II to V.

The distribution of inequality is important because it will, or at least should, influence the kinds of policies that would have most impact. If the inequalities take the form of a polarity between top and bottom, then redistributional measures would have to be highly concentrated and accurately targeted. If, on the other hand, the object was simply to reduce the number of 'excess deaths' occurring – that is, over and above the numbers that would have died if the death rate for social class I was applied to other social classes – the appropriate redistributional program might be different because the largest number of deaths are occurring in social class III, which also contains the largest proportion of the population (Snaith, 1981). At the heart of this observation lies a dilemma that is not explicitly tackled by the Working Group. The elimination of inequalities may be a valid long-term objective, but in the short-run resource constraints will make it necessary to select priorities. Is it, therefore, better to greatly reduce the inequalities experienced by a small part of the population, or to effect a smaller improvement for a larger number of individuals? No choice, of course, will ever be quite so stark, but the issue of weighting different degrees of inequality remains crucial.

Thirdly, the discussion of relationships between health and economic activity, which open up a way of potentially integrating the findings of the Report, is not pursued as far as it might have been. The 'materialist' explanation of the sources of inequality, and the references to the nature of Britain's economic system, might logically have led to a categorization of class based not on occupation but rather on the relationship of classes to economic ownership and control in society as a whole. This kind of approach, more fully documented elsewhere (see, for instance, Doyal, 1980, and Navarro, 1978), might have afforded more detailed structural insights into the causation of inequality. In particular, such an approach might have permitted the Working Group to discuss *why* inequalities have been so persistent and so difficult to reduce. This point is especially apt in relation to the recommendations of the Report, and will be discussed further below.

Finally, the Working Group's analysis fails to consider the many aspects of sexual inequalities in health that cannot be understood solely on the basis of sex-specific mortality rates. For instance, the variations in access to NHS abortion services across different regions are extraordinarily large, and it is difficult to believe that they would be tolerated in services which affect the population as a whole. Similarly, many women are known to be dissatisfied with the attitudes of the health service to their health problems and needs, particularly in primary care consultations and in the tendency to treat pregnancy and childbirth as illnesses. These factors suggest that there is a pattern of health experience based on sex which overlays the social class patterns the Report considers, and which may be a futher important dimension of inequality. Similar arguments might be made with respect to racial discrimination.

Turning to the recommendations made by the Working Group, comments can be made at a number of different levels. These comments can be traced to two sets of seeming contradictions contained within the Report. The first relate to the role of the health care system. In chapter 6 of the Report, the discussion of causes of inequalities does not even consider the possibility that they might be attributable partly to an unequal provision of health care facilities and resources. Yet the recommendations contained in chapter 8, by stressing the importance of resource allocation formulae, appear to be based on an opposite conclusion, albeit while acknowledging the greater importance of a 'wider strategy'.

The 'wider strategy' contains the second, and perhaps most important, set of contradictions. The Report notes the important role of 'economic and associated socio-structural factors', the persistent and deep-rooted nature of unequal income and wealth distribution, indeed the possibility that the present economic system may promote inequality, yet assumes that nevertheless a number of major changes are capable of being enacted to reduce substantially or eliminate inequality while leaving the framework of these 'economic and socio-structural factors' unchanged. The recommendations, for instance, that trade unions and CBI representatives should participate in drawing up 'minimally acceptable and desirable standards of work; security; conditions and amenities; pay; and welfare or fringe benefits' either flatly contradict the implicit conclusion of the 'materialist' explanation that conflicting interests are part of the economic system, or amount to what would be virtually a revolutionary change in that economic system. This is not to deny that scope exists for making changes that might help to reduce the severity of inequalities and their origins; it is rather to suggest that there are limits beyond which such changes would be resisted. The lack of discussion of the process by which such changes might be made, the assumption that a favorably inclined government initiating legislation might suffice to effect these changes, are perhaps an alternative context in which to place the 'unrealistic' charges levelled by Mr. Jenkin. It was perhaps an unspoken acknowledgment of these problems that led the Working Group finally to describe their recommendations on the abolition of child poverty as 'a modest first step which might be taken toward this objective' (DHSS, 1980, p. 366).

One of the more original contributions of the Report is the willingness to see health care as only one (perhaps not very efficient) way in which health can be influenced, and to discuss the possibility of focusing health programs on other areas of social policy such as housing or income maintenance. Such a strategy would be 'preventive' in a much wider sense of the word than is currently employed, and there is still a need to emphasize that in this definition a prevention program should not necessarily be viewed in the same way as a health care program: that is, a specific bundle of services whose effect can be increased by increasing expenditure to provide more of them. Rather, a preventive strategy as outlined by the Working Group is interventionist: it requires changes in policy across many government departments, and not foremost a budget of its own to spend on its own programs. A more detailed outline of the way in which such a prevention 'agency' could operate without undermining government autonomy would therefore be a valuable contribution.

In this framework of broad changes in the distribution of responsibilities for health across public policy programs, a likely outcome would be a perception of the National Health Service as, more correctly, a National Illness Service with responsibilities restricted to care, cure, and medical services. Nevertheless, the Report does envisage some redistribution of resources taking place within the NHS budget away from acute care and toward preventive health care and community care. The suggestion raises a problem which apparently led the authors of the Report to disagree: in changing the emphasis of expenditure from acute care to prevention, is it sufficient to cut back or freeze one budget and expand the other, or is it in the short-run necessary to spend more on the preventive services and not cut back on acute spending until the effects of increased preventive work can be felt? The answer to this question is dependent upon judgments concerning the potential effects of a cut in acute services, or possible wastages that might be eliminated. The issue, however, does demonstrate the much more limited scope than is sometimes argued for short-run savings in expenditure resulting from restructuring long-term objectives.

A final point to be made in relation to the recommendations of the Working Group is the need for evaluation. It would be wrong to suggest that detailed evidence of the effects of all the recommendations is an essential precursor of their implementation. The central theme of the association between inequalities in health and general socioeconomic inequalities is, as Illsley (1980) pointed out in his Rock Carling lecture, a century-old commonplace among Registrars-General, epidemiologists, and social reformers. It is incontrovertible in its totality if not its details, and controversy is more accurately attributable to the policy and political implications than to any doubts about the overall relationship. In addition, as Sir Douglas Black has himself pointed out (Black, 1981), it is in the nature of the different kinds of service involved in a reorientation of health policy that the present caring and curing services are tangible, familiar, in high demand, and more open to measurement than a comprehensive prevention strategy, which would inevitably be in large part an act of faith, albeit based on soundly reasoned expectations.

Nevertheless, the Report has highlighted the lack of information about the precise causes of health and ill-health, not least in the relative importance of the health service as opposed to other aspects of the socioeconomic system. There is little discussion of the comparative consequences of implementing chapter 8's recommendations on the health and personal social services and chapter 9's wider strategy. A starting point for the evaluation of proposals to reduce inequalities in health might therefore be an attempt to estimate accurately the effects of inequalities of health care provision and the consequences of making health care distribution, access, and/or impact more even. To this end, the proposed program of action in ten special areas would, if implemented, yield a mass of valuable information.

The likelihood remains, however, that such studies would confirm the limited extent of change that could be induced through the health service, and some way would have to be found to use evaluative techniques to decide priorities for a wider strategy. To date, discussion of these wider proposals (Morris, 1980; Deitch, 1981c) has focused almost entirely on costs, and has virtually ignored the benefits that could result from an improvement in health and a reduction in the unequal distribution of ill-health and death. Cost-benefit analyses have earned themselves a rather poor reputation, in many instances quite justified, by their attempts to place money values on all sorts of intangible costs and benefits and their often value-laden selection of the costs and benefits to be included in an analysis. The cost-benefit approach, however, has performed the useful role of establishing that costs and benefits are not simply the direct financial consequences of a project or program, but encompass such things as waiting-times, anxiety, uncertainty, as well as effects on production, employment and consumption. Moreover, it is clear from the discussion surrounding the costs of the Report's recommendations that the 'costs' are in many instances not costs as defined in a cost-benefit study (additional use of resources) but rather are transfers that do not result in any net additional use of resources. There are compelling reasons, therefore, for placing discussion of the recommendations in a framework that would comprehensively evaluate their overall economic implications. Economists in particular should be encouraged to pursue research in this area.

A concluding assessment of the Report must acknowledge the extremely useful compilation of data which the Working Group has prepared, and their willingness to step outside the bounds of traditional medical models of ill-health and consider the socioeconomic factors that have led to their wider strategy. If they have at some times found themselves ensnared in ambiguities and at others been unable to produce causal evidence, it does not follow that they are heading in the wrong direction nor that their recommendations should be ignored. Rather, these shortcomings are the consequence of a laudable attempt to shake off the traditional attitudes toward ill-health that still permeate health policies. The Report's detailed documentation of thirty years of static or widening inequalities is eloquent testimony to the need for change in thought and action.

Acknowledgments. Her Majesty's Stationery Office Crown Copyright graciously gave permission to quote freely from the original Black Report.

References

Black, D. (1981) The Black Report. *Lancet*, **1**, 1379

BMJ (1980a) News and notes. *British Medical Journal*, **281**, 690

BMJ (1980b) Equalities and inequalities in health. *British Medical Journal*, **281**, 763

Deitch, R. (1980) Commentary from Westminster: unwanted legacy from Mr. Jenkin's predecessor. *Lancet*, **2**, 545

Deitch, R. (1981a) Commentary from Westminster: Mr. Jenkin on the Black Report. *Lancet*, **1**, 735

Deitch, R. (1981b) Commentary from Westminster: the debate on the Black Report. *Lancet*, **2**, 158

Deitch, R. (1981c) Commentary from Westminster: a debate for the new session. *Lancet*, **2**, 428–429

DHSS (1980) *Inequalities in Health: Report of a Research Working Group*, Department of Health and Social Security, London

Doyal, L. (1980) *The Political Economy of Health*, Pluto Press, London

HMSO (1946) *A National Health Service Bill*, Cmnd. 6761, Her Majesty's Stationery Office, London

Illsey, R. (1980) *Professional or Public Health? Sociology in Health and Medicine*, Nuffield Provincial Hospitals Trust, London

Lancet (1980) Inequalities in health. *Lancet*, **2**, 513

Morris, J. N. (1980) Equalities and inequalities in health. *British Medical Journal*, **281**, 1003

Navarro, V. (1978) *Class Struggle, the State, and Medicine*, Martin Robertson, Oxford

Snaith, A. H. (1981) Debate on the Black Report. *Lancet*, **2**, 308

Reprinted by permission of the Baywood Publishing Company, New York. Alastair McIntosh Gray (1982) Inequalities in health. The Black Report: a summary and comment. *International Journal of Health Services*, **12**(3), 349, 372–377. © 1982, Baywood Publishing Co., Inc.

Chapter 52

Women, the NHS, and the control of reproduction

Lesley Doyal

The dramatic changes which have taken place in the lives of women during the twentieth century have been closely related to the development of various aspects of reproductive technology. It is now technically possible for all women to control their own fertility, either through contraception or abortion or more permanently through sterilization. Moreover, when a woman does have a baby, giving birth is now safer than it has been at any other time in history, and the baby is less likely to die in infancy or childhood. It is often believed that we have modern medicine to thank for these developments, but serious reservations need to be expressed about any such assumption. Although medical intervention played some part in improving infant and maternal mortality rates in the late nineteenth and early twentieth centuries, it is now generally accepted that improved standards of housing and nutrition probably played the most significant role. Similarly, doctors had very little to do with the development of new methods of birth control, while few were in the vanguard of attempts to bring contraceptive knowledge to women who needed it.

Nevertheless, the medical profession (and through it the state) has increasingly taken control of reproductive technology, and this has had at least two important consequences. The first is that decisions relating to research and practice in this field have often failed to take the interests and feelings of women seriously into account. Thus, doctors have tended to glorify the contraceptive pill – the most 'scientific' method of birth control – while paying almost no attention to the development of a male contraceptive. They have consistently played down legitimate anxieties about the pill and its possible side-effects, whilst emphasizing its ease and reliability. Secondly, the medical domination of reproductive technology has meant that the technical potential for women to control their own fertility has not been realized. Doctors – and through them the state, the church, and even particular sectors of industry – are able to influence issues such as whether or not a woman becomes pregnant, whether she continues an existing pregnancy, and even the conditions under which she will give birth. For women, the development of reproductive technology has therefore been a contradictory process. Technically, it has given women more control over their own bodies, but at the same time it has increased the capacity of others to exercise control over women's lives. We can explore these contradictions in more detail through looking at developments in contraception, in abortion and in childbirth.

The NHS has always been characterized by an ambivalent attitude towards the provision of contraceptive advice. Immediately after the war, the emphasis was on 'building-up' the population, so that birth control clinics were not made an integral part of the new NHS. Despite a growing emphasis during the postwar period on 'family planning' and on improving the quality of family life, the bulk of contraceptive advice has, until recently, been provided by the Family Planning Association (FPA) and other privately-run clinics such as the Brook Advisory Centres. As a result, working-class women in particular have often had difficulty in obtaining the advice they needed. In fact, it was not until 1976 that Area Health Authorities completed the takeover of the FPA clinics and integrated them into the NHS. Moreover, 'family planning' was until very recently available only to those who were already married. Sexuality outside marriage was not to be encouraged, and it was not until the late 1960s that clinics were prepared to offer birth-control advice to unmarried women. GPs were formally incorporated into the 'family planning' network in 1975,[1] but many problems still remain. Clinics are often extremely crowded, there are not enough of them, they are often not open at times which are suitable for working mothers, and the vast majority do not provide child-care facilities. Moreover there is increasing evidence that because of the particularly low priority given to services for women these shortages and inadequacies are being exacerbated as expenditure on the NHS is reduced.[2]

Problems in obtaining adequate contraception are not, however, limited to difficulties in physical access to advice and supplies. The knowledge gap between doctor and patient has widened so that it has become increasingly difficult for women to make an informed choice between different methods of contraception. The new techniques of birth control are much more complex than those of the past – the IUD needs to be inserted by trained personnel, while the pill, a chemical rather than a mechanical means of contraception, has far-reaching effects on body chemistry. Most women do not know the advantages and disadvantages of existing types of contraceptive device, and doctors themselves are often inadequately trained for their expanding role in family planning. Most spend very little time in discussion with women and provide very little information about possible alternatives. Indeed, with the encouragement of the drug companies, most doctors are themselves inclined to favour the oral contraceptive, despite recent research findings that on safety grounds the pill should be used much less frequently than it is at present.[3] Moreover, doctors are also inclined to choose a method which *they* believe to be most appropriate for the woman concerned, so that 'feckless' women may for example be given the injectable contraceptive Depo-Provera, without being adequately informed about the dangers involved.

The postwar period has, therefore, seen an expansion in the availability of contraception, as well as the introduction of new techniques. For women, these developments have brought significant advantages, but, as we have seen, they have also brought new problems. Hence, while contraception is a prerequisite for women's liberation, it has all too often created new forms of oppression through the way in which it has been provided. Moreover, it is important to recognize that the extension of 'family planning' was not just in the interests of individual women, but was at the same time in the interests of capitalism in a broader sense.[4] Women became more easily available for paid work; the nuclear family was strengthened, and 'problem families' which might have to be maintained by the state at great expense could be induced not to have any more children by the availability of free contraceptive supplies.

Attempts to liberalize the abortion laws have faced even greater opposition than attempts to extend the provision of contraception. The fight for the legalization of abortion really gained strength in Britain in the 1920s, and many of the early pioneers were feminists and socialists – women like Stella Browne, Dora Russell and Janet Chance. The Abortion Law Reform Association (ALRA) was founded in 1936, but made little headway in the inter-war period, and the church, the state, and the medical profession remained united against abortion. ALRA took up the campaign again after the war, working mainly through parliamentary channels, and during the 1960s the cause of abortion reform became part of the more general reform movement of the period. The greater aura of social confidence meant that abortion was no longer perceived as a threat to the existing social order, and the eventual reform of the abortion law in 1967 must be understood as part of a wider process of social change. As Greenwood and Young have commented,

> The 1960s could be characterized as an era of social reform. Legislation in the areas of juvenile delinquency, poverty, divorce, capital punishment, drug use, homosexuality and criminal justice came in for a radical re-appraisal (e.g. Murder/Abolition of the Death Penalty Act 1965, Sexual Reform Act 1967, Criminal Justice Act 1967, Divorce Reform Act 1969, Misuse of Drugs Act 1971). The political base for such a catalogue of reforms was the dominant bloc within the Labour Party which viewed a mixed economy as desirable and argued for state intervention backed by expert guidance. Problems abounded in society but these could be eliminated by selective social engineering and piecemeal reform.[5]

These general pressures for reform were strengthened by a growing awareness that the existing abortion law was being widely disregarded – it has been estimated that anything between fifteen thousand and one hundred thousand illegal abortions were being performed each year. Moreover, it was evident that many of the women who were deemed to need abortions most – particularly those with low incomes and large families – were not obtaining them. 'Problem families' of this kind were defined as a matter of serious concern by the new breed of social workers, and hence some of the support for the 1967 act had considerable eugenic undertones. The majority of doctors (GPs in particular) supported the proposed reforms, although they continued to express the fear that the 'social clause' in the bill would take away their 'clinical freedom', by making decisions about abortion a non-medical issue. However, other sections of the medical profession joined with the Roman Catholic church in forming part of a very vociferous opposition.[6]

Despite this opposition, the bill was passed and the new Abortion Act came into force in 1967. As a result, it was no longer illegal for a registered medical practitioner to perform an abortion if two doctors were of the opinion that to continue the pregnancy would be a greater risk to the life or health of the woman or her existing children than an abortion would be, or if there was a substantial risk that the child would be physically or mentally handicapped. After generations of repressive legislation, the effect of the act was to produce a sudden increase in the number of abortions. By 1973, the number of legal abortions performed on British residents had risen to nearly one hundred and twenty thousand, approximately half of them taking place within the National Health Service.[7] The 1967 act was, therefore, a very important step in widening the availability of abortion, but access still remains seriously limited. The difficulties faced by women seeking abortions reflect both the low level of resources allocated to abortion within the NHS, and also the control exercised by individual doctors over access to abortion.

When the 1967 act was passed, no extra resources were provided for abortion facilities. The legislation, therefore, represented an acceptance of the idea of more freely available abortion, but without the financial backing to implement this commitment. As a result, a form of implicit rationing has developed, and a large number of abortions continue to be performed outside the NHS.[8] This general lack of resources is exacerbated by the policies of individual consultants who are able to determine how many abortions will be performed in a given area. These various pressures have resulted in a situation where in 1973, for example, 79 per cent of women seeking an abortion in Oxford were able to obtain one from the NHS, while the corresponding figure in Leeds was 25 per cent and in Walsall only 10 per cent.[9] Moreover, individual consultants are also able to choose what type of abortion to provide, and as a result abortions are rarely available on an out-patient basis, as many women would prefer.[10]

At an individual level, doctors also make judgements about specific women, and whether or not they should be allowed to have an abortion. These judgments are an important illustration of orthodox medical ideas about the nature of female sexuality and reproduction, and particularly about the moral aspects of these questions. Other things being equal, it is more difficult, for example, for a married woman than for an unmarried woman to obtain an abortion, since doctors assume that having babies is a normal part of being married. Increasingly they are prepared to abort women who already have large families, and whose incomes are not adequate to support more, but few doctors will be prepared to recommend termination for a 'normal' married woman on the grounds of what the doctor may regard as 'mere convenience'. Similarly, Sally Macintyre has suggested that when doctors deal with abortion requests from *single* women, they classify them into three categories – 'normal as-if-married'; the 'nice girl who has made a mistake'; and the 'bad girl'.[11] The 'normal as-if-married' woman is someone who is in a stable relationship and who plans to get married – she has simply 'anticipated' the wedding. It is assumed that she will continue with the pregnancy as a married woman should, and that the pregnancy does not present a problem. The good girls and the bad girls are differentiated on the basis of their past sexual history and their present attitude towards the pregnancy. Doctors will ask their patients about their relationship to the father of the child (is it 'serious'?), their use of contraception, and any previous sexual experience. How the woman relates to the doctor, and how she makes her request, are also very significant. Jean Aitken-Swan came to the following conclusions from her study of the attitudes of a sample of Scottish doctors:

> Not unnaturally, the doctor does not like it if he and the help he can give seem to be taken for granted. The wording of her request, the wrong manner, too demanding or over-confident, even her way of walking ('she comes prancing in') may antagonise him and lessen her chances of referral. On the other hand, too passive an approach can be misinterpreted. 'You get the impression with a lot of these lassies that you could push them one way or the other and in a situation like this I tend to say keep the baby. ...' The doctors respond best to a concerned approach and tears are never amiss.[12]

It seems then, that a woman needs to treat her doctor very carefully if she is to obtain an abortion. Good girls may be successful, because they just 'made a mistake' and are duly contrite, but bad girls are likely to be denied an abortion because their doctor believes it would encourage them in their 'promiscuity'.

Increasingly, doctors have come to control not just the means to *prevent* pregnancy but also the conditions under which children will be born. Reproduction is assumed to be the most 'natural' of female functions but giving birth has now become a medical event. As Ann Oakley has put it – 'it has lost its character as a taken-for-granted aspect of adult life'. Certainly, medical intervention has played some part in improving rates of infant and maternal mortality, but its importance is often greatly over-estimated.[13] Indeed, it is now being argued that, although certain obstetric techniques have clearly added to the comfort and safety of mothers and babies, the 'medicalization' of childbirth and of antenatal care is now going beyond what is necessary or desirable.[14]

Notes

1. They are, however, paid an additional fee for each item of service performed, indicating a continued reluctance to define contraceptive provision as a 'normal' part of the GP's job.
2. *The Guardian*, 6 April 1977; and *Women's Report*, vol. 4 nos. 4 & 5, 1976.
3. Royal College of General Practitioners (1974) *Oral Contraceptives and Health*, Pitman Medical, London; and Mortality among oral-contraceptive users. *Lancet*, 2, 1977, 727–731.
4. The relationship between 'population control' and 'family planning' is discussed in Gordon L. (1977) *Woman's Body Woman's Right, A Social History of Birth Control in America*, Penguin, Harmondsworth.
5. Greenwood, V. and Young, J. (1976) *Abortion in Demand*, Pluto Press, London, pp. 15–16.
6. Hindell, K. and Simms, M. (1971) *Abortion Law Reformed*, Peter Owen, London: Macintyre, S. J. (1977) The medical profession and the 1967 Abortion Act in Britain. *Social Science and Medicine*, 7(2), 121–134; and Greenwood and Young, *op.cit.*
7. Abortions – public and private facilities. *Labour Research*, May 1977.
8. *Ibid.*
9. OPCS Registrar General's *Supplement on Abortion* in 1973 (1974) HMSO, London.
10. Hindell, K. and Graham, H. (eds) (1974) *Outpatient Abortion*, Pregnancy Advisory Service.
11. Macintyre, S. J. (1977) *Single and Pregnant*, Croom Helm, London.
12. Aitken-Swan, J. (1977) *Fertility Control and the Medical Profession*, Croom Helm, London, p. 65.
13. Baird, D. (1975) The interplay of changes in society, reproductive habits and obstetric practice in Scotland between 1922 and 1972. *British Journal of Preventive and Social Medicine*, 29, 135–146. Also DHSS (1975) *Report on Confidential Enquiries into Maternal Deaths in England and Wales*, 1970–72, HMSO, London, p. 124; Oakley, A. (1976) Wisewoman and medicine man: changes in the management of childbirth. In *The Rights and Wrongs of Women* (Mitchell, J. and Oakley, A., eds), Penguin, Harmondsworth.
14. Haire, D. The cultural warping of childbirth. In Ehrenreich, J. (ed.) (1978) *The Cultural Crisis of Modern Medicine*, Monthly Review Press; Arms, S. (1975) *Immaculate Deception: A New Look at Childbirth in America*, Houghton Mifflin, Boston; Stoller Shaw, N. (1974) *Forced Labour: Maternity Care in the United States*, Pergamon Press, New York; and Rich, A. (1975) The theft of childbirth. *New York Review of Books*, 2 October.

Reprinted by permission of Pluto Press, London. Lesley Doyal (1979) Women, the NHS, and the control of reproduction. In *The Political Economy of Health*, Pluto Press, London, pp. 228–234.

Chapter 53

Health and deprivation: inequality and the North

Peter Townsend, Peter Phillimore and Alastair Beattie

The publication of the Black Report in 1980 provided emphatic confirma-
tion that the years since the establishment of the National Health Service
had not seen a decline in social inequalities in health in Britain. Indeed, it
produced evidence of widening inequalities and not just vivid statistical
illustrations of big differences in health experience. Perhaps partly fuelled
by the Government's dismissive response to that report, and faced with the
implications for health posed by the deepest economic recession since the
1930s, public and scientific interest in health inequalities has continued to
grow during the 1980s. The swelling number of papers on the problems of
resource allocation for health care and area studies of health are just two
relevant examples. The present study epitomizes this recent development,
and provides, perhaps for the first time, an analysis of the health of small
areas across an entire region of the country.

The Northern Region is not a microcosm or reflection of the country as a
whole, either in health or social and economic terms: rather, it is one of
its most deprived constituent parts. The areas of highest mortality and
morbidity in Britain are overwhelmingly to be found in the North and
North-West, in Scotland and in Wales; they are almost entirely absent from
southern England, except for one or two areas of inner London. These are
also areas where the recession and its human dimension of unemployment
and reduced living standards have been felt most severely. An analysis of
inequality in health in the North is, therefore, biased towards the worse end
of the health spectrum in Britain.

Concepts and models of health

In all this work what must we understand by 'health'? In rich countries the
concept of health has come under fierce scrutiny in the late twentieth cen-

tury. Part of this has been due to a reaction against what has been perceived to be the dehumanizing effects of medical ideology and technology when carried to extremes – as in features of the modern practice of chemotherapy, surgery and obstetrics (see, for example, Powles, 1973; Illich, 1975; Navarro, 1976; Ehrenreich, 1978; Stark, 1982). Medicine is felt to be too narrowly concerned with diseases, rather than with people. Another aspect of the scrutiny of health stems from a different reaction – against the artificial, clamorous and manufactured nature of modern urban life. The search for 'the good life' has become as important as the critique of medicine in changing attitudes to health and preparing people to consider different perspectives.

Scientifically there are two alternative modes of explanation. These were reviewed in the Black Report (1980, pp. 5–9). Firstly, there is the medical model. This is an engineering approach to health, built originally upon the Cartesian philosophy of the body conceived and controlled as a machine, and dealing essentially with the cure of diseases in individuals. We mean that the idea is carefully structured in terms of cure rather than prevention, disease rather than the promotion of health and welfare, and the examination and treatment of individual rather than of social conditions – whether of couples, friends, families, groups, communities or populations. The curious fact here is that in trying to escape the social and political controversies which are necessarily involved in, say, pursuing unremittingly the reasons for differences in rates of mortality or morbidity between populations, or promoting the health and wellbeing of unemployed groups, or families living in poverty, or the population as a whole, the professional servant of medicine has accepted a circumspection of the scope of his or her work and a set of values which permits more than three-quarters of his or her potential scientific expertise and work to be drawn off and reconstituted as areas of political and bureaucratic responsibility. The restricted definition of responsibility for health has implications of which everyone should become aware. The development of knowledge to enlarge health is constrained. Some major social causes of ill-health and death are underestimated or ignored; and faith in the capacity of human beings to control the problems of life and liberate their potentialities is needlessly diminished.

The medical model is of course embodied in organizations and in the everyday analysis of fresh events. Ideas and meanings are not just disembodied abstractions; they are reflected in practice and structures. This means that priority is given in the allocation of resources to the prestigious departments of the practice of acute medicine, to specialized hospital treatment rather than general practice, and to casualty treatment instead of screening, prevention and health education. The use of the word 'ancillary' to denote someone whose work is defined to fit in with, but is clearly of lesser status than, that of medicine itself, is significant. Therefore the particular forms of the organization and practice of health care in Britain and in other countries reinforces the meaning of health central to the medical model. This is liable to be forgotten: even the critics of medicine will constantly be presented with examples of the re-affirmation of its principles which seem to deny any alternative.

Two qualifications have to be made to this summary representation of the medical model. One is that it is not unambiguously consistent and clear-cut. The social is accommodated to the medicalized meaning of health. There are specialities which introduce the social aspects of health, like psychiatry, paediatrics and social medicine or epidemiology, but there is a degree of necessary intellectual subordination or self-imposed submission. Thus, for example, epidemiology itself has generally been interpreted restrictedly as the study of the distribution of disease as the aggregate of individual phenomena (McMahon and Pugh, 1970; and see the critical discussion of Paterson, 1981). In addition, some critics of medicine, who have argued that most of the decline in premature mortality in the nineteenth and twentieth centuries has been due to social changes like improvements in diet and living standards generally (in particular McKeown, 1976; but see also Winter, 1977 and 1981 for a valuable historical illustration), have sought more to call attention to the complementary features of an 'environ-mentalist' approach than to reconstitute medicine within an alternative model of health. The same is true of certain penetrating evaluations of medical care – using social factors, including class as a form of standardization (for example, Charlton et al., 1983). They do not situate medicine as just one of the social institutions in an alternative model which seeks to explain the distribution of health. There are other ways in which medicine cannot be said to be 'monolithic'. There are forms of fringe medicine, like osteopathy, which are acceptable to many in the medical profession as well as to the public, as well as those forms which are unacceptable. Moreover, some conceptions of preventive action – albeit narrow or limited, and particularly when related to individual conditions or behaviour, such as check-ups or education about the risks of smoking or eating a diet heavy in cholesterol – are approved if not universally pursued.

Another qualification is equally important. Criticism of the medical 'model' which has developed must not be interpreted as cavalier rejection or disregard of certain benefits it has to offer. The challenge is in pursuing the larger questions about health to which medicine can offer only a partial or fragmented answer. Specialized features of medicine must therefore be incorporated into a larger model, parts of which are currently ill-developed. Certainly they are far less developed than some justly admired and honourable technologies and procedures of medicine. In contradistinction the social model of health takes as its basis the fact that human behaviour is ultimately social in its origin and determination, and depends upon social organization and convention to encourage or restrain. People perform roles, have relationships and observe customs which are socially defined (including those which are made compulsory in an authoritarian state) and this provides the means of identity and activity. This is not to say that people conform greyly to a uniform pattern: there are divergencies of age, background, environment and stage of family development which permit wide variation in personality and behaviour within any social structure, but the 'social' is what provides the necessary framework for observed health. It defines the pattern of daily life, diet, shelter, work and form of reproduction, upbringing and care; and it defines the variations between communities in adjoining areas as well as between cultures or nations. The vitality, endurance and freedom from disease, disability and stress – of individuals as much as of groups – can only be defined, explained and enhanced in that context.

The social approach to health is illustrated historically in the work of Virchow (1958) and Dubos (1959). Thus, in 1848 at the age of 27, Rudolf Virchow founded a journal entitled *Medizinische Reform*. He argued that poverty caused disease and that doctors had a duty to support social reforms to improve health. He believed that the treatment of individuals was only a small part of the practice of medicine and that the major part was the control of crowd diseases. This necessarily involved social and, if called for, even political measures. For him medicine was a social science. Dubos traced the origins and adoption of different ideas of health. He pointed out that before the late nineteenth century disease was generally regarded as resulting from a lack of harmony between the sick person and his or her environment, but with the work of Louis Pasteur, Robert Koch and their followers, medical opinion changed radically. They identified the virulent micro-organisms and through laboratory experiments they demonstrated that healthy animals could be made ill (see O'Brien, 1982, for an account of changes of direction in the history of medicine).

The definition of health adopted upon the foundation of the World Health Organization is often quoted as a modern illustration of the social model of health as an alternative to the medical model. In fact it represents a rather lame compromise. The WHO defined health as 'a state of complete physical, mental and social well-being and not merely the absence of disease or infirmity'. (This theme was confirmed in the Alma-Ata declaration – Alma-Ata, 1978.) In fact, while emphasizing positive in contrast to negative aspects of health, this definition conveys a curiously passive, steady-state idea of 'well-being' instead of one grounded in more active fulfilment – whether of productive work or useful and satisfying social roles and relationships. The definition implicitly favours an individual rather than a social orientation towards health, which may be said to perpetuate the wrong order of priorities in understanding and gaining control over the phenomenon. A more thoroughgoing social and dynamic conceptualization has to be sought.

What are the implications of adopting a social model of health? Trained personnel would continue to work within the traditional practices of medicine but more of them would begin to work on prevention, on the early stages of disease and on recovery and rehabilitation. Of course it is not only 'health' but the social context of health which requires clarification to develop better theory to explain the distribution of health. We say 'social context' because the two traditions of research which we have identified –

those of inequalities of health by area and by class – are imperfect representations of the population variations experienced in social structure and organization and need to be better synthesized. Although some points will be discussed in ensuing chapters, certain introductory comments are required.

A 'social' model of health must reflect the pervasive characteristics of social institutions and state organization. This means that society and not location must be treated as providing the causal mainspring of any local variations which may be observed in, say, health. Indeed some characteristics of 'location' are themselves socially rather than naturalistically derived – such as form of industry, enclosure and non-enclosure, waterways and roadways, afforestation or deforestation, vegetation and housing – and some of these features will ultimately be related to the history and present configuration of the ownership and price of land. So while there will be 'naturalistic' elements like climate or rock and land formation, many of them will have been adapted, reconstituted or overlaid by human use and will relate to, if not strictly conform with, social structure. The same points apply to the development of a concept of 'environment' to explain some of the effects of location upon health. Our necessary implication is that the *social* factors which themselves lie behind geographical, area or environmental variations in the distribution of health require identification.

A second necessary step is to accept that social class must not be regarded as just another social indicator, like employment status, tenure, race or overcrowding, but as *the* social concept which is fundamental to the explanation of the distribution of health – to which the listed indicators are secondarily related. In key respects this is a matter for scientific judgement (on the basis of empirical observation, experiment, statistical correlation, and theoretical consistency and integrity) and not mere ideology. As such, class must not be unnecessarily restricted to one aspect of social life, like occupation, but must be defined (operationally as well as in general principle) as a total reflection of differences in rank in economic and social position. This explains the Black Report's insistence on re-interpreting the usage of 'social' class in many commentaries on health as 'occupational' class (Black Report, 1980, p. 18).

The Registrar General has traditionally used an occupational classification as a basis for defining social class. A specific occupation may indeed denote, within narrow limits, what a person's earnings are likely to be, and therefore what income he or she and the household are likely to have, and the kind of home and the area they are likely to live in, as well as the amount of wealth they are likely to possess, the education they are likely to have had and even the kinds of customs and leisure activities they are likely to pursue. This is why in many studies of the past, occupational categorization has 'worked' so well. It is because occupational status has borne an approximate correspondence, albeit a rough one, with class structure that explains its widespread use. However, that does not presuppose either that social class should be reduced to occupational status or that occupational status continues to be as good a proxy for social class as formerly. Both require contemporary attention. People's social class is fundamental to the opportunities in, and experience of, life. This can be demonstrated at each of the stages of pre-natal development, infancy, childhood, education, occupational career, marriage, child-rearing, post-family maturity and retirement.

The fact that it is more difficult to categorize people by social class than, say, by race or age does not mean that it is any less important or fundamental. Neither is the problem just one of methodological procedure – of finding how a population can be ranked in relation to an amalgam of resources, status, power situation and disposition – it is in obtaining the necessary information in the first place; it is in appreciating that there are interests in society which are not particularly keen that such categorizations should be made, because questions would inevitably be raised about positions of wealth, power and privilege. Thus, it is difficult, for example, to take inherited wealth and the advantages of certain physical resources into account as factors in children's development and later recruitment to the grade as well as kind of jobs held. Perhaps the single most important component of 'class' which social scientists need to address is income – or a wider definition of income to include wealth and resources in kind, including fringe benefits (Townsend, 1979, Chapter 6). There is evidence that when successively more comprehensive and exact definitions of income are applied to a survey population, correlations with ill-health and disability are markedly more significant (*ibid.*, p. 1176).

References

Alma-Ata (1978) *Primary Health Care. Report of the International Conference on Primary Health Care, Alma-Ata, USSR, 6–12 Sept. 1978*, World Health Organisation, Geneva

Black Report (1980) *Inequalities in Health: Report of a Research Working Group*, Department of Health and Social Security, London

Charlton, J. R. H., Hartley, R. M., Silver, R. and Holland, W. W. (1983) Geographical variation in mortality from conditions amenable to medical intervention in England and Wales. *The Lancet*, 1, 691–696

Dubos, R. (1959) *Mirage of Health: Utopias, Progress and Biological Change*, Harper and Row, New York

Ehrenreich, J. (ed.) (1978) *The Cultural Crisis of Modern Medicine*, Monthly Review Press, New York

Illich, I. (1975) *Medical Nemesis: The Approximation of Health*, New York

McKeown, T. (1976) *The Role of Medicine*, Nuffield Provincial Hospitals Trust, London

McMahon, B. and Pugh, T. F. (1970) *Epidemiology: Principles and Methods*, Little, Brown and Co., New York

Navarro, V. (1976) *Medicine Under Capitalism*, Prodist, New York

Paterson, K. (1981) Theoretical perspectives in epidemiology – a critical appraisal. *Radical Community Medicine*, 8, 21–29

Powles, J. (1973) On the limitations of modern medicine. *Science, Medicine and Man*, 1, 1–30

Stark, E. (1982) Doctors in spite of themselves: the limits of radical health criticism. *International Journal of Health Services*, 12(3), 419–455

Townsend, P. (1979) *Poverty in the United Kingdom*, Penguin, Harmondsworth, Middlesex

Virchow, R. (ed. Rather, L. J.) (1958) *Disease, Life and Man: Selected Essays of Rudolf Virchow*, Stanford University Press.

Winter, J. M. (1977) The impact of the First World War on civilian health in Britain. *Economic History Review*, 30, 487–507

Winter, J. M. (1981) Aspects of the impact of the First World War on infant mortality in Britain. *Journal of European Economic History*, 11, 713–738

Reprinted by permission of Croom Helm, London. Peter Townsend, Peter Phillimore and Alastair Beattie (1988) *Health and Deprivation: Inequality and the North*, Croom Helm, London, 6–11, 151, 152.

Chapter 54

Justice and allocation of medical resources

Raanan Gillon

In the last chapter I indicated the wide range of issues concerning justice that are relevant to medical ethics. Even within the sphere of distributive justice the range is dauntingly broad. At one end of the range are what economists call microallocation decisions, of which the most dramatic deal with the allocation of scarce lifesaving resources such as haemodialysis between competing claimants. At the other end are macroallocation decisions taken at a governmental level on the division of the national 'cake' between, for instance, health, other welfare, education, arts, and defence budgets. In between are varieties of what one might call mesoallocation decisions. These include decisions on how to distribute the allocated national health budget – the subject matter of the Black report (Black *et al.*, 1982), which showed so clearly and so shockingly the statistical correlations throughout the nation between poverty and low social status on the one hand and adverse health outcomes on the other. (In doing so it also showed the inadequacy of assuming that overtly 'health care' decisions are the only or even the most important ones in determining the nation's health.) They also include decisions on how to allocate medical resources at health authority level between the competing medical and other health care claims and decisions within a hospital on how to allocate between competing specialties and firms. More specific still are decisions for allocation among the different members of a hospital firm or health centre; and then come the microallocation decisions of each doctor or health worker distributing his or her available resources among particular patients. Although this range of decisions is exceedingly broad and disparate, all are based on some moral assessment of how competing claims can be fairly adjudicated. They are all thus explicitly or implicitly based on some theory of justice.

Which moral principles should take precedence?

Once one turns to substantive theories of medical resource allocation –

answers to the question 'What are the relevant inequalities that justify giving more to some and less to others?' – one meets the same sort of disagreement and complexity about which moral principles should take precedence (see bibliography) as one does with theories of justice generally. The main alternatives, however, are straightforward enough, as my 8 year old daughter briskly reminded me when I was getting into my usual tangle over these impossible questions. How should I choose one out of three dying people to have the only available lifesaving machine?

'Well', she told me, sparing a minute or two from her television programme, 'you could give it to the youngest because she'd live longer (welfare maximization), or you could give it to the illest because she needs it most (medical need), or you could give it to the kindest because kind people deserve to be treated nicely (merit). No, you couldn't give it to the one you liked best (partiality), that wouldn't be fair'. Nor, she decided, would 'eenie meenie minee mo' (lottery) be fair because the one who needed it most, or the youngest, or the kindest might not get it. Nor did she (much to my surprise) think that the Queen should get it in preference to the poor man (social worth) – 'because she's got so much already and the poor man hasn't'. Of all the methods, her preferred one was to choose the illest because he needed it most – but, not surprisingly, she could not say why that was a better option than the others. Her list of options, however, is remarkably standard, and she joins many doctors in preferring medical need as the criterion of choice.

Perhaps unexpectedly medical need correlates most obviously with the Marxist criterion for justice – 'to each according to his need'. (I should add that this criterion is not exclusively Marxist, that few doctors are Marxists, and that few would accept the first half of the Marxist slogan – 'From each according to his ability'.) Unfortunately, the concept of a need – as distinct from a desire, for example – is not at all clear (Daniels, 1981). Furthermore, it is at least plausible to argue that assertion of needs entails assertion of implied value or values, in which case what are the implied values of the criterion of medical need? Prolongation of life, elimination of disease and attainment of health, and improved quality of life, in the sense of both reduction of suffering and enhancement of flourishing, are all candidates as values correlating to medical need but how are they to be chosen or ranked and what precisely do we mean by these terms? (Their complexities recall the World Health Organisation's definition of health as a state of complete physical, mental, and social wellbeing or the controversies over 'sanctity of life', which I outlined in earlier chapters.) Thus the apparently straightforward criterion of medical need, whilst it is undoubtedly a necessary criterion for just distribution of medical resources (Williams, 1973), in no way evades the need to make explicit the moral criteria it encompasses. Nor does it make any easier the choice between competing candidates agreed to be in medical need.

Medical success as a criterion

A related but by no means identical medical criterion is that of medical success. Medical resources should, it is often claimed, be allocated according to probability of medical success. This adds to the criterion of medical need one of efficiency and, like my daughter's criterion of maximal prolongation of life, corresponds roughly to the welfare maximizing objective of utilitarian theories of justice. There are, of course, straightforward cases when the criterion is unproblematic: it would be absurd and wrong to give the only three available pints of a rare blood group to the patient with an incompatible group rather than to the patient with a compatible group. But the criterion of medical success is plagued by all the moral evaluative problems of medical need as well as by additional problems of how to determine medical success: what criteria are appropriate and how is success to be measured? (In this regard the economists' methods of comparing different techniques in terms of 'quality adjusted life years' (QUALYs) (Williams, 1983) seem to offer conventional methods of clinical trial considerable additional precision for comparative purposes.)

The third plank of my daughter's analysis concerned merit and desert – save the life of the kindest because kind people deserve to be looked after. Other merit related criteria are forward looking rather than backward looking. A consultant physician would select 'a man who would be able to continue regular work in suitable employment or a married woman with young children ... in preference to an unemployed labourer with no fixed abode' (Nabarro, 1967). A consultant in clinical renal physiology, also writing about selection for renal dialysis, believed that '[g]ainful employment in a well chosen occupation is necessary to achieve the best results; only the minority wish to live on charity' (Parsons, 1967) (even when the alternative is death?). More recently a man described as demented, intermittently violent, uncooperative, dirty, doubly incontinent, and with a tendency to expose himself and masturbate while being examined was taken off dialysis treatment 'in the patient's best interests' (Brahams, 1985). How much were the patient's dementia and discomfort the reason for stopping treatment and how much his objectionable behaviour?

How much, in general, should a patient's merits and demerits, personal and social, affect his being selected for lifesaving medical treatment? Certainly in the medical triage of wartime return to combat duty has been an established medicomilitary criterion for treatment (Winslow, 1982). In peacetime, however, allocation of medical resources on the basis of a patient's non-medical merits is widely regarded as repugnant. How are we to account for such differing intuitions? And what about extreme cases such as Shackman's (1967) hypothetical choice between Fleming and Hitler, where only one of them could be treated?

A possible approach

Given the fervent disagreement about which moral values should take priority in allocating medical resources it is hardly surprising that doctors on the whole tend to avoid the issue and try to concentrate on doing their best for their individual patients. Two methods of trying to cut the Gordian knot are notable. One commentator, in a different context, has argued that if not all who need scarce lifesaving resources can have them then none should (Cahn, 1978). Two American theologians, Ramsey and Childress, have argued that once a preliminary assessment on broad medical suitability has been made allocation should be by randomization, either by a lottery or on a first come first served system (with steps taken to ensure that people could not unfairly 'use' the system by having inside knowledge) (Ramsey, 1979; Childress, 1970).

I have not yet discovered an acceptable way to give consistent moral priority to any of these substantive criteria for allocation of scarce medical resources (and do not really expect to do so). Calabresi and Bobbitt (1978) plausibly suggest that societies tend to try to 'limit the destructive impact of tragic choices between fundamental moral values by choosing to mix approaches over time'. Within such temporal cycles first one value and then another is emphasized, but 'none can, for long, be abandoned'. Be that as it may, it would be a mistake to suppose that either the possibility or the need for justice is undermined by such variability and disagreement about which fundamental moral value to abandon when, in a particular situation, not all can be retained. After all, justice is precisely a method for moral resolution of conflicting claims. Provided one or other fundamental moral value is given priority after due consideration of the different claims in the light of all of the agreed moral values and in accordance with the formal principle of justice then justice, it seems to me, is done.

Thus if, in the context of allocating scarce medical resource, practical systems were set up for resolving conflicts about which value, in a particular case, should have priority, and if those systems took account of the fundamental moral values of respect for autonomy, beneficence, and non-maleficence, and if their deliberative structures incorporated Aristotle's formal principle of justice with its demands of formal equity, impartiality, and fairness then they would be just systems and their deliberations could be expected to yield just results despite (perhaps because of) the conflict within them. I doubt if better than that is achievable. Is less acceptable?

References

Black, D. A. K., Morris, J. N., Smith, C., Townsend, P. and Davidson, N. (1982) *Inequalities in Health: the Black Report*, Penguin, Harmondsworth

Brahams, D. (1985) When is discontinuation of dialysis justified? *Lancet*, i, 176–177

Cahn, E. (1978), cited by Calabresi, G. and Bobbitt, P. *Tragic Choices*, Norton, New York, pp.188, 234

Calabresi, G. and Bobbitt, P. (1978) *Tragic Choices*, Norton, New York, p.196

Childress J. (1970) Who shall live when not all can live? *Soundings: An Interdisciplinary Journal*, 53(4), 339–355 [Reprinted in *Moral Problems in*

Medicine, 2nd edn (Gorovitz, S., Macklin, R., Jameton, A., O'Connor, J. and Sherwin, S., eds), Prentice-Hall, Englewood Cliffs, N.J., 1983, pp.640–649]

Daniels, N. (1981) Health-care needs and distributive justice. *Philosophy and Public Affairs*, 10(2), 146–179

Nabarro, J. D. N. (1967) Who best to make the choice. *British Medical Journal*, i, 622

Parsons, F. M. (1967) A true 'doctor's' dilemma. *British Medical Journal*, i, 623

Ramsey, P. (1979) *The Patient As Person*, 10th edn, Yale University Press, New Haven, Conn., pp.239–275 *passim*

Shackman, R. (1967) Surgeon's point of view. *British Medical Journal*, i, 623–624

Williams, A. (1983) The economic role of 'health indicators'. In *Measuring the Social Benefits of Medicine* (Teeling-Smith, G., ed.), Office of Health Economics, London, pp.63–67

Williams, B. (1973) The idea of equality. In *Problems of the Self* (Williams, B., ed.), Cambridge University Press, Cambridge, pp.230–239

Winslow, G. R. (1982) *Triage and Justice*, University of California Press, Berkeley, p.8

Bibliography (See also cited references)

Boyd, K. M. (ed.) (1979) *The Ethics of Resource Allocation*, Edinburgh University Press, Edinburgh

Campbell, A. (1978) *Medicine, Health and Justice – The Problem of Priorities*, Churchill Livingstone, Edinburgh

Childress, J. (1981) *Priorities in Biomedical Ethics*, Westminster Press, Philadelphia

Engelhardt, H. T. (1984) Shattuck lecture: allocating scarce medical resources and the availability of organ transplantation. *New England Journal of Medicine*, 311, 66–71

Klein, R. (1984) Rationing health care. *British Medical Journal*, 289, 143–144

Maxwell, R. J. (1981) *Health and Work*, Lexington Books, Lexington, MA

Mooney, G. (1984) Medical ethics: an excuse for inefficiency? *Journal of Medical Ethics*, 10, 183–185

Parsons, V. and Lock, P. (1980) Triage and the patient with renal failure. *Journal of Medical Ethics*, 6, 173–176

Rescher, N. (1969) The allocation of exotic medical lifesaving therapy. *Ethics*, 79(3), 173–186

Shelp, E. (ed.) (1980) *Justice and Health Care*, Reidel, Dordrecht

Wolstenholme, G. E. W., and O'Connor, M. (eds) (1966) *Ethics in Medical Progress, with Special Reference to Transplantation*, Churchill, London

Reprinted by permission of John Wiley and Sons, Chichester. Raanan Gillon (1985) Justice and allocation of medical resources. In *Philosophical Medical Ethics*, Wiley, Chichester, pp.94–99.

Chapter 55

The NHS – an assessment

A. J. Culyer

This book has been about need and how best to meet it. It is, perhaps, unfortunate that we should be lumbered with such a term, which both has prominent persuasive overtones and lends itself to vague and various interpretations. Our own interpretation has been to emphasize that need is not, nor ever was, purely a technical matter, and that it does indeed require the exercise of moral judgements in defining what the needs are and which of them are, at the margin, more important than others. The crucial question at the heart of the politics of the NHS is who should be making these judgements? Certainly not the author, or social scientists in general, or the medics; for while there does exist a school of thought that argues that, because 'experts'' opinions about the facts, the history, the technology etc. involve both expertise *and* judgement, their moral judgements also have some special authority. Nothing could be more dangerous than this view to democracy in general in a technical age of large organizations, and nothing could be more alien to the idea of the NHS. Admittedly, however, such a view is – predictably – popular among the professionals (and not only in medicine) and their trade unions, whose deplorable arrogance is a feature of our producer-oriented times.

In the NHS, the experts can help first of all in making clear the differences in the kinds of judgements that have to be made, and in devising concepts and presenting information that helps them to be made in a more effective and aware way. If, then, in this book we have focused a great deal on this kind of interpretation of 'need', that is because such a focus has been long overdue. We have muddled through for long enough.

Our unashamedly economic approach has also had the great virtue of encouraging a broader concentration on the social aspects of decision-making in the NHS, rather than on the financial aspects, while at the same time retaining the ends–means approach that is essential for proper management and proper policy formation. Only the end can justify the means. The end of the NHS is not the NHS. In Britain the end – effective, efficient and fair health care – is to be served by the means of the NHS. It is of course possible that this means is contrary to or inconsistent with the end.

But we have tried to present a large number of reasons why this is not the case, all of which can be ultimately classified under two broad heads: the public nature (via spill-overs and the like) of the objectives on the one hand and the appropriateness of alternative institutional forms in achieving the objectives on the other.

Much of the argument about the NHS in the 1950s and 1960s focused on the latter. In our judgement, this mostly *a priori* argument about what is essentially an *empirical* question was largely misplaced. The evidence, we believe, suggests that health care is an area where public ownership and a substantial diminution of the role of consumer prices is more effective a way of organization than others. ... But the reasons for this lie less on the demand side (as the NHS defenders of the 1960s argued) and more – much more – on the supply side. The NHS has, of course, failed notably to realize many of the potential benefits of 'rationalizing' supply, and the revolution – or evolution – to come will be concentrated here. At the same time, however, it must be acknowledged that a residuum of the political issue underlying the NHS debate of the 1960s remains an inherent danger in the NHS structure, for central to either a Marxist or a liberal philosophy is the view that the State is an instrument of oppression; that for Marxists it serves to entrench the position of the ruling class and that, for liberals, it does both this and removes power, discretion and freedom of action and choice from the individual citizen. In health care, with its traditions of authority and hierarchy within its professions and in its relation with the public, these dangers are real and have recently been confirmed dramatically in the NHS especially with regard to long-stay patients (Robb, 1967; official reports on hospitals at Ely, 1969; Farleigh, 1971; Whittingham, 1972; Ockendon, 1974). Nursing, where contact with the patient is often most intimate, is famous for its harridans. Haywood (1974) reports a typical story: ' "We did way with restrictions ages ago", said one matron, weightily propelling me past a large notice: Visiting from 4.30 to 5.0 p.m. daily. Identical placards hung outside all the wards. "We keep them up", Matron smiled at my naive mystification "because otherwise visitors [to a children's ward] would think they could pop in any time." '

These dangers are also, of course, present in more decentralized and competitive systems but are probably more real in a state-owned system that is heavily dominated by the medical professions. Against them the patient, either individually or collectively in a market situation, has little effective countervailing power, for though profit is clearly the driving force of many medical practitioners, their incomes and the patient's satisfaction with the competence and considerateness of care are tenuously related. The NHS organization does, however, have the potential to control the professionals and to monitor their performance in the light of socially, not merely medically, determined objectives. It is this element that at once both 'justifies' the NHS and which has, sadly, been largely lacking in its performance to date.

In the anti-medicine brigade, Ivan Illich (1975) must be the arch *advocatus diaboli*, for in his view the medics (as well as the industrial state) are destroying man's very humanity:

> The true miracle of modern medicine is diabolical. It consists not only of making individuals but whole populations survive on inhumanly low levels of personal health. That health should decline with increasing health service delivery is unforeseen only by the health managers, precisely because their strategies are the result of their blindness to the inalienability of life. ... Medical nemesis ... is the expropriation of man's coping ability by a maintenance service which keeps him geared up at the service of the industrial system.

The arcadian remedies implicit in Illich's diagnosis of 'structural iatrogenesis' (iatrogenetic disease is that induced by medical practice) are neither generally desired in modern societies nor would they seem particularly desirable. But the remedies that our economic analysis implies are pretty far-reaching, and amount to a substantial erosion of what is often called 'clinical freedom'. Our analysis suggests: that the definition of health, or ill health, is not mainly a matter for doctors; that the establishment of social trade-offs is not mainly a matter for doctors; that judgement about the proper size of the NHS relative to other public and private spending categories is not mainly a matter for doctors; that judgement about which cares and cures are to be available under the NHS is not mainly a matter for doctors; that judgement about the resource inputs, including manpower, required to provide these cares and cures is only partially a matter for doctors; that the monitoring of medical inefficiency, incompetence and carelessness ought to be much more the concern of doctors (and others too); and that evaluation of the clinical and social effectiveness of clinical procedures should be very much more the preoccupation of doctors (Culyer, 1975).

Much of the book has, of course, been devoted to the problems that arise in trying to formulate methods by which better decisions about all of these things may be made. In total, they do not warrant the conclusion that Britain's health has been badly served by the NHS compared with other countries, nor that we spend too little on health care. But neither do they warrant the reverse condition. What, in total, they do warrant is a massive research programme into the effectiveness of unvalidated clinical procedures and further development and application of the efficiency evaluation techniques we have sought to indicate in this book, with special attention being given to objectives: the meeting of needs.

The politically most challenging aspect of all lies not so much in the inculcation of notions of effective use of means for defined ends at the *management* level – though there are battles here to be fought and won – as in ensuring that efficient management decisions are carried out at the level of clinical practice. In the very short term, effective monitoring of results at this level (or indeed most others too) is difficult because of the absence of routine status measurement data of the sort described in chapters 4 and 8. But in the fullness of time we can envisage monitoring at, say, the GP level that might take the following form: a periodic sample is taken of the ten or so most frequent conditions constituting the bulk of the GP's routine work and of how the outcomes for patients treated differed at some appropriate statistical level of significance from those of norms established by, say, studies of 'best practice'. A marked adverse deviation would warrant the GP being called to explain this. There may, of course, be perfectly legitimate explanations (e.g. poor support facilities), which themselves would then become the object for further examination. There may also, however, be incompetence in the sense that the individual himself is operating in a way inconsistent with the objective of the NHS in maximizing, out of given resources, the reduction in need. As Michael Cooper has pointedly observed: 'the aircrews of passenger air services are given Ministry approval checks every thirteen months. Cabin crews are given yearly survival and emergency checks. Are surgeons really any less susceptible to obsolescence, sickness or incompetence?' (Cooper, 1975).

Even in the shorter term, however, some progress in the spirit of effectiveness monitoring could be made. Today it would be fairly easy to compare crude outcome variations as between different GPs and different hospitals (and hospital doctors) in terms of death rates, hospital fatality rates, re-admission rates, speed of return to work. Practitioners and institutions with marked deviations from a middle range could (after relevant associated data concerning population age and sex structures, hospital case mix, etc.) be called upon to explain. Often, advice and information about the procedures adopted by others might be sufficient a corrective in those cases where no satisfactory explanation for the divergence can be offered. But in some cases more ultimate sanctions of a financial sort or, in the limit, of even being struck off the medical register for incompetence may have to be used.

In the longer term, much finer measures of effectiveness and cost effectiveness will be developed, related not only to the treatments actually given but also to the impact of medical care in each area's needs. At this stage the processes of planning, monitoring and controlling will have become highly complementary.

For some (perhaps the professionals), the vision will appear to be an authoritarian nightmare – despite the fact that most researchers (for example) manage to cope quite capably with the period reviews and inspections that government research councils make of programmes they sponsor. To others (who focus more on the clients of the system) the NHS appears already to be a highly authoritarian institution.

The charge has frequently been made against the NHS (especially by the libertarians and others who are not easily fobbed off with assurances about the social responsibility of managers, professionals and scientists in large organizations, both public and private) that it is a quintessentially paternalist organization. Indeed, we have already discussed the Titmussian arguments for denying any kind of rationality to individuals as patients.

More generally, it is a measure of the generation gap that, in an age when the young intelligentsia is becoming increasingly libertarian and 'small-is-beautiful' in its social outlook, their elders having positions of power in society persist in unimaginative attempts to assuage these reasonable sceptics by assurances about their social intentions – despite the absence of social accountability. Thus the high priests of capitalism seek to correct its 'unacceptable' face by averring that the job of businessmen is to serve the interests of society (usually and conveniently left undefined), whereas their job is quite plainly to serve the interests of their shareholder/owners (subject to whatever social controls *Parliament* imposes on their activity). It is also quite plain that in pursuing profit and so serving these interests they may also serve (though this is merely instrumental) the wider community.

If there are lamentably few these days, however, to argue that profit-seeking may sometimes serve a useful social function, so there are even fewer around to explain what it is, especially in the public sector, that is to replace 'profit' as the general objective and as the general indicator of 'success'. There are, indeed, good reasons to view the paternalists with disquiet, for whenever they appear on the scene, clarity of objective, efficiency of means of achieving it and accountability to those on whose behalf it is supposed to be being achieved all tend to fly out of the window.

Yet there is a quite specific case for a paternalism of sorts in the NHS. It is not a negative case built upon the alleged irrationalities of individuals as patients (which is hardly an argument *for* anything at all!), but a positive case built upon the simple observation of what seems a quite indisputable fact: that in many (but not necessarily all) matters of health care, individuals wish to delegate decisions to others to act on their behalf. From this flows the argument for public ownership (as opposed merely to subsidy) as we saw in chapter 7, the definition of the NHS objective as reducing need efficiently, the definition of need and the meaning of efficiency. From it also flows the desirability of monitoring and controlling those to whom these important decisions have been delegated.

It is arguable, of course, that the framework we have developed here is not at all paternalist – at least in the traditional 'merit good' sense common in economics, or in the sense of beneficent coercion in political theory. In practice these traditional uses of the term invariably turn out to be merely fancy names for a more or less muddled, and more or less inefficient authoritarianism. By contrast, our vision is of an NHS serving individuals' unambiguous needs, with an unambiguous procedure for evaluating such needs and establishing priorities, and with an unambiguous procedure for ensuring that the producers in the system are the properly monitored and controlled servants of their clients.

While the word 'need' has been prominent in the rhetoric of the NHS, its effective utilization as a concept to produce the results the NHS aspires to has been notably absent. In this book we have tried to reformulate the old questions in such a way that they suggest practical means by which these aspirations may be realized. Much work remains to be done, of course, but done it must be, as must the objections of the vested interests be resisted and refuted, if the NHS is truly to live up to any testable claim that it is the 'best in the world'. The job cannot be one for the faint-hearted, and if this book can help rationally to persuade the unconvinced of its necessity as well as rallying the faithful to stand by the ideals of the NHS as they really are – and as they can be implemented – then its writing will have been more than worthwhile.

References

Cooper, M. H. (1975) *Rationing Health Care*, Croom Helm, London/Halstead, New York

Culyer, A. J. (1975) Health: the social cost of doctors' discretion *New Society*, 27 February

Ely Report (1969) *Report of Committee of Enquiry into Allegations of Ill-treatment of Patients and Other Irregularities at the Ely Hospital Cardiff*, Cmnd, 3975, HMSO, London

Farleigh Report (1971) *Report of the Farleigh Hospital Committee of Inquiry*, Cmnd. 4557, HMSO, London

Haywood, S. C. (1974) *Managing the Health Service*, Allen and Unwin, London

Illich, I. (1975) *Medical Nemesis: The Expropriation of Health*, Calder and Boyars, London

Ockendon Report (1974) *Report of the Committee of Inquiry into South Ockendon Hospital*, H.C. 124, HMSO, London

Robb, B. (1967) *Sans Everything: A Case to Answer*, Association for the Elderly in Government Institutions, London

Whittingham Report (1972) *Report of the Committee of Inquiry into the Whittingham Hospital*, Cmnd 4861, HSMO, London

Reprinted by permission of Blackwell Publishers, Oxford. A. J. Culyer (1976) The NHS – an assessment. In *Need and the National Health Service*, Martin Robertson, London, pp.145–151.

Chapter 56

Ambiguous past, uncertain future

Rudolf Klein

Health care reform was one of the international epidemics of the 1990s (Hurst, 1992). A series of health care reform initiatives swept across the globe driven by much the same concerns and shaped by much the same set of ideas as those which launched the Thatcherite enterprise and shaped Britain's 1991 NHS. There were significant differences in the way in which countries reacted to these concerns and adapted the ideas (Jacobs, 1994); the reform debate in each country spoke with a strong national accent (Saltman and von Otter, 1992). However, even though common themes tended to be translated into rather different policy prescriptions, depending on local circumstances and preoccupations, there was also much agreement. Almost all countries engaged in reforming their health care systems were concerned to improve efficiency by changing the incentives to providers and saw some form of market-like competition as the tool for achieving this aim. Similarly, there appeared to be an international consensus about the need to strengthen primary care, if only to cope with the burden of managing chronic illness in ageing populations (Fox, 1993), and to move towards the public health paradigm of health policy (Evans *et al.*, 1994). In all these respects, Britain was not so very different from other countries: a warning against trying to explain changes in health care policy exclusively in terms of the political, social or economic situation in any one country.

In one respect, however, Britain was different. The British Government not only initiated health care reform but succeeded in implementing it. In the United States, the Clinton attempts to reform health care foundered on the rocks of Congressional opposition; in Sweden a succession of local experiments and committees of inquiry failed to create a national consensus about the direction of health care policy; in the Netherlands, an ambitious plan of reform was agreed in principle but its implementation subsequently became a casualty of coalition politics and it suffered both amendment and delay. Only New Zealand, another country with a Westminster-type constitution, successfully introduced radical change quickly (Salmond *et al.*, 1994). The contrast underlines the extent to which political institutions and conventions determine the ability of national governments to implement new health care policies (Immergut, 1992). In Britain the Thatcher administration was able to transfer the debate about reform from the restricted health care policy arena – largely dominated by providers – to the wider parliamentary arena where it commanded an automatic majority. In other countries, however, the lack of any such automatic majority forced governments to submit their reform initiatives to the slow and frustrating politics of compromise and bargaining: a process which, in some cases, proved fatal.

There appears, however, to be an inverse relationship between the ability of different political systems to bring about changes quickly and the capacity to evaluate the impact of those changes. The Thatcher Government was able to impose its reforms so decisively and speedily precisely because it did not feel itself bound by the inherited consensus about the NHS and because it did not perceive any need to create a new one. But lacking any such consensus, there is no agreed currency for evaluating the impact of the reforms. Inevitably, therefore, the changes in the NHS since 1991 have to be assessed from a variety of perspectives with only one element common to them all: which is that the evidence needed to come to any firm conclusions is usually lacking.

A solution – but what was the problem?

The first step in trying to assess the impact of the 1991 changes is to come to some understanding of the nature of the NHS's problems to which the reforms were supposed to be the answer. Previous chapters have identified the political and economic imperatives driving government policy. But the fact that the Government perceived its reforms to provide a solution to these problems does not mean that its definition of the situation necessarily has to be accepted as a starting point for any exercise in evaluation. Any assessment of the situation after the 1991 reforms must therefore start by drawing up a balance sheet of the NHS's achievements – and failures – before the changes were introduced. Measured against the aims of the NHS's original architects – reaffirmed by the 1979 Royal Commission – how had the NHS performed?

The first aim of the NHS, as spelled out by Bevan in 1948 (see Chapter 1), was achieved by the act of creation itself. The introduction of a free health service automatically meant that the ability to get treatment was divorced from the ability to pay. The financial barricades having been torn down, the way was open for achieving equity in the use of health services: of ensuring that the only criterion for treatment or care was need, as defined by service providers. In the outcome, equity of access to the NHS (though not, of course, to the private sector) has indeed been achieved.[1] The poorest members of the community – who are also likely to be those with the greatest need for health care – also make a proportionately greater use of the NHS. However, the NHS appears to have been somewhat less successful in achieving equity in terms of the quality of care provided once access to the system has been achieved. The evidence on this point is not clear cut. Many of the studies cited in support of the 1968 view of Titmuss[2] that the more prosperous and better educated 'know how to make better use of the service' are now themselves out of date. But it would be surprising if differences in the ability to manipulate a complex bureaucratic environment – and to deal with high status professionals – did not affect the way in which the NHS is used, once access has been achieved. Inequalities in the distribution of articulacy, knowledge and social confidence (which is not necessarily identical with social class) may therefore play at least as important a part in determining the way the NHS is used as inequalities in the distribution of income. The NHS remained a multi-tiered service, accurately mirroring the multi-tiered nature of the society in which it operated.

Turning to Bevan's second aim, 'to provide the people of Great Britain, no matter where they may be, with the same level of service', the NHS can only be rated a qualified success. In this respect, the single most important achievement of the NHS was perhaps to bring about a better distribution of specialist manpower by maintaining strict central control over the creation of new posts (Godber, 1975). But geographical equity in the distribution of resources, and access to services, still remained to be achieved by the end of the 1980s. The RAWP formula (see Chapter 3) did, indeed, bring about a very considerable reduction in the inherited inequalities of funding between the regions. But inequalities *within* regions remained large. And variations in the services provided to the population were even more gross than variations in funding, since differences in the level of resources were compounded at the local level by differences in clinical practices and budgetary priorities. The point can be illustrated by the measures of access – service use per 1,000 population – provided by the NHS Performance Indicators.[3] At the beginning of the 1990s, the ratios of service availability between the best and worst provided districts were 57:22 for general surgery, 56:20 for general medicine, 24:10 for trauma and orthopaedics, 11:3 for ophthalmology and 21:4 for paediatrics. For the treatment of specific conditions, the variations were even more dramatic. Rates for removing cataracts varied by a factor of 7 and for hip replacements by a factor of 40. Some of the extremes in the distribution may be statistical flukes; other variations could no doubt be explained, in part at least, by differences in the composition of the population. But, even allowing for such problems in the interpretation of the figures, the conclusion is clear: more than 40 years after its birth, the NHS had yet to offer everyone the same level of service. Similarly, significant regional variations remain in the number of 'avoidable deaths' for conditions amenable to health service intervention, either preventive or curative. In the case of cancer, the range is from 59 per cent above the national average to 44 per cent below it. In the case of hypertension and stroke, the range is from 32 per cent above the national average to 26 per cent below it (The Chief Medical Officer, 1988).

The NHS's failure to ensure that everyone has the same level of services or access to the same range of treatment must not be exaggerated. The problem of achieving an equitable distribution of resources is international; if money is mobile, medical manpower is not. And compared to most other countries, Britain's record is a striking success story. However, the inability to eliminate variations within the NHS provides an illuminating footnote to the 1946 Cabinet debate between Bevan and Morrison (see Chapter 1). Bevan's main argument, it will be remembered, was that a national service was required if inequalities between the poor and rich parts of the country were not to be perpetuated; local government control, he maintained, was incompatible with this objective. Yet ironically central government has, in the outcome, proved more successful in reducing variations in the distribution of resources in at least some local authority services, such as education, than in the NHS (Buxton and Klein, 1978). This would suggest that institutional factors may be less important than the ability of the medical profession to control the number of doctors being trained. By maintaining strict limits on the number of medical students graduating every year – and relying on doctors from overseas to cope with any shortages – the British medical profession in effect ensured full employment for its members and a tight medical labour market. In turn, this meant that the less popular specialties in the less attractive parts of the country often found it difficult to attract the best qualified doctors: whereas the centre could control the distribution of posts, it could not control either the quantity or the quality of the candidates applying for them.

To make this last point is to underline that Bevan's most ambitious aim – which was to 'universalize the best' – was incapable of realization. In retrospect, the NHS's achievement lay not in universalizing the best – a flamboyant piece of political rhetoric devoid of any real meaning – but in universalizing the adequate. The NHS was an instrument not for ensuring that everyone got the best conceivable treatment – that the technological magic of modern medicine would be on tap without any budgetary constraints or that everything possible would be done for the chronically ill – but for rationing scarce resources. Political decisions about the NHS's budget were translated and diffused, as we have seen, into clinical decisions about whom to treat and how. By international, and in particular by American, standards this often meant that British patients received less than optimal treatment.[4] This conclusion must be interpreted with some caution: the more conservative approach of the British medical profession towards the use of new technology reflects not just resource constraints but also a proper scepticism about over-heroic treatment or the use of as yet untested procedures. However, even bearing this reservation in mind, there are some clear examples where the NHS has been slow – compared to other health care systems – to make potentially life-saving treatments available to all who might benefit from them. The case of renal dialysis in the 1970s ... is one example; that of coronary artery by-pass surgery in the 1980s is another. The same point could be made, even more forcibly, about treatments designed to improve the quality of life rather than to save lives, such as joint replacement and other forms of elective surgery. If the NHS offered no incentives to its providers to rush into the adoption of new technologies, or to increase their incomes by multiplying the number of diagnostic tests carried out, neither did it offer any incentives to maximize their activities in providing effective treatment. The pathology of the American health care system – and others based on item of service payments to doctors – is the risk of over-treatment. Conversely, the pathology of the NHS is the risk of under-treatment.

So far this attempt to draw up a balance sheet for the NHS, in its pre-1991 incarnation, has taken as its starting point the aims of the service's architects. But what if we change the perspective of evaluation to ask whether the NHS was satisfying the expectations of the population? The 1970s, as argued in Chapter 4, saw the rise of a more aggressive consumerism, both in the health care policy arena and more generally. The trend was continued in the 1980s; indeed one of the criticisms of the Thatcher administration was precisely that it encouraged the public to regard themselves as consumers seeking to maximize their individual welfare rather than as citizens seeking to maximize the collective welfare. It would therefore be logical to expect increasing evidence of consumer frustration with the NHS: rising resentment of the fact that (as the Griffiths report had accurately pointed out) the NHS was provider-dominated. And if that were the case, then one way of interpreting the 1991 reforms would be as a response to the failure of the NHS to respond to the changing environment and rising consumer expectations.

Intuitively plausible though this interpretation may be, it is surprisingly difficult to back it with evidence. The evidence of public opinion surveys in the 1980s (reviewed in Chapter 5) is ambiguous. Support for the NHS remained rock-solid, as we saw, while dissatisfaction with the service provided increased. But the meaning to be given to rising dissatisfaction – particularly among members of the general public who did not necessarily have first-hand experience of the NHS as patients – is not self-evident. Did it reflect frustrated expectations or was it induced by the providers? One finding, common to almost all surveys, was that dissatisfaction tended to rise with education but fall with age. This might indeed suggest that by the 1980s the NHS was exhausting the capital of deference and gratitude which had sustained it over the decades: that a younger, better educated generation increasingly saw health care as a consumer good. But it could also be argued that a fatalistic resignation to low standards is one of the by-products of ageing and will therefore characterize successive generations.

More substantial evidence about the NHS's lack of sensitivity towards consumers is provided by a survey carried out in 1988 based on the experience of patients (rather than the views of the general public) in four health districts (Prescott-Clarke et al., 1988). Overwhelmingly, the people were given no choice of date when offered an outpatient appointment;

between 15 and 37 per cent described the outpatient department as depressing; between 18 and 32 per cent considered the length of time spent waiting to see the specialist as unacceptably long; between 75 and 85 per cent reported that the specialist offered no choice of treatment and made all the decisions; over 50 per cent, in all four districts, agreed with the statement that 'hospital appointment systems are designed to suit hospital staff, not patients'. Yet, illustrating the ambiguity of public attitudes, a much higher proportion – well over 80 per cent – considered that 'hospitals do as well as they can considering their financial problems': the providers, clearly, had managed to convince the great majority of the public that any shortcomings were attributable to under-funding. The experiences, and attitudes, of people as inpatients were much the same. Between 21 and 37 per cent would have preferred a single room to a bed in a ward (but less than half actually got one); over 50 per cent, in all four districts, considered that 'doctors talk in front of you as if you weren't there'; between 14 and 29 per cent were bothered by the standard of hygiene on the ward; between 36 and 52 per cent were only told that they were going to be discharged on the day concerned.

More difficult to interpret is the increasing propensity to complain that characterized the 1980s and the start of the new decade. The fact that there was such a tendency is incontrovertible. It affected all parts of the NHS. In the period 1983 to 1991 the number of complaints about primary care rose from 1,313 to 2,205 and about hospital services from 16,218 to 44,680 (Williams, 1994). The number of complaints to the Health Service Commissioner (1994), over the same period, rose by some 50 per cent. Similarly, the General Medical Council (1994) reported a rising tide of complaints about the performance of doctors. One interpretation of this trend is that rising complaints simply mirrored falling standards. But equally plausibly it can be argued that the greater readiness to complain reflected increasing consumer assertiveness: a decline in deference towards the professional providers and a decreasing willingness to accept shoddy or incompetent treatment. On this view, if there was a gap between consumer expectations and the NHS's standards, it was because the former were rising more rapidly than the latter: the problem was not that the NHS was deteriorating – all the evidence pointed in the opposite direction – but that its rate of improvement did not match the rate at which expectations were increasing.

The most conclusive, and least ambiguous, evidence about the NHS's failure to meet expectations remains that provided by the growth of the private sector. Even the recession of the early 1990s did not stop the expansion of private health care insurance: by 1991, some 6,500,000 people were covered by such schemes, an increase of 1,500,000 over five years (*Laing's Review*, 1994). This, as noted in Chapter 5, did not represent people voting with their feet against the concept of the NHS. Exit did not imply disloyalty: in many cases, those using the private sector did so reluctantly and only occasionally. But it did demonstrate the NHS's failure to respond to consumer demand. A service predicated on the assumption that its function was to give priority to professionally determined need inevitably did not respond quickly or easily to the demands of consumers. Collective, medical priorities were in competition with individual consumer priorities within tightly constrained budgets. If waiting lists were an inaccurate measure of the NHS's failure to meet demand (as distinct from need) – if they reflected as much the inefficiency with which resources were used as inadequacies of funding – they were a politically powerful symbol of the NHS's inability to satisfy consumer expectations. And the fact that they had become so politically salient in itself suggests that those expectations had risen. The phenomenon of waiting lists was as old as the NHS itself. The political unacceptability of waiting lists was, however, comparatively new: the product of the 1970s and 1980s. In the early days of the NHS, the waiting list was part of a culture of queueing bequeathed by wartime experience: it was acceptable because bolstered by a sense of social solidarity and shared hardship. By the end of the 1980s, the waiting list had become an anomaly: the queue was seen as a sign of failure.

Remarkably, though, this failure was not blamed on the design of the NHS. Similarly, as we have seen, any shortcomings were not put at the door of the doctors and staff running the service. Perhaps the most outstanding achievement of the NHS at the end of the 1980s – just before the reforms were introduced – was therefore that it had established itself as Britain's only immaculate institution. If there were flaws, these were attributable to government interference. If there were complaints about falling standards and mounting inadequacies, the blame fell on ministerial niggardliness. If there was rising criticism it fell on the heads of politicians, not providers. It is this which explains an apparent paradox. For the rest of the world, Britain's NHS offered a model of how to contain costs while still offering a universal, equitable and reasonably adequate health service: why, then, change it? But for British Governments it was precisely the political costs of this success in containing costs that impelled, as argued in Chapter 6, the drive towards reform.

The balance sheet of the NHS's achievements and failures, before the introduction of the 1991 reforms, is therefore complex. In a global sense, the NHS provided a most efficient service: compared to most other health care systems, it provided a remarkably comprehensive service at a remarkably reasonable price. But in detail, the NHS provided endless examples of inefficiency.[5] In evaluating the reforms, the first question must thus be whether they can both build on past achievements *and* remedy past inadequacies. In trying to transform the dynamics of the NHS model, do the reforms risk also changing the nature of the model itself? If the virtues and vices of the NHS spring from the same source – i.e. the institutional design chosen in 1948 – then could the Siamese twins be separated without killing the patient?

Notes

1. Collins, E. and Klein, R. (1980) Equity and the NHS: self-reported morbidity, access and primary care. *British Medical Journal*, **281**, 1111–1115. The originally controversial finding of this study, that equity in access had broadly been achieved, was subsequently confirmed by a succession of other analyses. See, especially, O'Donnell, O. and Propper, C. (1989) *Equity and the Distribution of National Health Service Resources*, School of Economics, London, The Welfare State Programme Discussion Paper WSP/45.
2. Titmuss, R. (1968) *Commitment to Welfare*, Allen and Unwin, London. For a recent critical and illuminating review of the evidence, see Powell, M. (1994) *Social class, equality and the National Health Service*, Division of Social Sciences, University of Hertfordshire, Hatfield, Mimeo.
3. Department of Health (1992/1993) *Health Service Indicators for 1990/91 and 1991/92*. Both sets were published on computer discs (in 1992 and 1993, respectively) available from the Department.
4. Aaron, H. J. and Schwartz, W. B. (1984) *The Painful Prescription*, The Brookings Institution, Washington D.C. But note the more recent evidence that, in some sophisticated forms of intervention, Britain is actually ahead of the United States: see, for example, General Accounting Office (1994) *Bone Marrow Transplantation: International Comparisons of Availability and Appropriateness of Use*, GAO, Washington, D.C., GAO/PEMD-94-10.
5. The scope for improving productivity by universalizing best practices was documented in a series of reports from the Audit Commission: for example, *Lying in Wait: the Use of Medical Beds in Acute Hospitals*, HMSO, London, 1992; *A Short Cut To Better Services: Day Surgery in England and Wales*, HMSO, London, 1990. It was also acknowledged by one of the many American critics of the 1991 reforms: Light, D. W. (1992) Embedded inefficiencies in health care. *The Lancet*, **338**, 102–104.

References

Buxton, M. and Klein, R. (1978) *Allocating Health Resources*, Royal Commission on the National Health Service Research Paper no. 3, HMSO, London

Evans, R., Barber, M. and Marmor, T. R. (1994) *Why are Some People Healthy and Others Not?*, Aldine de Gruyter, Hawthorne, N.Y.

Fox, D. M. (1993) *Power and Illness*, University of California Press, Berkeley

General Medical Council (1994) *Annual Report, 1993*, GMC, London

Godber, Sir George (1975) *The Health Service: Past, Present and Future*, Athlone Press, London

Health Service Commissioner (W. K. Reid) (1994) *Annual Report for 1993–94*, HMSO, London, H.C. 499

Hurst, J. (1992) *The Reform of Health Care: A Comparative Analysis of Seven OECD Countries*, OECD, Paris

Immergut, E. M. (1992) *Health Politics: Interests and Institutions in Western Europe*, Cambridge University Press, Cambridge

Jacobs, A. (1994) *The politics of markets*. MSc Dissertation, University of Bath

Laing's Review of Private Health Care, 1994 (1994) Laing and Buisson, London

Prescott-Clarke, P., Brooks, T and Machray, C. (1988) *Focus on Health Care: Surveying the Public in Four Health Districts*, Royal Institute of Public Administration, London

Salmond, G., Mooney, G. and Laugesen, M. (eds) (1994) *Health Care Reform in New Zealand*, Special issue of *Health Policy*, **29**(1–2)

Saltman, R. and von Otter, C. (1992) *Planned Markets and Public Competition*, Open University Press, Buckingham

The Chief Medical Officer (Sir Donald Acheson) (1988) *On the State of the Public Health for the Year 1987*, HMSO, London
Williams, A. (Chairman) (1994) *Being Heard: the Report of a Review Committee on NHS Complaints Procedures*, Department of Health, London

Index